AF515790

Public Service Delivery: Does Accountability & Local Institutions Matter?

A Comparative Perspective of Child Nutrition Programmes in India

Public Service Delivery: Does Accountability & Local Institutions Matter?

A Comparative Perspective of Child Nutrition Programmes in India

JAYA GOYAL

Report of the Research
Sponsored by ICSSR, New Delhi

Indian Council of Social Science Research
Aruna Asaf Ali Marg,
Jawaharlal Nehru University, New Delhi 11006

Motilal Banarsidass Publications
4741/23 Ansari Road,
Daryaganj, New Delhi 110002

MOTILAL BANARSIDASS
PUBLICATIONS
4741/23, Ansari Road, Daryaganj, New Delhi - 110002 (India)
Email: *mlbd@mlbd.com* | *sales@mlbd.com* | *exports@mlbd.com*
Website: *www.mlbd.com*

Public Service Delivery
by
Jaya Goyal

First Edition Published in 2023

Published in India by
Motilal Banarsidass Publications
&
Indian Council of Social Science Research

ISBN : 978-93-91759-33-9 (HB)

Printed and bound in India

Contents

Foreword

'*The care of human life and happiness ... is the first and only legitimate object of good government.*' So told Thomas Jefferson (1743–1826), the third President of the United States of America to the republican citizens of Washington County, Maryland on 31 March 1809. Notwithstanding the endless political rhetoric and academic tomes on the so called 'good governance', Jefferson's prescription remains the touchstone of a good government.

The way a government takes care of the life of its citizens is premised upon the efficiency and effectiveness with which it provides them health services. The governments in India, the central government as well as most state governments, can hardly claim to have done much in this regard. Despite the increase in budgetary allocations, numerous schemes and interventions, and various agencies working to tackle it, child malnutrition remains a major health concern in the country. According to UNICEF's 'The State of the World's Children 2019' report, malnutrition is the main reason behind 69 percent of deaths of children below the age of five in the country. Moreover, every child in that age group is affected by some form of malnutrition like stunting (low height for age) or wasting (low weight for height). One doubts if India can realise the United Nations' Sustainable Development Goal 2 (ensure zero hunger) and Goal 3 (good health and well-being for all) by 2030.

What ails the public health service delivery in India and how can it be improved? In this book, which is based on her doctoral thesis, Dr Jaya Goyal attempts to answer these questions. The merit of her book lies in the incisive investigation that she has carried out through a skilful combination of quantitative and qualitative methodologies. She has meticulously collected secondary data from official sources and painstakingly collected primary data from fieldwork in two villages. Unlike most doctoral thesis-based books, which are no more than a report of a fact-finding exercise, this book presents empirical data in the background of theories of public policy and administration.

As a background and guide to her empirical study, Dr Goyal analyses the official data on the Government of India's ICDS (Integrated Child Development Services) schemes. Notwithstanding the question of reliability that is often raised about governmental data, this is the only credible source that one can tap on the subject. Moreover, this data is available at different levels of aggregation – state, district, block, and village. Based on two indicators from the ICDS Management and Information System – the percentage of eligible population receiving the benefits and the percentage of children malnourished (moderate and severe) of those weighed – Dr Goyal identified two districts in Maharashtra, namely, Satara and Osmanabad, for her empirical study. Using a multi-stage area sampling method, she selected Surli village in Koregaon block in Satara district and Nanduri village in Tuljapur block in Osmanabad district for intensive fieldwork. The choice of the districts, blocks, and villages were purposive and based on appropriate development indicators.

Dr Goyal's study exposes the rhetoric about accountability in policy and development discussions. It questions the assumption that increased accountability and engagement of the users enhances the quality of public service delivery. Dr Goyal's analysis of the choices that people make between services provided by public and private agencies, and the reasons therefor, show how these agencies influence the choice of the users, on the one hand, and how these choices, in turn, affect the performance of the agencies, on the other. Accountability, it is argued, is not a one-sided idea; it is posited on the relationship between service provider and the intended user of the service.

Substantively, Dr Goyal's findings challenge the widely held belief in policy circles that improvement in socio-economic status and enhanced food security would result in a reduction in the prevalence of stunting, wasting, and underweight among children. Alternatively, Dr Goyal finds that institutional factors, other than economic, social, and developmental, influence child malnutrition outcomes. Invoking Harvard University scholar Michael Walton, she argues that malnutrition is not only an aspect of current or future socio-economic inequalities, but is also causally related to unequal institutional structures. This takes her back to the relationship between service providers and the intended users.

This book deserves to be read because it critiques the dominant neo-liberal model of governance and management of public service delivery, especially the idea of accountability, through a systematic empirical investigation of a persistent health crisis, namely, child malnutrition. It makes out a case for moving beyond techno-managerial solutions to unresolved public health issues. While the book does not provide any quick-fix solutions to the problem of child malnutrition, it seeks to explain what has gone wrong with our efforts at public health service delivery and what could be done to rectify it.

N. Jayaram
Institute of Public Policy
National Law School of India University
Bengaluru

Preface

You must have come with some expectations that this book may have the answers to the question about linkages between governance and public service delivery outcomes, for nutrition programmes in India. I would use the word 'explanations' and not 'answers' as an expectation from this book. It is so because I believe that 'explaining' a phenomenon is a key contribution of a research study like this. Explanations may emerge, not instantly, but gradually and piece by piece, like in a jigsaw puzzle, or when or as one opens up layers and layers of complexities of one inquiry that leads to another like a mystery.

Research literally means to re-search. This monograph, starting from the first page of the first chapter, asks moot questions. Asking questions is the only way in which a body of knowledge progresses in any discipline. This in turn, shifts paradigms. The term 'Paradigm Shift' was coined by Thomas Kuhn, an American physicist and philosopher in his influential work 'The Structure of Scientific Revolutions' (1969). According to Kuhn, paradigm shifts arise when the dominant paradigm under which normal science operates is rendered incompatible with new phenomena, facilitating the adoption of a new theory or paradigm.

This book asks questions, rethinks and reconstructs possible explanations, to contribute to a shifting of paradigms or theories about public administration, including public service delivery, local institutions, accountability processes, and child nutrition programmes in India. Although quick fix answers or solutions on the issue of child malnutrition may not be apparent or explicit, this book will provide explanations to questions set out in the beginning. The book's key contribution is also presenting a framework in which new questions on accountability can be asked and explained, rooted in a reality, while factoring all assumptions of that reality.

The theme of this book is derived from my doctoral work, 'Accountability Processes in Public Service Delivery: A Study of Child Health & Nutrition Services in Maharashtra'. The idea emerged when I grew interested in social audits as tools to reduce corruption in public services, especially in nutrition programmes. I was fortunate that during my early career days, I was part of TISS action research called, 'The Outcome Budget' which the Government of Maharashtra had set out in 2007. I experienced social audits, first-hand, during a public verification exercise on a health programme called Jeevandai Araogya Yojana and the Integrated Child Development Scheme (ICDS), a national, community nutrition programme in Maharashtra. I documented these experiences in the form of two papers in a special issue of the Indian Journal of Social Work's, titled 'Outcome Budget: Concepts, Experiences and Lessons'.

Early on, I had gained insights on the political economy of health & nutrition programmes while working on another monograph in 2005, during my stint at the Observer Research Foundation (ORF). The study was titled 'Public Private Partnerships in Reproductive and Child Health Services in India', although the monograph remained unpublished for a while as I moved between jobs. Eventually, the study was published as a chapter in an edited book 'Medical Anthropology' in 2015. This book chapter was titled, 'Role of State in Public Private Partnerships in Reproductive and Child Health Services'. I used both these experiences while teaching masters students at TISS and had created training modules on Child Health and Nutrition Programmes for the UNICEF District Facilitators Training Programme, which later became popular as the Prime Minister's Rural Development Fellows.

My training in Home Science, while pursuing my Bachelor of Science (Honours) and Master of Science (in Community Resource Management and Extension or Human Ecology), provided me with a firm foundation on community nutrition, development communication, and extension education. During post-graduation in 2001, I had also competed a thesis on 'Information needs of adolescents on reproductive health issues in municipal schools in Delhi'. This monograph that you are reading, is therefore, a culmination of more than a decade of impressions, influences, and experiences from academic and professional training on the subject.

Coming back to the initial idea of social audits, I realised that doctoral work is not a fact-finding or solution-oriented project, but a contribution to philosophy and existing theories or paradigms on a subject. This is the mandate of a thesis. There has been a time lag of more than five years since I concluded this thesis in 2015 and time lag of 10 years since I collected data in 2012 and release of this published monograph. Therefore, I will present some recent trends to provide a sense of continuity and context for the readers to bridge the time gap. The global pandemic crisis of Covid-19 and the Indian State's response to it, followed by delivery measures and their impact, also has linkages to Public Health challenges and the conceptual framework presented in this study.

A World Bank report in 1999, 'Wasting Away: The crisis of malnutrition in India", mentioned that India accounts for forty percent of child malnutrition numbers in the world, despite progress in food production, disease control, and economic and social development since independence (World Bank, 1999). The trend has continued to be unabated in 2020, even in view of increased budgets, advancement in technology, and numerous agencies working to tackle the issue. According to a Global Burden of

Disease Study published in Lancet in 2019, malnutrition continues to top the list of risk factors, driving most deaths and disabilities in India at 35.3%, a statistic that is much higher than tobacco-use or any other health risks like cancer or diabetes (Times of India, 2019). Malnutrition is a much bigger health and economic risk for India, even in wake of Covid-19. In fact, the ongoing pandemic has exacerbated malnutrition crisis in the country.

From the time this study was initiated in 2009 till today, I still see and wonder if this challenge has remained same, improved, or deteriorated for children in India. NFHS or the National Family Health Survey is one of the most authoritative sources of nutrition trends. Between NFHS-1 (1992-93) and NFHS-4 (2019-21), the percentage of wasted children (weight-for-height) actually increased from 17% to 19.3%. Malnutrition numbers change year on year but are not going down fast enough. Issues have remained more or less same or have worsened. Observations from the Comprehensive National Nutrition Survey (2016-18) by the Ministry of Health and Family Welfare (MoHFW) were also similar to NFHS-4.

In Maharashtra's tribal belts of Palghar and Melghat located about 100 kms from Mumbai, the commercial capital of India, infant deaths continued unabated due to malnutrition, even in 2018-19. There were 348 infant deaths in Palghar and 309 in Melghat in 2018-19. In response to a PIL (Public Interest Litigation), the Bombay High Court asked categorically, that as a progressive state, should Maharashtra be proud of reduced deaths in the state or be ashamed of even one death? This was despite the fact that Maharashtra has been running Rajmata Jijau Nutrition Mission since 2005; Bombay High Court has been monitoring malnutrition deaths for 13 years; and for more than 5 years Maharashtra's Chief Minister Devendra Fadnavis hailed from the affected Vidharbha region (Times of India, 2019).

In addition to malnutrition deaths, wasting rates for Maharashtra (like for India) increased alarmingly from 16.5% as per NFHS-1 (2005-06) to 25.6% as per NFHS-4 (2015-16) and reduced to 19.3% during NFHS-V (2019-2022). This is an increase of almost ten percentage points during the said period. In actual terms, starting was only reduced to 35.5% as per NFHS-V (2019-22) and was no where close to achieving the target of 25%. Although wasting has a lower prevalence in India than stunting or underweight, it indicates that chronic malnutrition is more prevalent in India than acute malnutrition. These indicators have substantially increased in the last decade – which is quite alarming.

In response to this challenge, Prime Minister Narendra Modi inaugurated POSHAN (Prime Minister's Overarching Scheme for Holistic Nutrition) Abhiyan or National Nutrition Mission on International Women's Day on 8th March 2017 from Jhunjhunu in Rajasthan. With a war-like mission to tackle the issue of malnutrition, POSHAN proposed a three year budget of Rs. 9046.17 crores, covering all districts in a phased manner and benefitting almost ten crore people, in a bid to reduce stunting from 38.4% in NFHS-4 to 25% by 2022.

As mentioned on POSHAN's webpage on the Ministry of Women and Child Development's website, the idea behind the programme was based on three assumptions. First, that there were a number of schemes that were directly or indirectly affecting the nutritional status of children under six, pregnant women, and lactating mothers. In spite of these, the ministry admits that malnutrition levels in the country is high. According to the Scheme document, there is a lack of connected synergy among the various schemes, resulting in failure to achieve common goals. Therefore, POSHAN is aimed at ensuring convergences between various government schemes and departments to achieve outcomes. This book provides insights on how this convergence and synergy was already designed within the ICDS at the frontline of service delivery, in the form of Village Health Nutrition and Sanitation Committees, to analyse its implementation. The only difference here being that the POSHAN scheme made this more explicit and is applied at all levels of governance.

The second assumption of the POSHAN scheme is that real time monitoring of nutrition indicators remains poor and has not fed into the need of making quick policy and programme decisions. There is, however, a scope to question why the POSHAN scheme chooses stunting (height for age) as an indicator or a marker of success when the other two indicators of underweight (weight-for-age) and wasting (weight-for-height) were more robust markers of chronic malnutrition. These two indicators - weight-for-age and weight-for-height have been either constant or have increased in the last decade (2010-2020). and have been either constant or have increased in the decade. This however is a separate debate altogether. For now, the use of ICT (information, communication and technology) for real time growth monitoring of mothers and children, was a key intervention proposed. The book provides much evidence on the culture of bureaucratic monitoring as a means, when ends are not clear.

The third assumption was to make child nutrition a public movement, with emphasis on the first 1000 days of an infant. This book provides compelling evidence on the nature of public participation in nutrition programmes, the role of frontline functionaries of anganwadi workers (AWW), ASHA (Accredited Social Health Activist) workers, ANMs (Auxiliary Nurse Midwife) and the how they play into poor or better service delivery.

Therefore, the theme of this book is quite timely, and even more so, in the current context. Despite the years since its data was collected, the finding and methodology still are much relavant.

Here, I would like to quote Albert Einstein, that "*we cannot solve problems with the same thinking that caused them*". Although numerous reports, articles, papers, books may have been written on the subject of child nutrition, the framework used in this book, with interplay of factors of accountability, local institutions, service delivery and child malnutrition, is an innovation and an original attempt. This is despite the case that the subject matter is quite over-studied. A tangible tool like social audit could not be studied by itself as it might be anecdotal and not a pervasive or standardised phenomenon. The same applies to the case of many other tools of accountability like Citizen Report Cards, Citizen Charters, or Ombudsman, which were replicable in select contexts and regions only. There was a need to study a *sui generis* social reality. Therefore, a broader sociological construct of accountability and local institutions was used to theorise in a sandpit of arguments and counter-arguments, using a mix of qualitative and quantitative data in a comparative methodology.

I chose to question the idea of accountability itself in this monograph. *Hence, I would like the reader to not dismiss arguments in this book, on basis of its data being dated back to 2012. As seen above, the numbers related to malnutrition in India or Maharashtra has remained somewhat similar since the last two decades. The ideas discussed in this monograph remain highly relevant, and even more so today.* This monograph can provide much needed explanations with evidence to evaluate existing assumptions of nutrition policy and programmes, which if not disrupted with a paradigm shift, may continue to result repeatedly in similar regressive nutrition outcomes.

As a developing country and an emerging economy, India can do much better to secure a healthy present and future of all its children. Hence, there is a need to go beyond the techno-managerial prism or a lens of looking at technical solutions for a challenge which is far from technical. This is deeply socio-political and hence requires socio-political paradigms to make sense of this reality.

Chapter Plan

I have structured the book into six chapters. The first chapter titled 'Accountability of Service Delivery: Simultaneity of a Rhetoric and a Paradox', begins with moot questions that this monograph proposes to ask. These are derived from existing gaps in theories on accountability and public service delivery. The chapter provides readers with a rationale of this research, its objectives, and the context of public health, in order to locate this study with all its complexities. This is the most critical piece as it lays down and bare all possible questions on the table, for the reader to get an idea of the complexity.

The second chapter titled as 'Studying Accountability: Methodological Concerns' enlists reasons for choosing the conceptual framework for the study. Being a scientific work, this is critical as the method or process of discovery is equally important as the discovery itself. The chapter includes definitions of the main terms used like accountability, service delivery and public health. This is followed by a description of the analytical framework used for this study. The chapter then discusses the emergence of the research design that best suits the analytical framework, followed by the geographical and empirical context of the study. Finally, the chapter ends with methods of data collection including sampling, tools, and techniques of data collection – all of which are inextricably linked to the previous steps, starting from analytical framework.

The third chapter, titled 'Under-nutrition and Local Institutions: Insights from the Two Cases', provides a profile of the two case villages – one located in a district with high Human Development District (HDI) rank and another in a district with a poor HDI rank. This chapter will provide readers with a view of the community, people, and context of this study. Readers can imagine a typical Indian village in its nature and organisation. This attempt is not novel. Important point to note however, is that the questions asked and answers unearthed, to this context, are generalizable to any such context. It is for this significant reason, that I had no heart to put this chapter as part of back pages of this book.

The chapter presents an in-depth socio-economic and demographic profile of the sample (termed as the universe, it being a case study). Household composition, state of public services, gender, sex ratio, caste, occupation, literacy, education, and economic class are all discussed. This profiling is followed by a critical discussion on the politics of measurement of child under-nutrition both at the macro and micro levels, in comparison between both case villages. Lastly, the chapter analytically and statistically discusses the status of child malnutrition in both the cases to identify the change in the nutritional status of the children over a period of time. Such a change is also analysed in the context of the asset class and socio-religious class, to understand how these variables impact child malnutrition. The chapter concludes with summaries of key observations, dismissing at the same time a long held notion about the relationship between service delivery improvements like a well-functioning anganwadi centre and better nutrition outcomes.

The fourth chapter is titled as 'Providers and Users: Nature of Engagement'. The chapter explores answers to the first objective of the study while comparing the two case villages of the study. The chapter will attempt to understand the choices users make to access women and child health services, as well as their reasons behind those choices and how these choices define relationship of accountability between users and providers in the context of democracy and the rhetoric of accountability. The concept of choices is examined through the nature of engagement between users and providers, using indicators like access, level of trust, and ratings of services. With these concepts, the chapter argues that the nature of engagement between users and providers have a bearing on their capacities to demand accountability from the providers. The chapter also provides evidence to show that the mere supply of public health services, even if accessible and of good quality, may not be sufficient to guarantee use by the rural population.

The fifth Chapter is titled as 'Answerability and Sanctions: Getting Services Delivered'. The chapter deals with the commonalities and differences in the concept of answerability and sanctions, at the frontline of service delivery, in two study villages. This aspect is aligned with the study's second objective which is to analyse how users, especially the poor, demand or negotiate better services and entitlements through both formal and informal local institutional processes. The chapter delineates various formal mechanisms available to the users in both cases, exploring to what extent they are effective and the reasons if they are not. The chapter also discusses the commonalities and differences of providers' perspectives and the interpretation of how they are accountable to various stakeholders, within and outside the service delivery. The chapter critically discusses and compares the formal and informal mechanisms of accountability, arguing that institutional processes shape their practices and perceptions of accountability. The questions on how and why these processes were different between the two cases shed more insights on the key research question of this chapter.

The final chapter is titled as 'Rethinking Accountability'. The chapter threads together key observations and findings of the previous chapters to discuss the third and final objective of the study. It does so by two ways - first, by dismissing existing notions and practices of accountability using the empirical evidence presented in the previous chapters, and second, by summing up findings to strengthen the existing theoretical framework, thereby adding value to the knowledge on the subject. Such insights lead to enumerating implications for policy as well as the practice of public service delivery in general, and child nutrition programmes in particular. The chapter then ends by providing avenues for further research on the subject.

-Jaya Goyal, Ph.D.
Mumbai 2023.

Acknowledgements

Research is a solitary but self-engaging process. I often derived my motivation from this quote - *"it is not enough to take steps which may someday lead to a goal, each step must be a goal."*- Johann Wolfgang von *Goethe.*

At each step of this research, there were numerous people who helped me move forward. First and for most, I am deeply indebted to my family who were pillars of my perseverance. Our shared experiences from 2009 till 2016, of highs and lows of this journey, made it worth every moment.

I am deeply grateful to my doctoral thesis supervisor, Prof. Madhushree Sekher, at TISS for her mentorship for this research. I want to extend my heartfelt gratitude to Prof. N. Jayaram who had a lasting impression on me, as a teacher. As an advisory committee member of this research, he often placed the mirror me the mirror that forced me to pause, think, question, unlearn, and relearn the nuances of research. Prof. Jayaram also kindly agreed to write the foreword for this book. I am extremely grateful to late Prof. S. Parasuraman, former Director of Tata Institute of Social Sciences, for his valuable suggestions as a doctoral advisory committee member. His ability to see the big picture across perspectives helped me immensely in adding a new and much needed dimension to the study.

Over the course of field work and data collection, I remain heartily thankful to the help extended by my batch mate and friend Anagha who readily volunteered to help translate data collection instruments from English to Marathi. I offer my most sincere appreciation to Prof. R. Ramakumar who helped me with the estimation of asset values, data entry, and analysis in the MS Access software. My field work would not have been a great experience had it not been for Navnath and Ajay who accompanied me to translate at different points in time during data collection in Satara and Osmanabad.

My village volunteer friends Nikita, Ajay, Kumar, Pallavi, Vinod, and Archana need a special mention here. They greatly enriched my understanding of their village and context. I would also like to extend thanks to the officials of ICDS departments at Koregaon block in Satara and Tuljapur block in Osmanabad, especially Mrs. Inamdar and Mrs. Mahajan who cooperated in sharing block and village records. I owe deep appreciation to the people in both villages whose houses I visited and also my respondents of Anganwadi workers, ASHA workers, ANMs, Medical officers, Panchayat members, and others who shared their everyday lives with me. I also acknowledge and thank staff at the TISS Tuljapur Campus Guest House and Wathar Kiroli Gram Panchayat for ensuring my safe stay at these places during the field work.

I am grateful to Prof. John Cameron and Dr. C. Sathyamala whose critique on a paper presented at the 12th Development Dialogue at the Institute of Social Studies (ISS), The Hague, Netherlands, actually helped in strengthening arguments in this monograph. This experience was special because of friendship established with Nadira and Tejeshwar. This paper was eventually published in a well respected international journal called 'Development'. This paper id titled 'Acountability, Nutrition and Local Institutions in India'. Development: Rethinking' Demaracy, Society for International Development. 58(1). Palgrave McMillan. UK. was published in 2015 in a special issue on Rethinking Democracy. I would like to acknowledge and thank academics from The Graduate School, Geneva, Switzerland, Prof. Ricardo Bocco and Prof. Thomas Biersteker, for their suggestions on a paper presented at the Global South Doctoral Workshop at the University of Gadjah Mada, Yogyakarta, Indonesia. Special thanks go also to Shyam who critiqued my paper and fellow Suweon, Benny, Rajdeep, Meera, Mweso and Santana who made it a memorable experience. I am very grateful to ISS, Netherlands and The Graduate School, Geneva for awarding me Scholarships to present these papers.

My visit to the London School of Economics and Political Science (LSE) as a fellow was an unforgettable learning experience because of facilitation extended by Dr. Ruth Kattumuri at the Asia Research Centre and Dr. Mathijs Pelkmans from Department of Anthropology. This experience was made most worthwhile because of friends I found in Prerna and Krishna. I owe a deep gratitude to TISS, as an institution and my mentors there because of whom I was awarded the TISS-LSE fellowship to visit LSE. I would also like to thank discussants of my proposal and synopsis presentations, particularly Prof. Subodh Wagle, IIT Bombay, Prof. Manish Jha, Prof. Anil Sutar, and Prof. Mathew George of the Tata Institute of Social Sciences, Mumbai. Their thoughtful inputs helped improve arguments in the thesis in useful ways. I will also like to mention and sincerely thank the support of TISS librarians Dr. Satish and Dr. Mallikarjun and the entire library staff for attending to my research requests. My heartfelt appreciation to Prof. Surinder Jaswal, Prof. Laxmi Lingam, and the staff of the Doctoral Students Office at

TISS for facilitating the administrative requirements of doctoral thesis from which this monograph is based.

I am thankful to Supriya who painstakingly helped me to transcribe and translate all recorded interviews from Marathi to English. Words are not enough to express my appreciation for my friend and colleague, Dr. T. Laxmi, whose feedback on some of the arguments in this monograph was much timely. I offer great appreciation to Prof. D. P Singh and colleague Saritha C.T who helped me with SPSS and other statistical tests. I attribute the credit of keeping me in good humour during this research to my friends Poonam, Parul, Niharika and Uma.

My sincere thanks to ICSSR for funding this publication, without which this research would be gathering dust in a library. I am so grateful to Prof. Malhotra Member Secretary, ICSSR; Mr. Mahesh Madhukar and Dr. Ajay Gupta for expediting approvals especially during the pandemic. I am deeply thankful to the publisher Motilal Banarsidass Publications, especially Rajeev Jain ji and Pranav ji for their gentle nudges and warmth; and their entire team for a publishing a Social Sciences book, adding to their forte on Indian Philosophy.

Last but not the least I want to genuinely thank my house staff Ashwini, Sunita, Bhumika and Sheela at varying points in time, especially during my absence at LSE, field work in Maharashtra, and writing of this monograph.

I would like to acknowledge and thank my copy editors, Mr. Ismail Shogo from Singapore and Ms. Oluchi Emenike (Igbo) from United Kingdom for helping me proof-read this entire manuscript for easy flow of reading for readers.

Finally, I offer deep gratitude to my spiritual mentors Dr. Daisaku Ikeda, Late Dr. Vijaya Venkat, and Anju Venkat of The Health Awareness Centre (THAC) in Mumbai for making this learning a part of my human evolution and awareness consciousness.

List of Tables

APPENDIX I

APPENDIX II

List of Figures

APPENDIX II

APPENDIX II

List of Boxes

Abbreviations

ANC	Ante Natal Checkups
ANM	Auxiliary Nurse Midwife
ASHA	Accredited Social Health Activist
AWC	Anganwadi Cenetr
AWW	Anganwadi Work
BC	before Christ
BDO	Block Development Officer
BJP	Bhartiya Janata Party
BPL	Below Poverty Line
CAG	Comptroller & Auditor General of India
CBM	Community Based Monitoring
CBO	Community Based Organisation
CDC	Child Development Center
CDPO	Child Development Project Officer
CEHAT	Centre for Enquiry into Health and Allied Themes
CHW	Community Health Worker
CMO	Chief Medical Officer
CNSM	Comprehensive Nutrition Survey Maharashtra
CO	Community Organisations
CPR	Centre for Policy Research
DHO	District Health Officer
DMO	District Medical Officer
DPSP	Directive Principles of State Policy
ECCE	Early Childhood Care and Education
et al.	and others
FGD	Focus Group Discussion
GDN	Global Development Network
GDP	Gross Domestic Product

GPS	Geo Positioning System
GOI	Government of India
GP	Gram Panchayat
GP-WSC	Gram Panchayat's Water & Sanitation Commitee
GR	Government Resolutions
HDD	Human Development District
HDI	Human Development Index
HH	Household
IAC	India Against Corruption
IAD	Institutional and Development Framework
IAY	Indira Awas Yojana
ibid.	in the same source (referring to a previously cited work)
ICDS	Integrated Child Development Services
IDS	Intitute of Development Studied
IFPRI	International Food Policy of Research In Institue
IFPRI	International Food Policy of Research In Institue
IIPS	International Institute of Population Science
IMF	International Monetary Fund
IMNCI	Integtrated Management of Neonatal and Chuildhood Illness
INC	Indian National Congress
IPHS	Indian Public Health Standards
LHV	Lady Health Visitor
MAM	Modertae Acute Malnutrition
MCH	Maternal and Child Health
MCI	Medical Council of India
MDM	Mid Day Meals
MIS	Management and Information System
MKSS	Masdoor Kisan Shakti Sangathan
MNC	Multi National Corporation
MO	Medical Officer
MPR	Monthly Progress Report
MPW	Multi Purpose Workers
MS	Misrodoft
nd	no date
NFHS	National Family Health Survey

NGO	Non Govermental Organisations
NHM	National Health Mission
NPM	New Public Management
NREGA	National Rural Employeement Guarantee Act
NRHM	National Rural Health Mission
NSSO	National Sample Survery Organisation
OBC	Other Backward Class
ORS	Oral Rehydration Salt
PAC	Public Affairs Center
PDS	Public Distribution System
pg. or pp.	page
PHC	Primary Health Center
PIL	Public Interest Ligitations
PRI	Panchayat Raj Institution
PSE	Pre School Education
QoG	Quality of Govermance
RCH	Reproductive and Child Health
RKS	Rogi Kalyan Information
RTI	Right to Information
SAM	Severe Acute Malnutrition
SAP	Structural Adjustment Programme
SATHI	Support for Advocasy and Training to Health
SC	Schedule Caste
SNP	Supplementary Nutriotion Programme
SPSS	Statistical Package for Social Science
SSA	Sarya Shikha Abhiyan
ST	Schedule Tribe
TISS	Tata Institute of Social Sciences
THR	Take Home Ration
TMO	Taluka Medical Officer
TSC	Total Sensition Campaign
ULBs	Urban Local Bodies
UN	United Nations
UNICEF	United Nations International Children's Emergency Fund
UT	Union Territory

VCDC	Village Child Development Centers
VEC	Village Education Comimittee
VHNSC	Village Health Nutrition and Sanitation Committee
VHNWSC	Village Health, Nutrition, Water & Sanitation Committee
VHSC	Village Health Sanitation & Nutrition Committee
Vol.	Volume
WB	The World Bank
WFA	Weight for Age
WFLH	Weight for Lenght/Height
WHO	World Health Organisation
ZP	Zila Parishad

CHAPTER 1

Accountability in Service Delivery: Simultaneity of a Rhetoric and a Paradox

"Just as it is impossible to know when a fish moving in water is drinking it, so it is impossible to find out when government servants in charge of undertakings misappropriate money."- Kautilya (300 BCE) (Premchand, 1995: 21)

1.1 Rhetoric and Paradox

An old saying goes, "Power corrupts." Governments as custodians of the people's mandate in a democracy have the power and by that logic, can be corrupt unless checks and balances are strong. Throughout time, political thinkers have been contemplating the question of how to prevent governments' abuse of power. The first documented evidence was found as early as 300 BCE in Kautilya's *Arthshastra* on theories and principles of governing a state.

Accountability has emerged as an answer to this question (Schedler, 1999). Accountability is increasingly used in political, policy and development discourse, to convey an image of trans-parency, trustworthiness, and responsiveness to the needs of the citizens. It has come to assume a central place in contemporary governance discourse over the last ten years owing to an increased donor attention on the idea of 'good governance'[1] (Newell and Wheeler, 2006).

---

1 There are different definitions of 'governance' and 'good governance', but it could be said that 'good governance' essentially deals with the crucial issue of balance between the power of the state and the market (Wagle & Dixit, 2006). According to United Nations, good governance has eight major characteristics. It is participatory, consensus oriented, accountable, transparent, responsive, effective and efficient, equitable and inclusive and follows the rule of law. It assures that corruption is minimised, the views of minorities are considered, and that the voices of the most vulnerable in society are heard in decision-making (For more see Mander et al., 2004; United Nations Economic and Social Commission for Asia and the Pacific, 2015).

In policy and development debates, experts across board, have increasingly promoted accountability as an essential element in the concept of good governance. Reason being, that since more than a decade, international organisations like the World Bank, the International Monetary Fund (IMF) and the United Nations have focused on the importance of good governance and sound institutions. The broad assumption is that only with a high quality of government can a country reap the benefits of economic growth and social development (Holmberg et al., 2009).

The discourse on governance is also viewed by many critics as an attempt by the international financial institutions to establish indirect control over state institutions and policy-making processes especially in developing countries of the South (Wagle & Dixit, 2006). While this is debatable, the discourse on good governance supplied the criteria or standards necessary to call for political and administrative reforms in developing countries like India.

In fact, an evidence of this notion of accountability reaching rhetoric proportions was seen in the 2014 general elections in India, when the right-wing Bhartiya Janata Party (BJP) led the National Democratic Alliance and the incumbent Indian Prime Minister Narendra Modi won with sweeping majority through exploiting this notion of good governance in general and corruption in particular. People have now conveniently assumed that the notion of accountability holds government and society together like glue (Hodge & Coghill, 2007).

The commonly held notion is either we see accountability as simply a matter of periodic voting for political representatives or we view it as a longer and more complex chain of responsibility for decisions and actions (ibid.). In a democracy, holding political leaders and public bureaucracies morally responsible for apathy, harm or wrongdoing is significant in maintaining accountability of the government and it is imperative that citizens exercise that pressure (Sinha, 2006). Therefore, in contemporary governance discourse, accountability is brandished as the complete and final solution to all governance problems – the chief instrument for combating the 'three-headed monster of corruption, clientelism and elite capture' (Ackerman, 2004; Jayal, 2008).

Co-existing with this rhetoric simultaneously is the following paradox identified by many social scientists. India is hailed as the world's largest democracy, but it is rather curious that accountability levels are so low here, despite the country's strong democratic tradition (Dreze & Sen, 2002). Interestingly, a quality shared by the world's most mature democracies, is the ability to deepen democracy, that is, to make politics more inclusive and the state more accountable. In India, democratic deepening has undoubtedly been impressive, but it has progressed much further in terms of inclusiveness than with respect to accountability (Jenkins, 2007).

Harriss (2010) dismisses any argument that cites India as a 'failing state' and argues that it is quite clearly not so because the central functions of government are often performed with exceptional competence, but the delivery of basic services is generally very poor. In fact, according to Sen (2006), doubts on the merits of Indian democracy can be well addressed in the perspective of 'Development as Freedom' which was also the title of his 2004 book. He observes,

> *'It is important to examine the connection between political and civil rights, on one hand, and prevention of major disasters, such as famines, on the other. The availability and the use of political and civil rights give people the opportunity to draw attention forcefully to general dangers and vulnerabilities, and to demand remedial action....India has not had a real famine since independence (despite continued endemic under-nourishment and often precarious food situation) whereas, China had the largest famine in recorded history during 1958-61,when the ill-calculated public policies that led to the disaster were continued by the government without any substantial emendation for three years, while nearly 30 million people died' (Sen, 2006: 161).*

Sen (2006) also claims that the Asian economic crisis of 1997-99 that affected many economies especially those with undemocratic governance, could not impact India due to the protective power of its democracy. The common generalisations that the democracy tends to slow down economic growth is refuted by Sen (2006) where he cites extensive cross-country comparisons which have not provided any empirical support for this often-repeated belief. Some scholars also argue that,

> *'India's problem of democratic 'governability' is not the hollowing out of the state, or the decline of state's sovereignty, in the face of encroaching multilateral disciplines, but rather the success of democracy itself. It meant that the pent up demands by the formerly marginalized groups – for economic goods, for government jobs, for cultural recognition – began to overwhelm the capacity of India's democratic system to process them' (Goetz & Jenkins, 2005: 22).*

Therefore, the merits of Indian democracy need not be undermined. However, Sen (2006) argues that the limited reach of Indian social policies on education, basic nutrition, health care, land reform and gender equity reflects the weakness of the democratic practice. Pritchett (2009) has named this phenomenon as India being a 'flailing state' where the head which is well endowed with ideas is unable to coordinate with the limbs which actually act. It is true that there is also no dearth of successful initiatives in India since 'Vikram Chand (2006) in a World Bank study has documented more than a dozen case studies of successful initiatives in service delivery' (Pritchett, 2009). One is not denying an oasis of success stories, but the question is on that of services delivery being poor in general.

Therefore, one of the central paradoxes faced by India is this - There are enough successes and practices documented in the field, so why are services not improving at a pace they need to?

According to Centre for Policy Research (CPR), a public policy Think Tank working on governance and accountability, there is rampant corruption, absenteeism, indifference, incompetence, inefficiencies or outright failures across public services and this paradox is inescapable (Posani & Aiyer, 2009). The crisis of accountability manifests in chronic problems of service delivery for most public programmes like the teaching standards in government schools that have remained abysmally low, health centres have continuously provided dismal services, environmental plunder has gone on unchecked, the public distribution system has been extensively looted and resettlement programmes have routinely failed (Dreze & Sen, 2002).

Such a scenario becomes more challenging because a large proportion of households in India depend heavily on the government for a wide range of essential public services (Paul et al., 2004). Also, many of its public services like policing or preventive health are public goods from the benefits of which, no one can be excluded (ibid.). The government is responsible and accountable for implementing policies, deploying budgets and personnel towards these services, tasks that are within its control.

A people's audit of the basic five services by Public Affairs Centre (PAC) Bangalore was conducted across major states of India covering 37,000 households. This study revealed that governments have done more for extending access to services like drinking water, roads, primary education, public health and public distribution system (PDS), but much less to ensure their effectiveness and reliability (ibid.). Evidence from the field also demonstrates that basic public services have failed the poor. For instance, in terms of human development indicators such as literacy, schooling, morbidity and mortality, India ranks amongst the poorest countries in the world (Keefer & Khemani, 2004).

At the same time, the rhetoric of accountability has made in-roads in every aspect of public service delivery especially in the policy advocacy and human rights movements (Brinkerhoff, 2004; Potts, 2005). It was clear during the Anna Hazare[2] led Campaign Against Corruption. This was a civil society led mass mobilisation of Indians from all levels of society to support India's anti-corruption mood in 2011. In addition, the public policy discourse has zeroed in on weak accountability as one of the reasons for service delivery outcomes *still* being poor in India overall (Posani & Aiyer, 2009).

2 Anna Hazare is a social activist and a national leader who has launched a grass roots campaign to eradicate corruption in India. Both his style and his strategies are reminiscent of Gandhi and they have won him global recognition and many awards. https://www.huffpost.com/entry/anna-hazare-and-the-campa_b_3814120.

Eminent scholars believe that the heart of development failures in India is a systemic lack or crisis of accountability in the public sector. They also acknowledge that accountability has long been both a key theme and a key problem in constitutional scholarship (Scott, 2000). Therefore, there seems to be both simultaneity and co-existence of the rhetoric and crisis of accountability, which are evident in the discourse on the notions of public services, nature of state and its governance.

1.2 Moot Questions

The question that therefore, arise is, why is public service delivery outcomes poor in India, despite the considerable decentralisation and systems of monitoring and evaluation in place? How does one ascertain 'deficits' in accountability and how do these deficits manifest between actors?

Mounting evidence suggests that a country's economic status alone cannot entirely explain differences in public policy outcomes (Kumar, 2007; Ruger, 2005; Sen, 1999; Banerji, 1986). It is important to extend analysis to broader structural factors, such as political institutions and processes of public accountability for a better understanding of regional inequalities in service delivery.

These questions lead to the following research questions: How is accountability one of the determinants of improved or poor service delivery and hence good or bad governance? Answering these questions will not be possible unless one also understands various institutions of accountability and the actors involved in service delivery. Therefore, the central question of this book is how is accountability a significant idea in the everyday encounters of various actors in public service delivery? This question assumes importance especially in the context of high rhetoric of accountability in policy and development discourse.

Accountability processes are also more direct at the local level, if the democratic processes work. There is more vigilance on issues where more local stake is involved especially when stakeholders are conscious that it is their money being wasted or stolen. Electoral sanctions may be more effective at the local level, than at central level where multi-dimensionality of electoral issues dilutes responsibility (Bardhan, 2009).

Therefore, it is imperative to understand how users, especially the poor, interact and interface with accountability mechanisms especially the informal ones when the formal mechanisms of accountability fail or exclude them and how regional differentials in public service delivery shape local processes of accountability.

These are only initial probes that would direct the course of this research. It is worthwhile to understand how the idea of accountability emerged in history before it became rhetorical and critical for governance.

1.3 Indian State & Institutions of Accountability

1.3.1 Historical Linkages

Accountability was one of the four areas of governance identified for action for the first time, in the World Bank publication *Governance and Development* in 1992 (Joseph, 2001). The consecutive *World Development Report,* 1997 focused on 'operationalising' accountability and the focus was on bringing in popular 'voice' into decision making. It opened up channels to civil society and decentralisation of government (ibid.).

It emphasised that the citizens should be given a voice as 'consumers' in relation to different utilities - as taxpayers, as members of voluntary associations etc. This phase marked a peak in usage of the terms like transparency, accountability and decentralisation in international policy circles. Scholars feel that trailing in the wake of amorphous 'governance agenda', the elastic concept of voice and accountability have come to dominate not just the development discourse, but also the language of international politics, business and activism (Goetz et al., 2005). That is how during the last few years, despite being highly contested, the ideas of good governance in general and accountability in particular have earned the status of an international orthodoxy (Mander et al., 2004).

There were other global trends that led to building this orthodoxy. Accountability as one of the pillars of good governance became predominant from three perspectives – Neo-liberal and World Bank perspective, followed by other multi-lateral agencies like the United Nations; human rights perspective by civil society and people's movements, and finally by state's perspective as many democratic regimes wanted to portray an image of transparency, trustworthiness and responsiveness to its citizens. Essentially it meant that the governments, global financial institutions, markets and civil society, all led to the making of the rhetoric of accountability from their own positions and perspectives.

By the turn of the century, Structural Adjustment Programmes[3] (SAP) during liberalisation reforms of the 1990s did more ill than keep up with its promises in developing nations of Asia and Africa. It was at the same time when the political reforms demanded the need for state's intervention in the markets. And with the wave on 'Bringing the State back in', there was a renewed interest in strengthening institutional structures and practices for bottom up accountability mechanisms in public service delivery (Evans et al., 1985).

---

3 Structural Adjustment Programmes (SAPs) were economic policies for developing countries that were promoted by the World Bank and International Monetary Fund in the early 1980s. It allowed countries to get a loan but with conditionalities like significant policy reforms has to be complied with before getting the loan. These conditionalities included removing excess government controls and promoting market competition (For more see Joseph (2001); Structural Adjustment Programs (SAPs) (2015).

Good governance and administrative reforms of the New Public Management[4] (NPM) wave thus became part of the package of reforms which started being promoted in developing countries (Joseph, 2001). Consequently, democratic governments in developing countries came under pressure to improve effectiveness in the delivery of public services in terms of tangible outcomes or results that directly impact the poor. As a result, governments started responding to the international organisations' promotion on accountability and transparency as essential elements in the reforms that incorporate good governance.

Soon, the idea of good governance evolved to recognition of institutions and their role in shaping interactions between the State, market, and society, post-Washington consensus in 1990s. In the new millennium, the World Bank's reports – *Building Institutions for Markets* (2002) and *Making Services Work for the Poor* (2004) stressed the significance of various kinds of institutions in explaining paradoxes like 'poverty in the midst of plenty' (North, 1990 cited in World Bank, 2001: 1; World Bank, 2004).

The understanding that emerged was that accountability in service delivery is closely related to the role of institutions that shape these processes. According to Joshi (2006), while more financial resources are required for basic services, the main barriers to improved services are institutional ones. It is recognised that 'societies get locked into inefficient set of institutions because of the interest of the power holders in their reproduction' (Harriss, 2006: 23).

Therefore, consistent record of poor public services is not a matter of social policy or weak implementation alone, but about institutions of politics and relationships of power between various actors like the State, the beneficiaries, the market and the civil society. One of the key institutions that shape and implement policies, on which various actors interact in a social setting, is the State. Hence, it is imperative to understand how the Indian State's institutions have performed to begin with. Consequently one also needs to understand how the Indian Constitution, which is an apex institution of the country, has influenced performance of these institutions, which is the focus of the following section.

1.3.2 Indian Institutions: Status Quo

In addition to lack of accountability per se in public service delivery, experts have increasingly positioned the processes of accountability within the framework of various institutions that determine the outputs and outcomes in public service delivery. A direct impact of weak institutions, low accountability and hence poor public services is on

4 New Public Management (NPM) was a reaction to the traditional public administration theories. NPM involved a set of ideas to innovate public organisations. It is based on the neo-liberal paradigm, where public organisations were equated with private organisations. An entrepreneurial spirit was introduced into the public realm; however, the political dimension was left out (For more see De Vries, 2010).

majority of households in India that depend on the government for several essential public services (Paul et al., 2004).

However, public policy in India has often ignored the role of institutions especially for public services like health and education. It is for this reason there is a consistent pattern of either poor outcomes or low improvements in public services. For instance, as observed in the state of Tamil Nadu, despite a relatively good Integrated Child Development Services (ICDS) programme (as compared to the rest of the country) and significant improvements in the delivery of healthcare, these measures have managed to reduce the proportion of underweight children by a mere 4 percentage points over seven years – from 39 per cent in 1998-99 to only 34 per cent in 2005-06 (Kumar, 2007).

Another study of the two centrally sponsored schemes of ICDS and NRHM in a Union Territory of Andaman & Nicobar Islands (ANI) revealed similar findings (Goyal, 2014). The paper observed that despite well-functioning Anganwadi [5] Centres (AWCs) and presence of superior spending and infrastructure on health, child nutrition outcomes had deteriorated in the corresponding time period (ibid.). This suggests that reducing child malnutrition requires more than a well-functioning anganwadi centre (Kumar, 2007).

India's institutions of accountability have under-performed significantly. This includes the Judiciary that holds the Executive to account or the Legislature or the various oversight and regulatory authorities like the Vigilance Commissions, the Comptroller & Auditor General of India (CAG), Ombudsman or Lok Ayukts etc. (Posani & Aiyer, 2009). There is an environment of multiple institutional failures (ibid.). Amid this crisis, civil society led by Gandhian crusader Anna Hazare started a movement called India Against Corruption (IAC) on the Jan Lokpal Bill[6]. The movement reached euphoric proportions in 2011. The core idea behind this movement was the notion of public accountability, by way of setting up an independent sanctioning institution to punish the power holders charged with corruption.

To be fair, the Indian state has, in the past, initiated efforts to create newer structures for closer citizen engagement to strengthen accountability. The 73rd and 74th Amendment Acts of the Indian Constitution paved way for Panchayat Raj Institutions (PRIs) and Urban Local Bodies (ULBs) for rural and urban contexts, respectively. It decentralises powers and responsibilities to local governments to strengthen bottoms-up accountability. In recent years, the Indian state has also converted key socio-economic entailments related

5 Anganwadi is a courtyard generally located within a community or slum area, which serves as a platform to deliver services of the central government's Integrated Child Development Services (ICDS) scheme (Shastri, 2013).

6 The Jan Lokpal Bill is an act to create effective anti-corruption and grievance redressal systems at centre so that effective deterrent is created against corruption and to provide effective protection to whistle-blowers (For more see www.indiaagainstcorruption.org; http://www.annahazare.org/lokpal and NDTV, 2015).

to food, employment, education, and information to legally enforceable rights. These are the Right to Information Act (2005), National Rural Employment Guarantee Act (2005) (NREGA), the Right to Education Act (2009) and the National Food Security Act (2013).

There are few more pending provisions which can facilitate citizen mobilization around newer axes and create opportunities for the emergence of newer spaces and instruments through which citizens can engage with and scrutinise the state (ibid.). These are in form of pending bills[7] like the Citizen's Charter and Grievance Redressal Bill 2011 and the Whistle-blower Protection Law or the Public Interest Disclosure (Protection of Information) Bill 2011.

For service delivery, governments did introduce community based monitoring and social audits as institutionalised accountability mechanisms in many government schemes like National Rural Health Mission (NRHM), NREGA and Sarvya Shiksha Abhiyan (SSA). However, some recent studies suggest that community monitoring of public programmes can have only a small or insignificant impact on reducing corruption or improving the accountability of public officials (Banerjee et al., 2004; Afridi, 2008).

According to Harriss (2014), social welfare legislations like that of NREGA provides a promise of governance reforms through a new kind of democratic participation like social audits. However, evidence from Rajasthan on social audits showed that when panchayats and officials opposed it, the State Government stopped it. Similarly, in Tamil Nadu NREGA was successful in empowering *dalits* and women but there was hardly any action taken on social audit reports. Therefore, social transformation potential of social audits and NREGA does not extend to change rural people's relationship with the state (ibid.).

The serious paucity of accountability and transparency in the functioning of government institutions at bottom most levels of governance could render even the most primary level organisation, like a gram panchayat or a village development board, to be futile (Mukhopadhyay, 2005). Hence, decentralisation which was cited as a panacea to all the problems of governance is also losing luster in development debates owing to its failures in bringing about effective and inclusive development.

Mukhopadhay (2005) cites reasons like – low awareness on roles and responsibilities of elected representatives, minimum devolution of functional and financial powers to local bodies, and no systems for sharing information with the stakeholders. All these point to a fact that mere decentralisation for the sake of it without institutional capacity makes for nothing but, decentralised corruption (ibid.).

Therefore, it emerges that accountability is one of the democratic practices enacted through various institutions that influences public service delivery. Various accountability

7 These bills are pending in the Legislatures to be made into Acts.

mechanisms benefit both the service providers and their users. These include elections, right to information, citizen report cards, social audits, user satisfaction surveys, government audit reports etc. that can support interactions between communities and services. It is for this reason that experts cite that while both democratic institutions and democratic practice are important for good governance, the latter is not guaranteed by the former (Dreze & Sen, 2002; Vaddiraju & Mehrotra, 2004). It means just because democratic institutions exist, there is no surety that it will dish out democratic practices too.

This statement gives justification for the focus on practices and processes of 'accountability' in the framework of institutions in public service delivery.

1.3.3 Means or an End?

Despite being accepted as a crucial aspect of governance, there is a danger in studying the idea of accountability as an uncontested one and in isolation. For instance, 'in Nazi Germany and Fascist Italy, state's accountability was high, which is one of the key features of totalitarian regimes with 'total' control of the state' (Finer, 1970: 95). In hindsight one knows that such accountability was not justified on grounds of justice and equality. In fact, it had perpetrated gruesome and mass acts of violence against its own people. Some academics acknowledge the rhetoric of accountability and, instead of being carried away, want to steer this rhetoric in the direction of creating an egalitarian society. Scholars have argued,

> *'...while it is clear that questions on transparency and accountability are gaining ground in the current political system, it is also true that the neo-liberal order has made these ideas extremely privileged. Even the fascist orders in Germany kept their governance ideals extremely transparent. But, that in no way reflected on the nature of the state at that time. Therefore, the wider understanding should be to treat transparency and accountability not as an end in itself. The focus should rather be on the kind of society we envisage for ourselves and whether our nature of engagement and confrontation is adequate to bring about that change' (Praveen Jha quoted in Rath, 2014: 36).*

Therefore, a key question that I would like to propose is this: Are people's rights and 'social justice' met with prevailing accountability institutions and processes in a democratic state? That is, whether accountability is an absolute virtue in a state-society relationship that cannot be a given and is subject to critique. Also, in context of the Indian state, another question to ask is, what should be the nature of accountability that would deliver 'justice' for its people? The idea of social justice is relevant to accountability of public service delivery in order to secure improved welfare interventions through welfare systems and processes.

A section of academia led by scholars like Harriss (2014) argues that how can one talk of accountability when Indian State was never meant to give social justice in the first place. It is this reason that it is important to historically access the Constitutional provisioning that give policy directions to the Indian State. India is part of the sixty odd states that were created in between the two world wars, after 1945, out of the collapse of the British, French, Belgian and Dutch overseas empires, mostly in Asia and Africa. At the same time, India already had a tradition of statehood for centuries before it was colonised, other examples being, Egypt, Vietnam, Burma, Cambodia, Laos etc. Finer (1970) provides an account,

> *'...governments in these newly independent countries shared a common set of political presuppositions derived from three European events – the French Revolution, the Industrial Revolution and the Russian Revolution. The newly formed democracies wish or claim to wish to 'modernise'. But the very term implies that they regard their societies as non-modern. And being non-modern, their political, economic and social structures at independence did not readily support these liberal-democratic institutions or that meant 'Westernisation'. It is precisely from this confrontation that their political experiences and institutional experiences flow' (quoted in Finer, 1970: 98).*

The idea of social justice was well 'intended' when India got independence but got mired into structural confusion about its implementation. According to Harriss (2014), Nehru's address to the Constituent Assembly in 1947, on the country's vision of 'development', was of a 'just society that provides fullest opportunity for its people to develop according to their capacities' (Harriss, 2014). This is same as Sen's idea of social justice in his book 'Development as Freedom (1999)' (Sen, 1999). In the 1931 Karachi Session of Indian National Congress[8] (INC) and also, in the 1928 Motilal Nehru Committee Report[9], there was a strong commitment for social and economic concerns like economic freedom for starving millions, redistributive land reforms, improvement of agriculture, and right to well-being (ibid.). It is evident that long before independence there was a strong consensus among political leadership on a need for economic and social rights.

---

8 The Gandhi Irwin Pact was endorsed by the Congress in the Karachi Session of 1931 (March 26-31), which reiterated the goal of "Poorna Swaraj". In the Karachi session, presided over by Sardar Patel, the congress adopted a resolution on Fundamental Rights and Economic Policy which represented the party's social, economic and political programme. It was later known as Karachi Resolution. Nehru had originally drafted it, but some Congress leaders thought it was too radical and it was redrafted (For more see www.gktoday.in).

9 In 1928, a committee was appointed under the chair of Motilal Nehru, to draft the proposed constitution. The draft constitution was prepared and was called "Nehru Committee Report." The report had defined citizenship and fundamental rights for the first time (For more see www.gktoday.in).

However, while drafting the Constitution, only civil and political rights were included as Fundamental Rights in Part III of the Constitution, while the vital social and economic rights like right to work, education, nutrition, public health and welfare were transferred to Directive Principles of State Policy (DPSP) in Part IV of the Constitution. Such a move is attributed to the Advisory Committee on Fundamental Rights which cited reasons like 'practical ineffectiveness' and 'doubted capacity of state to be binding to this commitment' (Jayal, 2013 quoted in Harriss, 2014). The courts in India have no power to enforce them if citizens are denied the socio-economic rights mentioned in DPSP while Fundamental Rights are justiciable and enforceable by the courts of law. It meant that rights in the DPSP became non-justiciable and only 'desirable' directions for policy but with no legal backing as opposed to justiciable rights like right to life, liberty and property under fundamental rights.

There are 16 articles of the Constitution, from 36 to 51which deal with DPSP, covering a wide range of state activity embracing social, economic, legal, educational and international issues (Pylee, 1963). The Constitution directed the state that it 'should' promote these directive principles, without effectively requiring the state to do any of these things (Harriss 2014: 2). Further, Harriss (2014) argues that the Indian state never committed itself to social justice (as legal entitlements) in the first place. While saying so, Harriss (2014) dismissed the argument made by anthropologist Gupta (2012) that 'Indian State is attributed to two million avoidable deaths in a year', in his book titled, 'Red tape: Bureaucracy, Structural Violence and Poverty in India' (Gupta quoted in Harriss 2014). However, Dr. B. R Ambedkar could envisage this confusion and had mentioned,

> '*...establishment of political democracy is a fundamental aim of the constitution. But that in itself is not enough. If the fundamental rights guarantee a political democracy in India, the DPSP ensure the eventual emergence of an economic democracy to sustain the former. Thus, DPSP become the greatest guarantee for a genuine democracy in India' (Ambedkar quoted in Pylee 1963: 154).*

After 60 years of independence, the Government of India took route of legislations to convert some economic and social rights to legal entitlements like rural employment guarantee, right to education, right to food and right to information. Harriss (2014) critiques this legislation route, which is at the cost of investing in structural social transformation. For instance, though Right to Education was enacted in 2009, there was no corresponding increase in Gross Domestic Product (GDP) towards education and health in consequent Union Budgets, even as recent as the year 2014. Many more rights like health mentioned in Article 47 according to Pylee (1963: 143), such as 'To secure the improvement of public health and the prohibition of intoxicating drinks and drugs' or ones pertaining to land acquisition and forests rights are still out of the ambit of being legally enforceable right.

Therefore, while studying accountability for public service delivery in a democratic state, one needs to consider these qualifications and the goal of social justice before treating it as an end in itself.

1.4 Theoretical Perspectives: The Gaps

The accountability in a democratic society is a topic of long-standing interest (Robert, 2002). Accountability as a concept has evolved over the centuries from the traditional Kautilya's notion of state[10] to Rousseau's social contract[11] to Weberian theory of bureaucracy[12]. The discourse on accountability has been viewed as not only from the perspective of authority and representation but also in terms of delivery of public services by the state, as a principal provider.

And focusing specifically on the idea of accountability in public service delivery, three broad perspectives or theoretical positions can be traced (see Figure 1.1). Also, many studies mentioned in the discussion that follows on theoretical perspectives, have studied accountability theoretically and conceptually which has been discussed in detail in Chapter II. Hence such studies where there are no contestations have not been discussed at length here but mentioned as a reference.

1.4.1 Public Administration Perspective

In many studies, accountability was conceptually and theoretically rooted in the context of public administration. This includes works by Romzek & Dubnik (1987), Schedler (1999), Mulgan (2000), Scott (2000), Caseley (2006), Hodge & Coghill (2007), Bovens (2007), and Rubenstein (2007), to name key scholars (Also see section 2.3). In fact, academic discourse on accountability has conventionally belonged to the discipline of public administration, in which it acquired a meaning related to 'efficiency' within the government institutions and hence also termed as horizontal accountability[13], a term first coined by O'donnell (1999).

---

10 In 1928, a committee was appointed under the chair of Motilal Nehru, to draft the proposed constitution. The draft constitution was prepared and was called "Nehru Committee Report." The report had defined citizenship and fundamental rights for the first time (For more see www.gktoday.in).

11 "The heart of the idea of the social contract may be stated simply: Each of us places his person and authority under the supreme direction of the general will, and the group receives each individual as an indivisible part of the whole (Pelkmans, 2011)."

12 Weber's theory of bureaucracy mentioned that the responsibility of public servants is restricted to the execution of orders given by the legitimate power (Aiyar, 2012).

13 For classification on kinds of accountability, see Figure 2.4.

Horizontal accountability is also reflected in the studies that used the constitutional perspective aimed at studying corruption and audits, largely in the domain of financial accountability. This includes studies by Roberts (2002), Deininger & Mpuga (2005), Joseph (1986, 1987, 2001), United Nations Department of Economic & Social Affairs (2007), Thanjavur (1990), Bardhan & Mookherjee (2006), Mukhopadhyay (2005), Akella & Kidambi (2007) and Akcay (2006).

This framework works towards financial or legal accountability used in improving public service economics and financing. Thus, a large section of studies that focus on accountability takes a technocratic view emphasising disclosure of information, bureaucratic and legal processes (Mahmud, 2004). This is also the accountability that is the mainstay of public administration of service delivery in India with emphasis on bureaucratic and managerial reporting, checks and evaluations. However, such a kind of accountability is claimed to achieve varying degrees of quality assurances and improvements but has limited synergies with the citizens or the users of public services.

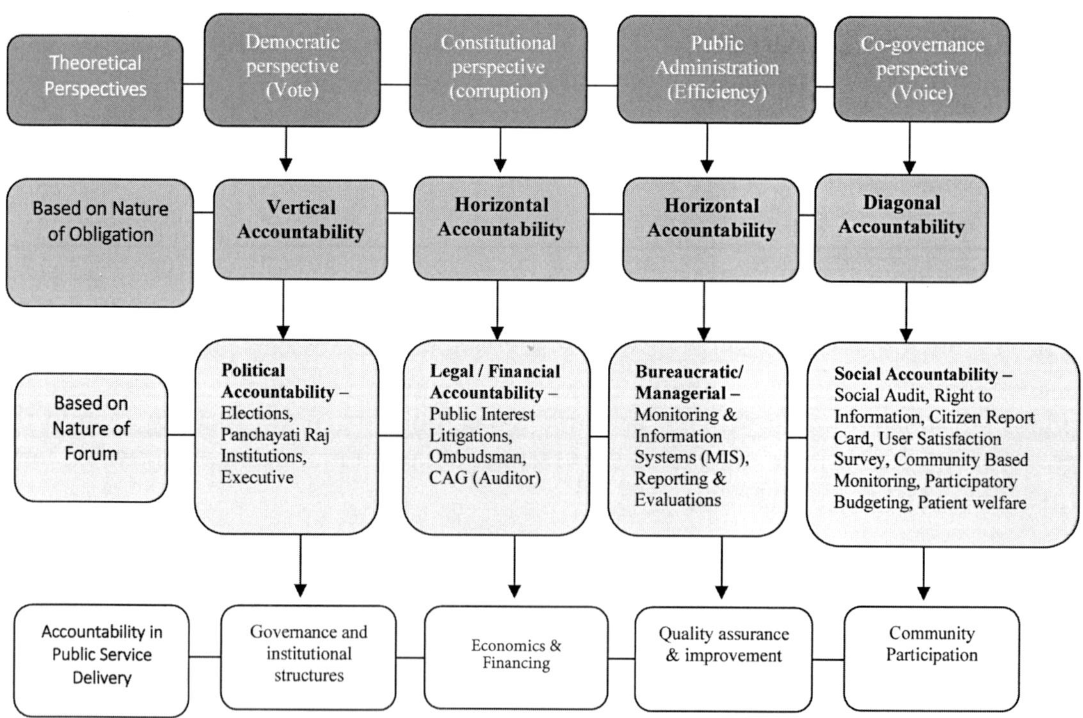

Figure 1.1: Unpacking Accountablity

Source: Compiled from Romzek & Dubnick 1987; Glynn & Murphy 1996; Roberts, 2002; George, 2003; Brinkerhoff, 2004; Rubenstein, 2007; Bovens, 2007, Hammer et al., 2007.
Illustration by Author

1.4.2 Co-Governance Perspective

Majority of studies on accountability in public services used the co-governance framework largely dominated by the World Bank. Co-governance means civic engagement within the state functions, also called social accountability, in which ordinary citizens, civil society organisations, and the media rise to improve accountability (Smulovitz & Peruzzotti, 2000). Social accountability is seen as a complement to electoral (or vertical) and horizontal accountability, with the assumption that society itself can be a powerful force for ensuring accountability (Ma, 2012). The World Bank's World Development Report 2004 drew on these emerging notions of accountability to articulate a basic three-actor framework for social accountability (Figure 1.2).

The World Bank's framework emphasises 'voice' (instead of vote) in empowering local governments in managing public services and the role of incentives that determine provider behaviour (Hammer et al., 2007). The framework is summarised as:

> *'...failures of service delivery are seen as failures of accountability. Market failures in this picture are the problems or risks with the "short route" of accountability. Government failures are problems with the "long route". There are two classes of government failures. The first is those associated with the policymaker not succeeding in hearing or taking cognisance of what people want. We call this "voice" though we could equally well call it "politics". It does not work well if policymakers – elected officials or the higher levels of the administrative bureaucracy – are not accountable to the citizens. The second assumes that politicians (policymakers) want to transmit the wishes of the people to the providers of services. The accountability of providers to policymakers is called the "compact". When working properly, the compact creates incentives such that the providers implement the wishes of the policymakers, who, in turn, accurately reflect the wishes of their constituents. Government failures associated with the compact are due to policymakers not being able to create these incentives and the provider again fails to satisfy clients/citizens wishes' (Hammer et al., 2007).*

Also, as per this literature, accountability gets reflected in the idea where market mechanisms transform citizens into consumers who extract accountability by choosing to 'exit' or 'demand' positive change from the providers (Paul, 2006, Hammer et al., 2007). The assumption is based on the 'Rational Choice Theory' and 'Game Theory' of the Neo-Classical economics which assumes that all individuals are rational and make rational choices on the basis of gains they perceive from that choice with existing information they have.

This framework marked a powerful endorsement of account-ability concerns into the NPM (New Public Management) literature. Studies in this framework included works by Paul (2006, 2002), Posani & Aiyar (2009), Hammer et al. (2007), World Bank Institute (2005), Public Affairs Foundation (2007), Mehrotra & Jarrett (2002), Ackerman (2004), Jayal (2008) among many others.

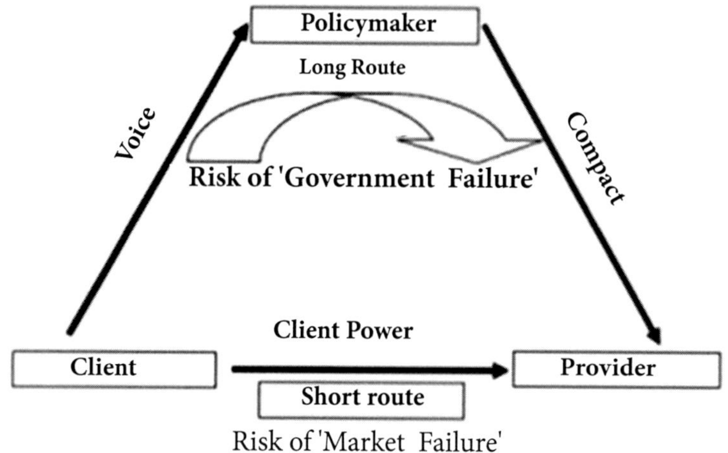

Figure 1.2: World Bank's Public Accountability Framework

Source: Hammer et al., 2007

Among the scholars that have professed increased role of the citizens in government within this framework, early literature included works of scholars like Paul (1992), Ostrom (1990), Evans (1996), Tendler (1997) and Rose-Ackerman (1999) to name a few. The notion of such a type of accountability was however on the fringes of the State and was referred to by these scholars as largely 'apolitical' at that time (Ackerman, 2004).

Samuel Paul (1992) in his paper 'Accountability in public services: Exit, voice and control', was the first to put forth this agenda that in addition to elections and horizontal accountability, societal actors can directly oblige government actors to answer for their actions and sanction them for wrongdoing (ibid.). As the work in this domain progressed especially on the realisation of the role of power of various actors, especially the state and citizens, another set of scholars began to term it **political co-governance** depicted in works of scholars like Smulovitz & Peruzzotti (2000), Cunill (2000) and Waisbord (2000). Their works involved studies on political forms of societal participation through mass mobilisation, media expose and courts to improve accountability (Ackerman, 2004).

In early 2000s, scholars re-named the citizen's ability to question the state as **diagonal accountability**, found in works of scholars like McGarvey et al. (2001), Gaventa (2002), Goetz & Jenkins (2001), Fox (2007), Newell & Wheeler (2006), Gupta & Khaira (2008) to name a few. It is called diagonal accountability as it confuses the boundary between the state and society. The RTI act and NREGS are two programmes where scholars have studied the role of accountability in improving services like Goetz & Jenkins (2001), Sinha (2008), Afridi (2008), to name a few. Also, many of these scholars used the rights framework to understand accountability in public service delivery. The financial component of accountability seems so dominant in accountability practice and research in India that even where there is people's participation in holding the State to account, usage of the term 'audit' is fixated even in social accountability mechanism called 'social audit'[14].

Mainstream critique of the World Bank's framework points to the fact that when service providers are responsive only to citizen-consumers, who 'vote' with their money, what happens to accountability to those with limited purchasing power or no voice in the system, like in the case of children, elderly, sick and disabled people (Joseph, 2001, Brinkerhoff, 2004, Novak, 2007). Also, scholars influenced by Marxists ideology and proponents of the rights-based framework critiques this framework on the ground that unless relationships of power are changed between users, state, and providers, exclusively boosting of material well-being will not help (Yamin, 2008; Harriss, 2014).

The assumption of this framework is that lack of people's voices is the reasons for accountability failures and poor services. It further continues that a civil society can aid mobilisation of people to let their voices be heard. This assumption is however, built on a shaky ground. I would like to provide reasons for my observations.

Firstly, the reason being that the role of civil society is inherent in this framework, but not stated upfront. Many scholars hold opinions that civil society is a contentious term, much debatable and cannot be an apolitical actor or devoid of vested interests. Therefore, the biggest critique of the World Bank's framework of good governance is that there is a failure to recognise this faulty assumption on which the relationship between civil society and accountability has been conceived. Scholars have argued,

> *'...the ability of civil society to contribute to accountable governance, especially in development – providing an informal and diffuse watchdog service – has been oversold, during the past 20 years, particularly since the end of cold war. This is the chimera that the aid industry has been chasing' (Goetz & Jenkins, 2005:20).*

There is a recognition that the World Bank's framework of accountability is techno-managerial in nature and it depoliticises development (meaning obscuring the need for political struggle) because it assumes that it is not possible to interfere with politics of countries and hence development should be free of politics,

14 Social audit is a tool first championed by the civil society organisation called Masdoor Kisan Shakti Sangathan (MKSS) in National Rural Employment Guarantee Act (NREGA) and Public Distribution System (PDS) to empower stakeholders to voice out concerns and demand justifications about their wages or rations from public providers and state authorities. In fact, social audits are institutionalised as a mandatory feature for participatory community-based monitoring in many public programmes like NREGS, NRHM, Mid-Day Meals (MDM) etc. In practice, it is largely confined to NREGS and that too in few states (For more see Goyal, 2011).

which is contrary to the theoretical and field evidences (Corbridge et al., 2005). In addition, on the philosophical grounds, proponents of 'Moral value theory' dismiss the World Bank's framework on grounds that many times one cannot explain the reasons for choices people make on rationality alone. For instance, despite a functional and accessible government PHC, rural people still flock to local quacks. This school of thought attributes such choices to familiar or community connections and conformity to ascribed rules[15]. Therefore, there is a need for a framework that accounts for all the existing actors, their contexts and local institutions while trying to understand how, why and when to hold poor service providers to account, from below.

1.4.3 Democratic Participation Perspective

Accountability has found a mention in many studies with links to democratic participation, decentralisation and Panchayati Raj Institutions (PRIs) in the works of Woelk (1992), Crook & Manor (1998), Ahmad (2009), Rifkin (2009), Holmberg et al. (2009), Moat & Yesudian (2009), Bergh (2004), George (2003), Murthy & Klugman (2004), Vaddiraju & Mehrotra (2004), Pal (2009), Kamat (1991), Kohli (1990), Harriss & Kohli (2009), Bardhan (1998, 2009) and Sebastian (2007).

Here accountability is understood in terms of democratic perspective where it flows vertically between various levels of governance. Studying accountability from democratic perspective has an inherent issue – that vertical channels of accountability found in the democratic system are inherently flawed (Goetz & Jenkins 2005). For instance, scholars have argued,

> *'...that observers of democracy now recognize elections to be, at best, very blunt instruments of accountability. Despite heavy anti-incumbent voting (in India and many other countries), elections seem to discipline politicians less than we would like' (Mehta quoted in Goetz & Jenkins, 2005: 18).*

Therefore, the question of why the spread of democracy over the past quarter century has not resulted in the degree of accountability for which many had hoped, arises. This question perhaps is not at all novel to the debate on democracy and accountability. However, the fact that it is still being asked confirms the observation by few scholars who argue that while in theory accountability is central to democracy, in practice the two are substantially de-linked (Goetz & Jenkins, 2005). This is a reason according to Goetz & Jenkins, why in many countries people increasingly seek channels of accountability beyond electoral system (ibid.). The idea here is not to dismiss decentralisation per se but know its limitations as a lens to study accountability relationships. The findings of one of the few empirical based studies on accountability in public services have shown that

15 Discussion with Prof. Madhushree Sekher, TISS on the assumptions on various theoretical frameworks, on October 10, 2013.

competitive local politics mattered. It mattered in districts where politics is competitive, political elites face stronger incentives to concentrate on satisfying community needs (Sebastian, 2007).

This study however could not explain the underlying sociological and institutional factors that resulted in competitive politics in the first place in some districts while not so in others. It was because the study focused only on the providers in a decentralised framework with large quantitative databases to allow for generalisations but fell short of explaining a large part of the whole. It could not explain the local power structures and kinds of relationships between the local power elites and community at large which are the building blocks of competitive politics or lack of it.

A topic of interest with many scholars is 'community participation' which is 'assumed' to result in improved accountability and better service delivery (Cornwall 2000, Rifkin 2009). Various scholars have worked on the theme of 'participation' of citizens in planning and implementation of public programmes that supposedly is linked to increased accountability and reduced corruption, which are yet to empirically established. Studies by Murthy and Klugman (2004), Rifkin (2009) and Afridi (2008) consider participation as a proxy to accountability and assume that communities would come together and participate when they have a common interest. This assumption has been proven erroneous by Mancur Olson in his much-acclaimed work titled 'Logic of Collective Action' in 1965. Olson (1965) argues and provides evidence that, 'existence of a large group with a common interest does not automatically give rise to collective action. There must be individual incentive to join in or there must be compulsion' (Olson, 1965: 24).

Further Olson's work show that communities are not homogenous entities and even if they are, they would not come together owing to power relations among its members, despite a common interest, unless either incentive or coercion is present. In most cases of community participation, there is elite capture. Further, empirical findings also suggest that the ability and effectiveness of the community groups to function as spaces for participation and provide means for developing capabilities is limited, constrained by poverty, social inequality and dependency relationships, invisibility, low self-esteem and absence of political clout (Mahmud, 2004).

In addition, there appears to be no clear correlation in the literature between democratic decentralisation and improved services in terms of quality, access, voice or sustainability. An examination of the impact of decentralisation of education and primary healthcare in India suggests that indicators of democratic decentralisation such as frequency of elections, political participation, and presence of NGOs have generally positive effects on services, although not statistically indistinguishable from zero (Mahal & Srivastava, 2000). Another study of the impact of decentralisation of primary healthcare centres in Kerala found that decentralisation brought no significant change to the health sector (Varatharajan et al., 2004).

This essentially means that all the studies that assumed accountability would automatically happen with people's participation and decentralisation, leading to improved service delivery, is theoretically and empirically weak.

Jayal (2008) points to the need for comparative research on accountability practices in various countries to know why certain types of initiatives are more effective in some contexts and which policy instruments enhance accountability. As mentioned by Brinkerhoff (2004), the frameworks presented here represent accountability from various theoretical perspectives, with the intent to respond to calls for attention to 'how best to regulate, supervise and monitor both public and private sector providers and how best to encourage them to act in the broader public interest'.

However, scholars have critiqued each framework on the assumptions it had about the nature of reality which may not match with everyday randomness of field situations. Hence, there is a need to study strategies that citizens take to claim accountability, particularly in public services, from below, within a framework of institutions. Thus, there is a high urgency for such a study to bridge the gap between the theory and practices of accountability in public service delivery.

In this chapter, I have discussed most studies on accountability in public service delivery in general, from main theoretical positions and perspective. There were only few studies on accountability in public health service delivery, which I am now discussing in the following section.

1.5 Context of Public Health

Governance and accountability can encompass virtually anything that is related to the public sector. Of the many public services, lack of accountability in health services has serious implications not only on people's ability for quality living but also for basic survival. Public health services produce "public goods" of incalculable benefit for facilitating economic growth and poverty reduction (Das Gupta, 2005). Growing evidence shows a disconnect between India's GDP growth and a corresponding decrease in child under-nutrition, a serious public health challenge. In a 2011 study in *PLoS Medicine,* Subramanian and his colleagues found "zero evidence that increases in economic growth led to any reduction in child under-nutrition (Baragona, 2014)."

Writing in the journal *The Lancet Global Health*, they found that when they compared the impact of GDP growth on indicators of child malnutrition - like stunted growth and being underweight - the effect was "practically zero to very, very small" (ibid.). For example, for every five percent gain in GDP, they found a less than one percent decrease in stunting. Study's lead researcher, Subramanian says reasons are that investments that raise GDP are not the ones that will improve child health (Subramanyam et al., 2011). Clearly, it is more to do with politics and governance than merely financing of public health programmes.

The World Bank's key concluding observations on the state of public health services in India reflects an equally high rhetoric about accountability in health policy and advocacy; and health and human rights movements. The World Bank in its World Development Report of 2004 said that health services are failing poor people not because of lack of knowledge for preventing and treating illnesses but because health systems are trapped in a web of failed relationships of accountability (The World Bank, 2004).

This observation had a snowball effect and soon recommendations on health systems development from international agencies and social movements increasingly started emphasising on strengthening accountability mechanisms in the wake of large public investments, high privatisation and governments entering into public private partnerships to deliver health services (George, 2003).

Scholars like Brinkerhoff (2004) started arguing that public health is one sector where improving accountability is often called for as an element in improving health system performance. They argued that a focus on accountability can lead to an increased understanding of health system operations, clearer identification of the pressures and incentives facing health system actors, and better reform design and implementation (Brinkerhoff, 2004). In addition, understanding how actors perceive accountability relationships can lead to designing better public health interventions and policies that are sensitive to both the people's needs and the providers' needs in a political and social context (ibid.).

The crisis of accountability too is evident across curative public health services. There is a widespread discontent among the people on various aspects of public health services like costs, quality assurance, service availability/access, fair distribution, abuse of power, financial mismanagement, corruption and lack of responsiveness. The World Health Statistics 2010 by the World Health Organisation (WHO) bears testimony to the fact that public health services in India are appallingly poor. According to this report, India is home to 23% of the tuberculosis patients, 86% of diphtheria patients, 54% of leprosy patients, 42% of polio victims and 55% of malaria patients in the world, affecting both the poor and the rich.

India has the highest percentage of underweight children below the age of five years (43.5%) and highest number of children aged 6-35 months who are anaemic (73 %) (WHO, 2010; Kumar, 2007). Also, every 15 seconds, a child in India dies from water-related diseases (Times of India, 2008). Furthermore half of malnutrition is attributable not to lack of food but to infections arising from poor sanitation (Das Gupta et al., 2010).

An editorial of a reputed Indian Journal Economic and Political Weekly (EPW) in its special issue on Health said forcefully, "Is it not time that the governments be held accountable for being incapable of reducing child deaths, whatever their immediate cause?" (Economic and Political Weekly, 2002). Sinha (2006) says that in a true democracy, every child must be regarded as indispensable and the government must be held accountable for the deaths of children and mothers.

Global level initiatives like The Global Nutrition Report launched by International Food Policy Research Institute (IFPRI) in November 2014 is reported to track worldwide progress for 193 UN countries in improving nutrition status and aim to contribute to country-led efforts to strengthen accountability and accelerate the reduction of malnutrition (Mishra, 2015). The literature on accountability in public health shows that analysis of health policies and strategies lacks focus on the study of accountability and its relationships among various actors as a central theme. Very few studies were found on the subject of accountability and the provision of public health services (George, 2009).

One of the few studies on accountability in public health services, by Garn (2010) argued the complexity of dynamics of accountability in the community-based monitoring (CBM) of health services programme in Tamil Nadu. The study assessed how accountability was perceived by various actors, mainly the providers like health service providers, institutional actors like VHSC (village health & sanitation committee) members, NGO representatives and state actors (public health officials, bureaucrats).

The crucial aspect of the relationship with the users and the reasons for their engagements, disengagements or coping mechanisms was missing in the study. Other studies on health system reforms treat accountability (if mentioned at all) as a secondary or corollary dimension (Brinkerhoff, 2004). Accountability features 'indirectly' in the literature on health economics and financing pertaining to public private partnerships, user fees etc. or is implicitly mentioned in areas of quality assurance and improvements (ibid.).

Most Indian studies on accountability seem to indirectly capture it through concepts like transparency, corruption, democratic decentralisation and participation, and the focus is rarely on public health. According to Ruger (2005), there are few studies on the relationship between political institutions (that shapes accountability processes) and health both at theoretical and empirical levels. Ruger (2005) accepted the hypothesis that lack of democratic institutions like free press and multi-party elections can have a disastrous effect on health. However, in the Indian context there are few studies that explain why despite decentralised democratic institutions, health service delivery remains poor. Thus, there is a dearth of knowledge in the Indian context that unpacks accountability relationships between various actors in the public health services.

1.6 Rationale for the Study

The abstract nature of the concept of accountability has not been studied adequately. Also, it is known to be a very elusive concept because it can mean many different things to different people (Bovens, 2007). As a result, accountability is seriously misunderstood to mean only 'naming and shaming' or 'blame and punishment' (Potts, 2005). As Bovens (2007) puts it, "accountability has become such an icon for good governance that the concept has grown less useful for analytical purposes and has turned into garbage filled with good intentions, loosely defined concepts, and vague images of good governance. We must move from a rhetorical or discourse analysis to a more descriptive, sociological analysis".

This means that most of the current perspectives on accountability in public policy and programmes are based on rhetorical and theoretical assumptions of accountability and good governance with minimal links with evidence. One cannot answer the empirical question on the relationship of accountability between actors in the dynamics of social reality from within the realm of theory alone. This book proposes to address this question empirically and then revisit the theoretical propositions in circulation.

It is clear that there is a high rhetoric about accountability in policies and public service delivery in general. It is assumed that with increased accountability and engagement of the users, public service delivery would improve. This book questions the assumptions behind this orthodoxy. Better outcomes such as literacy levels, medical services, state of law and order, civil society empowerment cannot be exclusively linked to quality of government or attributed to accountability processes. Such an approach runs the risks of equating good governance with anything that produces good outcomes (Holmberg et al., 2009).

However, there is evidence to show that certain Quality of Governance (QoG) variables like corruption perception, rule of law, and government effectiveness have a strong positive correlation with health indicators like subjective health, life expectancy at birth, infant mortality rate and child mortality rate (ibid.). In addition, the relationships between the QoG variables and measures of inequality like unemployment and relative poverty are reasonably strong (ibid.). Therefore, one can empirically examine how accountability (as a component of good governance) is being enacted at sites of service delivery of public health programmes.

Secondly, the link between governance and public service delivery has not been explored to the same degree and the 2004 World Development Report made important contributions in this regard (Global Development Network, 2009). Many studies have documented the relationships between governance indicators like accountability with other socio-economic indicators like poverty, equity etc. at the macro level. However, the complexity and heterogeneity of institutional setups across countries and sectors makes it difficult to study them in a comparative fashion at the macro level and there is a need to study these relationships at the frontline of service delivery.

Also, the literature on governance or accountability does not explain the differentials in service delivery outcomes within the context of the same region or state using its theoretical assumptions or empirical evidence. This book would seek to understand how local accountability processes work under differential public health service delivery outcomes using the accountability framework. This book would thus essentially test out the theoretical postulates of accountability (and good governance) with the evidence of empirical reality.

Furthermore, this book seeks to contribute a theoretical and conceptual framework for studying accountability processes and relationships in service delivery, in context of public health services, which could also be applied to studying other public services. This would be a significant theoretical contribution of this monograph.

Lastly, despite the critical importance of the role of accountability in governance, little work has been done to explore its meaning and content in context of public service delivery in general and public nutrition in particular. Scholars have mentioned,

> *'Finally, we need a new type of research programme around nutrition governance. It would use disciplines that are sensitive to power, voice and accountability with quantitative and qualitative methods to identify and learn whether innovations in institutional and governance arrangements can improve the capacity, responsiveness and accountability of the state and civil society to generate improved nutrition outcomes' (Haddad, 2009).*

A similar observation has also been made by the World Bank (2010),

> *'...the accountability linkages for rural service provision vary widely across countries, depending on the political system and the approach to decentralisation in service provision. Understanding these linkages is essential for identifying entry points to make rural service provision more responsive to gender needs' (The World Bank and IFPRI, 2010: xiii).*

Therefore, there is a need to understand the context-specific and bottom-up institutional processes on how accountability is realised at the frontline and grassroots by the people especially in context of public health services. Scholars like Sinha (2006) hope that public action involving local institutions, local bodies, and large support structures at the state and national levels, enabling community to question, negotiate and bargain with authorities to deliver services would pave a way for enhancing every child's access to ICDS and making it an institution for protecting the rights of children aged 0-6 years.

Experts like Dr. Shanta Sinha call for grassroots level accountability by means of making programmes like ICDS a site for contesting power. Hardly any scholars have unpacked accountability at the village level or have provided explanations on how communities cope up or reasons why they do not organise collective action against the authorities in case of poor services. This book encapsulates these ideas to a great extent and attempts to address these issues both theoretically and empirically.

1.7 Research Objectives

One of the core research objectives of this book is to understand how accountability, as an element of good governance, plays a role in service delivery of public health programmes at the frontline level. Accordingly, the book aims to identify relationships of accountability existing between various actors - providers, users, user groups, local politicians/PRI members and local NGOs, at the frontline of public health service delivery.

The objective of this empirical work is to help understand how accountability relationships are enacted between various actors on the frontline of public health service delivery to understand why users do not protest for poor services.

Second objective is to analyse how users, especially the poor, demand or negotiate better services and entitlements through informal mechanisms when the formal mechanisms of accountability fail or exclude them.

In the process, the arguments and evidence presented will aim to identify and compare various institutionalised formal accountability mechanisms with informal forms in order to assess if informal forms of accountability have a comparative advantage over formal ones or vice versa. Final objective of the book is to attempt to revisit the idea of accountability in governance in light of empirical findings.

The next chapter opens to various methodological approaches explored and finally selected to achieve book's objectives above. Research Methodology is critical as it provides a framework or the 'how' to arrive at explanations or 'why and what' of the moot questions and key objectives of this study. Hence, the following chapter on 'how to study accountability' is a critical link, that connects objectives with its findings and implications of this empirical work.

***

References

1. Aakella, K. V., & Kidambi, S. (2007). Challenging corruption with social audits. *Economic and Political Weekly*, *42*(5), 345–347.
2. Ackerman, J. (2004). Co-governance for accountability: beyond exit and voice. *World Development*, *32*(3), 447–463.
3. Afridi, F. (2008). Can community monitoring improve the accountability of public officials? *Economic and Political Weekly*, 43(42), 35–40.
4. Ahmad, E., & Brosio, G. (Eds.). (2009). *Does decentralization enhance service delivery and poverty reduction?* United Kingdom: Edward Elgar Publishing.

5. Aiyar, Y. (2012, March 2). Accountability failures mar NRHM. *Livemint*. Retrieved March 13, 2013 from http://www.livemint.com.
6. Akccay, S. (2006). Corruption and human development. *Cato Journal*, 26(1), 29-48.
7. Banerjee, A., Deaton, A., & Duflo, E. (2004). Health care delivery in rural Rajasthan. *Economic and Political Weekly, 39*(9), 944–949.
8. Banerji, D. (1986). *Social sciences and health service development in India: Sociology of formation of an alternative paradigm*. New Delhi: Lok Paksh.
9. Baragona, S. (2014, March 26). Rising wealth not enough to raise child health. *Voice of America*. Retrieved March 28, 2014 from http://www.voanews.com.
10. Bardhan, P. (2009). Governance dilemmas in service delivery. In Ahmad, E. & Giorgio B. (Eds.). *Does Decentralization Enhance Service Delivery and Poverty Reduction?* United Kingdom: Edward Elgar Publishing.
11. Bardhan, P. K. (1998). *The political economy of development in India*. Oxford, UK; New York, USA: Oxford University Press.
12. Bardhan, P., & Mookherjee, D. (2006). Decentralization, corruption and government accountability. In Ackerman, S. A., (Eds.). *International Handbook on the economics of corruption* (pp. 161–188). United Kingdom: Edward Elgar Publishing.
13. Bergh, S. (2004). Democratic decentralisation and local participation: a review of recent research. *Development in Practice, 14*(6), 780–790.
14. Bovens, M. (2007). Analysing and assessing accountability: a conceptual framework. *European Law Journal, 13*(4), 447–468.
15. Brinkerhoff, D. W. (2004). Accountability and health systems: towards conceptual clarity and policy relevance. *Health Policy and Planning, 19*(6), 371–379.
16. Caseley, J. (2006). Multiple accountability relationships and improved service delivery performance in Hyderabad City, Southern India. *International Review of Administrative Sciences, 72*(4), 531–546.
17. Chand, V. (2006). Reinventing Public Service Delivery in India. Selected Case Studies. The World Bank. SAGE Publications India Pvt. Ltd. New Delhi.
18. Corbridge, S., Williams, G., Srivastava, M., & Véron, R. (2005). *Seeing the State: Governance and Governmentality in India*. Cambridge, UK: Cambridge University Press.
19. Cornwall, A. (2000). *Beneficiary, consumer, citizen: perspectives on participation for poverty reduction* (p. 98). Swedish International Development Cooperation Agency, Stockholm. Retrieved on August 6, 2013 from http://www.alnap.org.
20. Crook, R. C., & Manor, J. (1998). *Democracy and decentralisation in South Asia and West Africa: Participation, accountability and performance*. UK: Cambridge University Press.
21. Cunill, N. (2006). Critical junctures of societal accountability: lessons from Latin America. *Enforcing the Rule of Law: Social Accountability in the New Latin American Democracies*, Pittsburgh: University of Pittsburgh Press.

22. Das Gupta, M. (2005). Public Health in India: dangerous neglect. *Economic and Political Weekly*, *40*(49), 5159–5165.

23. Das Gupta, M., Shukla, R., Somanathan, T. V., & Datta, K. K. (2009). How might India's public health systems be strengthened? *World Bank Policy Research Working Paper Series, Paper No. 5140*. Retrieved on March 14, 2013 from http://papers.ssrn.com.

24. De Vries, J. (2010). Is New Public Management Really Dead? *OECD Journal on Budgeting*, *10*(1), 1–5.

25. Deininger, K., & Mpuga, P. (2005). Does greater accountability improve the quality of public service delivery? Evidence from Uganda. *World Development*, *33*(1), 171–191.

26. Dreze, J., & Sen, A. (2002). *India: Development and participation*. USA: Oxford University Press. *Economic and Political Weekly* editorials. (2002). Healthcare: enforcing accountability. *37*(36), 3688.

27. EPW Editorials. (2002). Healthcare: Enforcing Accountability. *Economic and Political Weekly*, XXXVII (36), September 7.

28. Evans, P. (1996). Government action, social capital and development: reviewing the evidence on synergy. *World Development*, *24*(6), 1119–1132.

29. Evans, P. B., Rueschemeyer, D., & Skocpol, T. (1985). *Bringing the state back in*. UK: Cambridge University Press.

30. Finer, S. E. (1970). *Comparative government* (First). Harmondsworth, UK: Penguin books.

31. Fox, J. (2007). The uncertain relationship between transparency and accountability. *Development in Practice*, *17*(4-5), 663–671.

32. Garn, K. D. (2010). *Dynamics of Accountability in the Community Based Monitoring of Health Services Programme, Tamil Nadu, India*. (M.Phil dissertation). Copenhagen: Department of Public Health, University of Copenhagen.

33. Gaventa, J. (2002). Exploring citizenship, participation and accountability. *IDS Bulletin*, *33*(2), 1–14.

34. George, A. (2003). Using accountability to improve reproductive health care. *Reproductive Health Matters*, *11*(21), 161–170.

35. George, A. (2009). By papers and pens, you can only do so much: views about accountability and human resource management from Indian government health administrators and workers. *The International Journal of Health Planning and Management*, *24*(3), 205–224.

36. Global Development Network. (2009). Varieties of governance: effective public service delivery, concept note ninth global research project. Retrieved on March 28, 2014 from http://gdn.int.

37. Glynn, J. J., & Murphy, M. P. (1996). Public management: failing accountabilities and failing performance review. *International Journal of Public Sector Management, 9*(5/6), 125–137.

38. Goetz, A. M., & Jenkins, R. (2001). Hybrid forms of accountability: citizen engagement in institutions of public-sector oversight in India. *Public Management Review, 3*(3), 363–383.

39. Goetz, A. M., Jenkins, R., & Shaw, T. M. (2005). *Reinventing accountability: making human democracy work for human development* (First). London: Palgrave Macmillan.

40. Gopal, K.S. (2009). NREGA social audit: myths and reality. *Economic and Political Weekly*, 44(3), 70-71.

41. Goyal, J. (2011). Social audits in outcome budgeting: an experiment of accountability in Maharashtra. *Indian Journal of Social Work, 72*(4), 537–562.

42. Goyal, J. (2014). Centrally sponsored schemes in Andaman and Nicobar Islands: a governance paradox. *International Journal of Sociology and Social Policy,* 34(3/4), 196-213.

43. Gupta, A. (2012). *Red tape: Bureaucracy, structural violence, and poverty in India.* USA: Duke University Press.

44. Gupta, A., & Khaira, N. S. (2008). Flaws in child nutrition and health governance. *Economic and Political Weekly, 43*(17), 17–21.

45. Haddad, L. (2009). Lifting the curse: overcoming persistent under nutrition in India. *IDS Bulletin, 40*(4), 1–8.

46. Hammer, J., Aiyar, Y., & Samji, S. (2007). Understanding government failure in public health services. *Economic and Political Weekly, 42*(40), 4049–4057.

47. Harriss, J. (2006). *Power matters: Essays on institutions, politics, and society in India*. USA: Oxford University Press.

48. Harriss, J. (2010). Is Government in India becoming more responsive? Has democratic decentralisation made a difference? *Simons Papers in Security and Development (8)*. Vancouver: School for International Studies, Simon Fraser University. Retrieved on March 13, 2013 from https://www.sfu.ca.

49. Harriss, J. (2014, March 20). State of Injustice: The Indian State and Poverty. *ISAS Working Paper No. 182.* Singapore: Institute of South Asian Studies, National University of Singapore. Retrieved on February 4, 2014 from www.isas.nus.edu.sg.

50. Harriss, J., & Kohli, N. (2009). Notes on the differing states of child under nutrition in rural India. *IDS Bulletin, 40*(4), 9–15.

51. Hodge, G. A., & Coghill, K. (2007). Accountability in the privatized state. *Governance, 20*(4), 675–702.

52. Holmberg, S., Rothstein, B., & Nasiritousi, N. (2009). Quality of government: what you get. *Annual Review of Political Science, 12*, 135–161.

53. Holmberg, S., Rothstein, B., & Nasiritousi, N. (2009). Quality of government: what you get. *Annual Review of Political Science*, 12, 135–161.

54. Jayal, N. G. (2008). New directions in theorising social accountability? *IDS Bulletin*, *38*(6), 105–112.

55. Jayal, N. G. (2013). *Citizenship and its Discontents - An Indian History*. Cambridge, Mass: Harvard University Press.

56. Jenkins, R. (2007). Civil society versus corruption. *Journal of Democracy*, *18*(2), 55–69.

57. Joseph, K. P. (1986). Accountability of government audit in India. *Economic and Political Weekly*, *21*(22), M–59 to M–65.

58. Joseph, K. P. (1987). Public accountability and audit in India. *Economic and Political Weekly*, *22*(22), M–67 to M–75.

59. Joseph, K. P. (2001). Growing fraud in government. *Economic and Political Weekly*, *36*(7), 535–537.

60. Joseph, S. (2001). Democratic good governance: new agenda for change. *Economic and Political Weekly*, *36*(12), 1011–1014.

61. Kamat, V. R. (1991). *Political and Cultural Context of Primary Health Care Implementation: A Study in a Region of Rural Maharashtra* (PhD Thesis). Tata Institute of Social Sciences, Mumbai.

62. Keefer, P., & Khemani, S. (2004). Why do the poor receive poor services? *Economic and Political Weekly*, 39(9), 935–943.

63. Kohli, A. (1990). *Democracy and disorder: India's growing crisis of governability*. Cambridge: Cambridge University Press.

64. Kumar, A. S. (2007). Why are levels of child malnutrition not improving? *Economic and Political Weekly*, *42*(15), 1337–1345.

65. Kumar, S. (2007). *Parallel bodies & the Panchayati Raj Institutions: A study of village based special committees in three districts of Maharashtra* (Unpublished). Tuljapur: School of Rural Development, Tata Institute of Social Sciences.

66. Ma, J. (2012). The rise of social accountability in China. *The Australian Journal of Public Administration*, *71*(2), 111–121.

67. Mahal, A., & Srivastava, V. (2000). People's participation, decentralisation and delivery of public sector services in India. *National Council of Applied Economic Research Working Paper No. 71*. Retrieved on August 4, 2014 from https://ideas.repec.org.

68. Mahmud, S. (2004). Citizen participation in the health Sector in rural Bangladesh: perceptions and reality. *IDS Bulletin*, *35*(2), 11.

69. Mander, H., Asif, M., & Sasi, K. P. (2004). *Good governance: resource book*. Bangalore: Books for Change.

70. McGarvey, N., Goetz, A., Gaventa, J., Cornwall, A., Crook, R., Ehrichs, L., John, P. (2001). *Bringing citizen voice and client focus into service delivery.* Monograph. Institute of Development Studies. Retrieved on March 15, 2013 from http://strathprints.strath.ac.uk.

71. Mehrotra, S., & Jarrett, S. W. (2002). Improving basic health service delivery in low-income countries: voice to the poor. *Social Science & Medicine, 54*(11), 1685–1690.

72. Mishra, A. (2015, February 5). India is facing multiple burdens of malnutrition, says Global Nutrition Report. *Business Today.* Retrieved on February 12, 2015 from http://businesstoday.intoday.in.

73. Moat, K. A., & Yesudian, C. A. K. (2009, December 19). Analyzing the decentralization of health services in Maharashtra: decision space and district performance under the National Rural Health Mission (Unpublished). LSE/TATA Institute of Social Sciences MSc International Health Policy collaborative programme, Mumbai: TISS.

74. Mukhopadhyay, A. (2005). Accountability and Communicative Action: An Alternative Imaginary. *Economic and Political Weekly*, 40(52), 5463–5469.

75. Mulgan, R. (2000). Accountability: an ever-expanding concept? *Public Administration, 78*(3), 555–573.

76. Murthy, R. K., & Klugman, B. (2004). Service accountability and community participation in the context of health sector reforms in Asia: implications for sexual and reproductive health services. *Health Policy and Planning, 19*(1), i78–i86.

77. *NDTV*. What is the Jan Lokpal bill, why it's important? Retrieved on March 26, 2015 from http://www.ndtv.com/india-news.

78. Newell, P., & Wheeler, J. (Eds.). (2006). *Rights, resources and the politics of accountability* (Vol. 3). Institute of Development Studies. London: Zed books.

79. North, D. C. (1990). *Institutions, institutional change and economic performance.* UK: Cambridge University Press.

80. Novak, P. (2007). Accountability to whom? *Economic and Political Weekly, 42*(30), 3172–3177.

81. O'donnell, G. (1999). Horizontal accountability and new poliarchies. *Lua Nova: Revista de Cultura E Política*, (44), 27–54.

82. Olson, M. (1965). *The logic of collective action; public goods and the theory of groups.* Harvard Economic Studies. Cambridge: Harvard University Press.

83. Ostrom, E. (1990). *Governing the Commons: The Evolution of Institutions for Collective Action*. Cambridge University Press.

84. Paul, S. (1992). Accountability in public services: exit, voice and control. *World Development, 20*(7), 1047–1060.

85. Paul, S. (2002). New mechanisms for public accountability: the Indian experience. Oslo Governance Centre, Chr. Michelsen Institute Workshop, United Nations

Development Programme (Vol. 18) (pp. 1-18). Retrieved on April 12, 2015 from http://regulationbodyofknowledge.org.

86. Paul, S. (2006). *Who Benefits from India's Public Services? A Peoples Audit of Five Basic Services*. Public Affairs Centre, Bangalore: Academic Foundation.

87. Paul, S., Balakrishnan, S., Gopakumar, K., Sekhar, S., & Vivekananda, M. (2004). State of India's public services: benchmarks for the states. *Economic and Political Weekly*, 39(9), 920–933.

88. Pelkmans, M. (2011). AN226/451 Lecture 5 Studying the state anthropologically (power point presentation). Course on politics of anthropology during TISS-LSE doctoral fellowship. London: Asia Research Centre, London School of Economics and Political Science.

89. Posani, B., & Aiyer, Y. (2009). State of accountability: evolution, practice and emerging questions in public accountability in India. Accountability Initiative Working Paper No. 2 (pp. 1-45). New Delhi: Center for Policy Research. Retrieved on March 14, 2013 from http://www.accountabilityindia.in.

90. Potts, D. H. (2005). *Accountability and the right to the highest attainable standard of health*. Human Rights Centre, UK: University of Essex.

91. Premchand, A. (1995). *Effective government accounting*. Washington DC: International Monetary Fund.

92. Pritchett, L. (2009). Is India a flailing state? detours on the four lane highway to modernization. J. F Kennedy School of Government, Faculty Research Working Paper Series, Scholarly Paper No. ID 1404827 (pp. 1-46), Rochester, NY: Social Science Research Network, May 13, Retrieved on February 7, 2015.

93. Public Affairs Foundation, Sirker, K., & Cosic, S. (2007). Empowering the marginalized: case studies of social accountability initiatives in Asia. *WBI Working Papers*. Washington DC: World Bank Institute. Retrieved on November 26, 2013 from http://unpan1.un.org.

94. Pylee, M. V. (1963). *India's Constitution*. New York: Asia Publishing House.

95. Rath, P. (2014). *Transparency and Accountability in the Social Sector: Pedagogy, Theory of Change and Showcasing Key Success Stories* (Conference Report) (pp. 1–50). Pune: National Centre for Advocacy Studies, National Foundation of India and Centre for Budget and Governance Accountability.

96. Rifkin, S. B. (2009). Lessons from community participation in health programmes: a review of the post Alma-Ata experience. *International Health*, *1*(1), 31–36.

97. Roberts, N. C. (2002). Keeping public officials accountable through dialogue: resolving the accountability paradox. *Public Administration Review*, *62*(6), 658–669.

98. Romzek, B. S., & Dubnick, M. J. (1987). Accountability in the public sector: lessons from the challenger tragedy. *Public Administration Review*, *47*(3), 227-238.

99. Rose-Ackerman, S. (1999). *Corruption and government: causes, consequences, and reform*. UK: Cambridge University Press.

100. Rubenstein, J. (2007). Accountability in an unequal world. *Journal of Politics, 69*(3), 616–632.

101. Ruger, J. P. (2005). Democracy and health. *QJM, 98*(4), 299–304. Sakal Times. (2011, June 3). Sex ratio improves in three districts. Retrieved on November 2, 2014 from http://www.sakaaltimes.com.

102. Schedler, A. (1999). *The self restraining state: power and accountability in new democracies*. USA: Lynne Rienner Publishers.

103. Scott, C. (2000). Accountability in the regulatory state. *Journal of Law and Society, 27*(1), 38–60.

104. Scott, C. (2000). Accountability in the regulatory state. *Journal of Law and Society, 27*(1), 38–60.

105. Sebastian, E. (2007). *Accountability & decentralised service delivery: explaining performance variations across local governments in Indonesia.* Institute of Local Public Finance Working Paper 02-2007.

106. Sen, A. (1999). *Development as freedom*. Oxford University Press.

107. Sen, A. (2006). Development as freedom: an India perspective. *Indian Journal of Industrial Relations, 42*(2), 157–169.

108. Shastri, P. (2013, January 14). Anganwadi food poisoning: two suspended, two given show-cause notice. *Times of India.* Ahmedabad. Retrieved June 17, 2013, from http://articles.timesofindia.indiatimes.com.

109. Singh, R. R. (2004). Kautilya's conception of State. *The Indian Journal of Political Science, 65*(1), 41–54.

110. Sinha, S. (2006). Infant survival: A political challenge. *Economic and Political Weekly, 41*(34), 3657–3660.

111. Smulovitz, C., & Peruzzotti, E. (2000). Societal accountability in Latin America. *Journal of Democracy, 11*(4), 147–158.

112. Subramanyam, M. A., Kawachi, I., Berkman, L. F., & Subramanian, S. V. (2011). Is economic growth associated with reduction in child under nutrition in India? *PLoS Med, 8*(3), e1000424.

113. Tendler, J. (1997). *Good government in the tropics.* USA: Johns Hopkins University Press.

114. Thanjavur. (1990). Beyond true and fair. *Economic & Political Weekly,* 25(37), 2049–2051. *The Hindu.* Early childhood care and education policy proposed. (2012, March 26). New Delhi. Retrieved on March 26, 2012 from http://www.thehindu.com.

115. The World Bank and International Food Policy Research Institute. (2010). *Gender and Governance in Rural Services: Insights from India, Ghana, and Ethiopia.* Washington DC: World Bank Publications.

116. The World Bank Institute. (2005). *Social accountability in the public sector: A conceptual discussion and learning module.* Working Paper No. 37249, Washington

DC: The World Bank. Retrieved on March 15, 2013 from http://siteresources.worldbank.org.

117. The World Bank. (2001). *World Development Report 2002 Building Institutions for Markets: Overview*. Washington DC: The World Bank.
118. The World Bank. (2004). *World Development Report 2004 Making Services Work for the Poor*. Washington DC: The World Bank and Oxford University Press.
119. Times of India. (2008, January 14). Water borne diseases kill a child every 15 sec! Retrieved on March 14, 2013 from http://articles.timesofindia.indiatimes.com.
120. United Nations Department of Economic and Social Affairs. (2007). *Auditing for social change, a strategy for citizen engagement in public sector accountability*. Expert group meeting, 6th global forum on reinventing government towards participatory and transparent governance, Seoul: Republic of Korea. Retrieved on March 15, 2013 from http://www.scribd.com.
121. United Nations Economic and Social Commission for Asia and the Pacific. What is good governance? Retrieved on March 26, 2015 from http://www.unescap.org/sites/default/files/good-governance.pdf.
122. Vaddiraju, A. K., & Mehrotra, S. (2004). Making panchayats accountable. *Economic and Political Weekly*, 39(37), 4139–4141.
123. Varatharajan, D., Thankappan, R., & Jayapalan, S. (2004). Assessing the performance of primary health centres under decentralized government in Kerala, India. *Health Policy and Planning, 19*(1), 41–51.
124. Wagle, S., & Dixit, K. (2006). Revisiting Good Governance: Asserting citizens participation and politics in public services. *Beyond the Market: The Future of Public Services*. Amsterdam: TNI/PSIRU.
125. Waisbord, S. R. (2000). *Watchdog journalism in South America: news, accountability and democracy*. USA: Columbia University Press.
126. Woelk, G. B. (1992). Cultural and structural influences in the creation of and participation in community health programmes. *Social Science & Medicine, 35*(4), 419–424.
127. World Health Organisation. (2010). *World Health Statistics* (p. 177). Geneva: WHO. Retrieved on March 14, 2013 http://www.who.int.
128. Yamin, A. E. (2008). Beyond compassion: the central role of accountability in applying a human rights framework to health. *Health and Human Rights, 10*(2), 1–20.

CHAPTER 2

Studying Accountability: Methodological Concerns

2.1 Introduction

Research Methodology of the current study is guided by two main components. First, the research questions leading to corresponding research objectives and second, the theoretical (ontological and epistemological) assumptions that in-turn have briefed these research objectives.

Last chapter discusses the moot questions, laying out the context and discussing the theoretical assumptions of the study. This chapter begins with the research methodology that includes building a conceptual framework and finally an analytical framework that would guide the context, locale of the study, and methods of data collection.

2.2 Conceptual framework

The core research question of this book is to understand how accountability, as an element of good governance, plays a role in improving or hindering service delivery of public health and child nutrition programmes at the frontline level.

To operationalise the study, the first step is to define main terms and concepts used in the study. The three main terms of the study are: Public Service Delivery, Public Health and Accountability. The next step is to set up a relationship between study concepts which I have depicted in a conceptual framework, followed by operationalising the terms by converting them into indicators.

2.2.1 Definitions

Public Service Delivery: The provision of roads; clean drinking water; sanitation is easily recognisable as public services, as none, other than governments (more so, in Indian context), provide these to its people. But what about primary health care or school education? Are these public services too? If they are, then why there are huge heterogenous private providers who are also supplying same service for a fee, is a question to ponder on.

Humphreys (1998) defines public services as those services which are mainly or completely, funded by taxation. Most typically, public services would include areas of public management like central and local government, health, education, defence, justice/home affairs and non-commercial organisations.

Public services do not normally run for financial profit or require immediate payment for goods or services prior to delivery. If public services are charged for, then they are not usually sold to customers at commercial prices set to produce profits (Humphreys, 1998). According to a service delivery policy of Govt. of Kerala, titled 'A People Centered Service Delivery Policy (2004)', "the delivery of public service means the goods and services offered by govt institutions to the public and includes interface between citizen and government" (www.img.kerala.gov.in). I have used this definition while referring to public service delivery in this book.

Few other definitional features of public service delivery are important to discuss as it aids in the understanding of current challenges faced by Indian public service delivery while suggesting reforms or improvements. Key features of public services that are quite distinctive from private provisioning, according to Humphreys (1998) are:

- Lack of competition and monopolistic nature.
- Provider-customer relationship is often complex and indirect since payment is not made directly for service received.
- Consumer control and choice is weakened.
- Relationship between demand and supply (provision) of public service is perverse. Fall in demand is usually a relief while an increase in demand is not welcomed as it puts more pressure on staff and facilities without an increase in budget. In fact, excess demand can decrease the motivation of government employees to improve services.
- Large scale exit is unlikely because public providers occupy a monopolistic position. In such scenario, low-income consumers are hit the most as they are trapped in a monopolistic system which provides them with essentials like healthcare, education, food security, social security etc. They get used to the low standards and so do the service providers.(Humphreys, 1998; Pollitt & Bouckaert, 1995: 13).

Some examples of public services that would fit the above description, in Indian context, include water provision, roads & highways construction and maintenance, railways, waste disposal and sanitation, national security, policing, issuing identity and passports. Services like telecommunications, public distribution system, primary education, public healthcare, early childhood care have ceased to remain exclusively public in India and have seen private players enter.

Literature on 'public services' mentions terms such as client, customer, consumer and citizen, are often used interchangeably which can add to the confusion (Humphreys, 1998). Each of these terms has different meaning attached that varies with context and time (Figure 2.1). The term stakeholder or actor is also being increasingly used in literature on civil society's notion of citizen. However, depending upon the literature quoted in this study, I have retained these terms.

It is not possible to have a universally applicable definition but for this study, the term 'user' is used to denote an entire community of people eligible to access, utilise or even reject public services, including adolescents and children and not only those who have the power to influence through votes. Without going into the semantics of the terminology, where each term has a connotative meaning, the term 'user' denotes a factual image and yet is not completely apolitical.

Description of Member of the public	*The service relationship is strongly shaped by:*
Client	The dominance of the client by the professional
Customer	The experience of the customer in using the organisation
Consumer	The interest of the consumer in the product or service provided
Citizen	The concern of the citizen to influence public decision which affect the quality of life.

Figure 2.1: Users in Public Service

Source: Humphreys, 1998; Burns et al. 1994

Citizens delegate the democratic authority arising from popular sovereignty to government, but the implicit price is a suitable system of accountability (Hughes, 2003). Whether people relate to government as citizens, users, clients subject to regulation, participants, or litigants, they expect a strong accountability framework to exist (Hodge & Coghill, 2007).

Public Health: According to the World Health Organisation (WHO), "public health refers to all organized measures (whether public or private) to prevent disease, promote health and prolong life among the population as a whole" (www.who.int). Its activities aim to provide conditions in which people can be healthy focuses on an entire population, not on individual patients or diseases. Thus, public health is concerned with the total system and not only the eradication of a particular disease" (ibid.).

In another definition of public health by the World Bank, public health refers to the combination of the organisation of service delivery and stewardship or administration that culminates in the delivery of population-based services, e.g. infectious disease prevention, control and surveillance. It can refer to health programmes that target specific populations (e.g. children) or specific diseases (e.g. tuberculosis). Since there is no major debate over the definitions of public health, I have used the above definitions of Public Health.

Accordingly, the erstwhile National Rural Health Mission (NRHM) which is now National Health Mission and the Integrated Child Development Scheme (ICDS) are two of the largest and most significant public health programmes in India that are population based and deal with all three aspects of preventive, promotive and curative heath. Therefore, these two programmes form the context of the study.

Defining and Conceptualising Accountability: The idea of accountability means that when we are requested by others to achieve something, we report back to them on how we have performed (Hodge & Coghill, 2007; Hughes, 2003). In other words, it is answering for one's actions (Ott & Russell 2001: 355). Accountability can also involve "setting goals, providing and reporting on results and the visible consequences for getting things right or wrong, including rewards or sanctions as appropriate" (Funnell et al., 2012).

Bovens (2006) defines accountability as a social relationship in which an actor feels an obligation to explain and to justify his or her conduct to some significant other. Accountability is "a concept which is contingent on the context which gives rise to accountability relationships" (Glynn & Murphy, 1996)", "between an accounting and an accountable actor who is attributed different rights and responsibilities depending on their respective roles" (Garn, 2010). Broadly speaking, accountability is the institutionalized practice or a process of account giving, via which a person, or group of people, can be held to account for their conduct.

Scholars who have worked on the concept of accountability cite that it is a complex and hence often an ill-defined concept, despite its popularity and rhetoric. According to Schedler, "accountability represents an underexplored concept whose meaning remains evasive; whose boundaries are fuzzy and whose internal structure is confusing" (Schedler, 1999). Mulgan (2000) calls accountability a 'complex and chameleon-like term'. The ambiguity in defining the concept of accountability is because of its usage. People apply it to denote a variety of situations and alternately used to describe or prescribe behaviour of different actors.

Therefore, as Bovens (2007) said, accountability is a contested and contestable concept, because there is no consensus about the standards for accountable behaviour, and because they differ from role to role, time to time, place to place and from speaker to speaker.

One thing that clearly emerges from review of literature is that accountability involves unequal power between actors. Therefore, accountability is often theorised as a relationship between power wielders and accountability holders (Rubenstein, 2007) or between an agent (that has a responsibility and resources and does action/

service) and a principal (with rights and duties and bears effects of action/service) (Posani & Aiyer, 2009).

In the context of a democracy, or public administration and public services, some relationships of accountability can be between the state and its various agencies (as the power wielder) and citizens (as the accountability holders) (Figure 2.2).

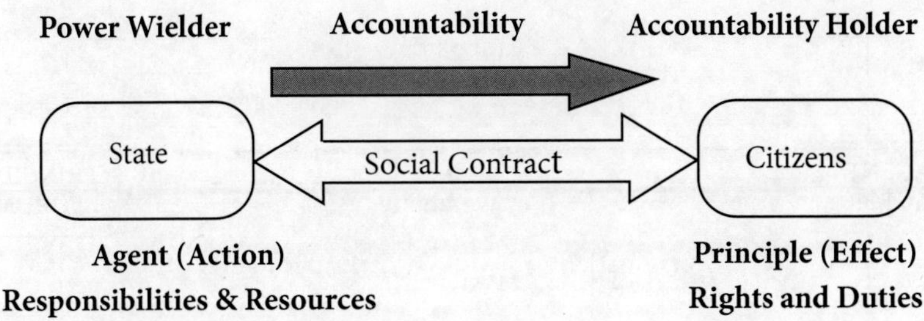

Figure 2.2: Public Accountability

Source: Compiled from Posani & Aiyer, 2009. Illustration by Author

The need for the state to be accountable to its citizens stems out of the 'social contract' that citizens share with the state. In a democracy, this contract gets operationalised when citizens elect a government and bestow the elected representatives with the power to govern them. The government on its part, is obliged to perform its duties of governance. Such an understanding answers a basic question on accountability - **who** is accountable to **whom**?

Another question that I have attempted to answer to an extent in the section on the theoretical frameworks on accountability (Figure 2.4) is – **accountability for what?** Further, readers will be able to understand accountability conceptually, with its essential elements as identified by scholars (Figure 2.3). In other words, the relationship between the actor and the forum, the account giving, usually consists of at least two elements or stages. Many scholars have recognised that accountability relationships are based on a set of implicit rules inherent in the processes of **'answerability'** and **'enforceability or sanctions'** (Schedler, 1999; Brinkerhoff, 2004; Goetz & Jenkins, 2001).

Answerability is the essence of accountability because to be accountable is to have to answer for one's actions or inaction and hence to be responsible for their consequences (Robert, 2002). This requires two steps – one is, sharing of **information**, which is usually one-way, from the accountable to the overseeing actor(s) for the purpose of basic monitoring. Accountability instruments like the Right to Information Act (RTI) or the Controller and Auditor General (CAG) report is an example of how government fulfils answerability, although 'partially' through sharing of information.

According to Brinkerhoff (2004), the second more crucial aspect of answerability is about **explanations or justifications** or reasons for one's actions. Justifications incorporate information dissemination but go beyond to dialogue and confrontation between those accountable and the overseeing actor (Brinkerhoff, 2004). There are various accountability instruments that enact the justification aspect of accountability through dialogue, like parliamentary hearings where a minister answers questions of the legislatures or community meetings where officials answer residents through events like social audits also termed as *jan sunwais*[1] or public hearings.

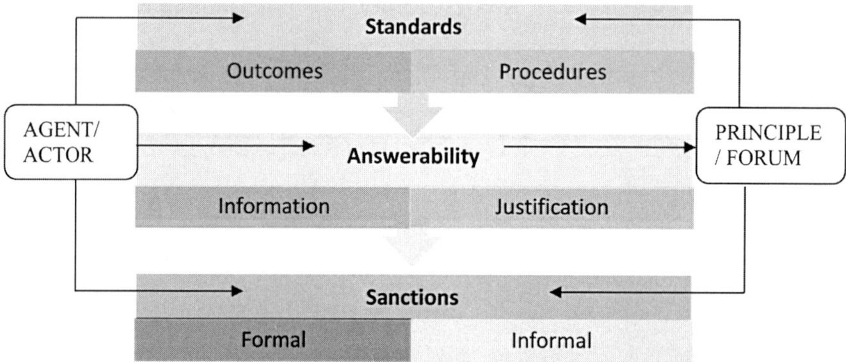

Figure 2.3: Elements of Standard Accountability

Illustration by Author

The most defining element of accountability is **enforceability** or **sanction** (Potts, 2008). Accountability holders, to whom a government owes an obligation, play a significant role in sanctioning or imposing punishment or giving incentives to those in power who are held accountable for failures or successes (Rubenstein, 2007; Brinkerhoff 2004).

Sanctions gives 'teeth' to accountability. Answerability without sanctions is weak accountability. Examples of sanctions are - constituents vote unresponsive representatives out of office, mistreated workers file complaints against their employer with the Department of Labour, groups wronged by an NGO report the situation to the media etc. (Rubenstein, 2007). Most health policy sanctions are based on regulatory power. An example is in the United States where Medicare is authorised to levy fines on hospitals that improperly code patient discharges.

In India, its apex medical council called the Medical Council of India (MCI) have cancelled registration of doctors and barred from medical practice owing to medical misconduct and negligently treating patients (Deb Roy, 2013). The courts too have intervened with legal sanctions to enforce accountability of a provider to the patient.

1 For more information on Social Audits, refer to Goyal, Jaya. 2011. Social Audits in Outcome Budgeting: An experiment of accountability in Maharashtra. The Indian Journal of Social Work. 72 (4), 537-562. hearings where a minister

The case in point is the Consumer Protection Act where patients have got relief from courts against hospitals or doctors on the grounds of medical negligence or malpractice.

Other regulatory frameworks range from formal sanctions like licensing and accreditation of physicians, nurses, other categories of health care providers; to quality assurance policies that establish standards and benchmarks; to practice guidelines and compliance mechanisms to improve quality of care; and to service utilisation and client satisfaction. There are informal sanctions documented as well like professional codes of conduct that do not have status of law (Brinkerhoff, 2004). This sanctioning aspect of accountability is the one that distinguishes itself from other similar concepts like responsibility, transparency responsiveness, participation and deliberation2.

Some scholars also have a term called 'rudeness' as a kind of an informal sanction that the poor use to negotiate and sanction public providers. Hossain (2010) while studying health services in Bangladesh observed that 'rude' forms of accountability are central to how poor people negotiate their entitlements on the frontline of service delivery. Rude accountability refers to the informal mechanisms widely deployed by citizens to claim public service and sanction service failures. These include shame and embarrassment, pressure to maintain reputation and status and threat of violence (Hossain, 2010). It is characterised by a lack of official rules or formal basis and a reliance on the power of social norms and rules to influence and sanction official performance (ibid.).

Rubenstein (2007) mentioned additional aspect of accountability which is the role of **'standards'** in the form of rules, norms, outcomes and procedures, as the first step to realizing accountability. It is against the 'standards' that accountable comply and are held responsible for their decisions and actions. Accountability holders endorse the standards, while the power wielder recognises the standards in an accountability mechanism (even if the power wielder does not endorse them). The kinds of standards to which power wielders are often held, include either formalised forms like "citizen charters" or other less formal messaging like 'promote constituents' preferences', 'obey the law', 'do not be racist' or 'using environment friendly' laws etc. (Rubenstein, 2007).

Thus the definition of accountability includes three main elements, which (Grant & Keohane, 2005) refer to as "standards, information and sanction" Accordingly, Bovens

2 See Bovens (2007) on Transparency, often used as a synonym for accountability, is not enough to constitute accountability. Open government and freedom of information are particularly important prerequi sites for accountability in the context of governance, because they may provide accountability forums with the necessary information. However, transparency as such is not enough to qualify as a genuine form of accountability, because transparency does not necessarily involve scrutiny by a specific forum. One needs to distinguish accountability from responsiveness and participation. Responsiveness to the needs and preferences of stakeholders and new forms of participation may be especially important to enhance the political legitimacy of an institution. But they do not constitute accountability. They provide proactive inputs into the policy process and one needs to classify and study them separately for what they are: forms of consultation and participation. They lack the element of justification, judgement and consequences.

(2007) defines accountability as a relationship between an actor and a forum, in which the actor has an obligation to explain and to justify his or her conduct, the forum can pose questions and pass judgement and the actor may face consequences (Rubeinstein, 2007). To elucidate the relationships among these elements, it is useful to consider a schematic model of standard accountability that explains all the three in Figure 2.3.

According to the 'standard model' of accountability, holding another actor accountable entail sanctioning that actor if it fails to fulfil its obligations without a justification or excuse. It gives the impression that the less powerful actors therefore cannot hold more powerful actors accountable, because they cannot sanction more powerful actors (ibid).

Hence, there is an emergence of other types of accountability mechanisms where there is a proxy actor like a civil society organisation (NGO) that mediates the accountability relationship. Standard accountability follows the traditional form of accountability where accountability flows upwards, from bureaucracy to elected representatives and then to public. However, with the spread of managerialism in the public sector, it has made traditional accountability less relevant as compared to other emerging forms of accountability like social accountability or managerial accountability (McGarvey, 2001).

2.3 Classifications of Accountability

Just like the State disperses power in a liberal democracy, so is accountability spread between multiple actors and institutions. However, because of the obscure nature of the concept, it can mean different things to different actors in different contexts. As mentioned earlier in Chapter I, a range of actors from social movements to the World Bank have voiced concerns about accountability (George, 2009; Goetz & Gaventa, 2001; World Bank, 2004). As a result, accountability mechanisms like patient charters, hospital boards, village or municipal health committees, right to information acts, consumer courts, contracting, accreditation and franchising are being implemented worldwide (ibid.). Accountability through these mechanisms serves mostly to regulate relationships between service providers and patients.

Diverse types of accountability may be distinguished depending on the relative positions of the actors involved in this relationship (Garn, 2010). For instance, applying classifications of types of accountability to health services delivery will develop a clearer picture of what accountability issues emerge and of where gaps, contradictions and conflicts may lie (Brinkerhoff, 2004).

To analyse what types of accountability are involved, various scholars have developed their own classification of accountability in general and accountability in government or public administration in particular (see Figure 2.4). Based on the sanctioning mechanism utilized between the accountability holders and power wielders, accountability can be categorised into 5 types – electoral accountability, legal accountability, market-based accountability, civil society based accountability and administrative accountability (Rubeinstein, 2007). There could be synonyms for these types of accountabilities, for instance, electoral accountability refers to political accountability and civil society accountability is another name for social accountability.

According to Glynn & Murphy (1996) there are several different, but well established, types of accountability in the public sector. These include:

a. **Public accountability**, which Glynn summarises as "those who are charged with drafting and/or carrying out policy should be obliged to give an explanation of their actions to the electorate".

b. **Financial accountability** – this is perhaps the longest established type of accountability concentrating on the regularity with which resources entrusted to an agent have been managed.

c. **Legal accountability**, i.e. accountability to a court of law, or equivalent, for the exercise of powers.

d. **Managerial accountability**, i.e. accountability by managers for the achievement of defined and agreed, resource utilisation objectives (Garn, 2011).

According to scholars from the Institute of Development Studies (IDS) University of Sussex, accountability is categorised as **political, social and managerial accountability** (Gaventa, 2002). Political accountability consists of checks and balances within the state through individuals in public office, responsible for carrying out tasks on behalf of citizens by either horizontal or vertical mechanisms. Social accountability focuses on citizen action holding the state to account using strategies such as social mobilisation, press reports and legal action. And lastly, managerial accountability focuses on financial accounting and reporting within state institutions judged according to agreed performance criteria like auditing.

In addition, there are also several '**binary**' classifications of accountability which are independent of one another, like the **horizontal accountability** (O'donnell, 1999) **and vertical accountability**According to Ackerman (2004), vertical accountability mechanisms such as elections, that require government officials to appeal 'downwards' to the people at large have been complemented by horizontal accountability mechanisms that require public officials and agencies to report 'sideways' to other officials and agencies within the state itself.

Examples of horizontal accountability are when the executive is accountable to the legislature and the legislature is accountable to corruption control agencies like the CAG (Comptroller and Auditor General of India), ombudsman, administrative courts, legislative commissions and parliamentary audit committees. Vertical accountability is between the state and the citizens enacted through mechanism like elections or PILs (Public Interest

Litigations), giving power to the citizens to ensure accountable governance (Posani & Aiyer, 2009)

Other binaries of accountability include - **upward and downward accountability; strategic and functional accountability; external and internal accountability; constitutional and democratic accountability** and **legal and political accountability** [3] (Rubenstein, 2007).

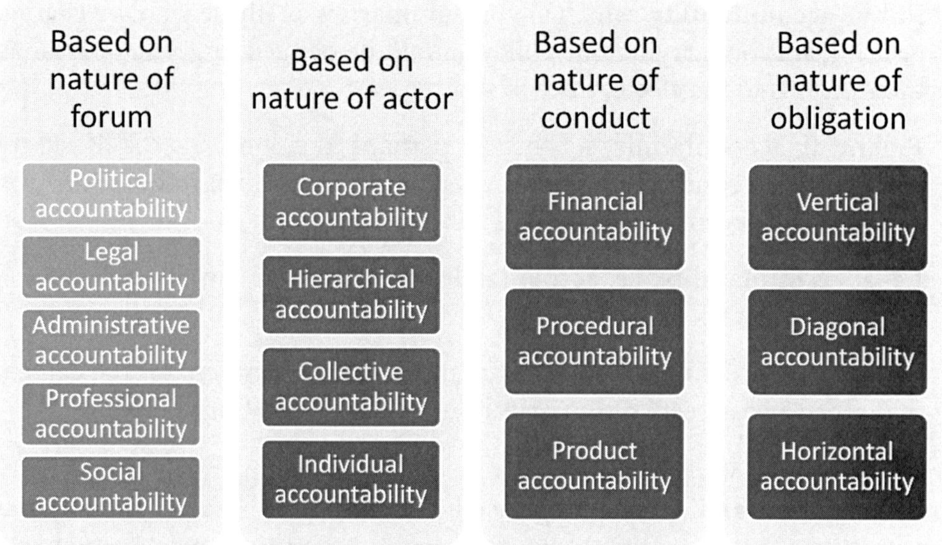

Figure 2.4: Types of Accountability

Source: Complied from Bovens (2007) Illustration by Author.

Romzek & Dubnick (1987) created finer-grained distinctions among accountability mechanisms that are derived from two dimensions: source of control (external or internal) and the degree of control (high or low) exerted over public agents (Roberts, 2002). Accordingly, four types of accountability are possible – legal accountability (external with high degree of control), bureaucratic accountability (internal with high degree of control), political accountability (external and low degree of control) and professional accountability (internal and low degree of control).

In the context of public health, scholars have perceived accountability to foster dialogue between providers and users and thus increase the responsiveness of the health system to the needs of its users (Cornwall, 2000). Brinkerhoff is one of the few scholars who have theoretically and conceptually explained accountability in public health. According to Brinkerhoff (2004), the accountability interests of actors in the health

3 For various frameworks of accountability, see Figure 1.1.

sector vary depending upon for what purpose actors will use accountability. There could be broadly three purposes of accountability:

a. for reducing abuse of power – misuse of public resources or authority
b. for assuring compliance with standards (legal and professional) and societal values
c. for improving performance and management through feedback and learning

These purposes provide the answer to the question on **accountability for what?** Brinkerhoff broadly classifies accountability in public sector as financial accountability, performance account-ability and political or democratic accountability in order of their purposes cited above.

George (2003) argues that accountability is needed for confronting unequal power relations between actors through use of information dissemination, monitoring, mediation and peer pressure between actors.

Actors in the health sector can be numerous, like - health service users or patients, Ministry of Health, funding agencies and international donors, parliament, NGOs, hospital boards, healthcare providers, professional associations, local government officials, health councils, unions etc. (Brinkerhoff, 2004). George (2003) lists accountability measures in the health sector like consumer charters, hospital boards, village health committees and publicity campaigns are being used to implement health policy and programmes worldwide. Others like Potts (2008) mentions legal types of accountability mechanisms in health sector such as judicial procedures, national human rights institutions, health commissions, local health councils, patients' committees etc. According to George (2003), accountability in the health sector can be administrative, legal, fiscal, political, constitutional, horizontal (within the government) and vertical (between other agencies like funders and government).

Mark Bovens (2007) gave a comprehensive and almost exhaustive classification of accountability in his work titled 'Analysing and assessing accountability: A conceptual framework". Bovens used four criteria to group various accountability mechanisms (Figure 2.4). The first classification is based on the nature of forum which means to whom is account given; to what type of forum; and which actor is required to being accountable? Accordingly, there are five types of accountability from political to social, wherein social forum includes the civil society.

The second is based on the question of who should render accountability or nature of actor. The third classification comes remarkably close to the first as it focuses on the objective or purpose of accountability or nature of conduct. Finally, the last group of accountability types deals with the nature of obligation or why the actor feels compelled to render accountability. The last classification defines the nature of hierarchical relationships between the actor and the forum Bovens (2007).

Unpacking the contestation. Scholars have recognised this complexity of various kinds of accountability in a range of typologies and frameworks of accountability from various disciplines (Figure 1.1). There is no consensus among scholars on these typologies which most feel is not mutually exclusive but overlap thus creating a web of multiple, overlapping accountability relationships (Romzek, 2000; Roberts, 2002). For instance, financial accountability aimed at uncovering malaise often creates tension with performance accountability which accepts role of errors, improvements, discretion and external factors as contributory factors. Also, both financial and performance accountability have implications on democratic or political accountability. Such classification of accountability is imperative to decode complexities of various mechanisms, tools, applications, relationships and their implications for democratic governance.

It also puts the World Bank's observation in perspective that the long route of accountability (political accountability) has failed people's expectations. As a result, there have been efforts to create newer spaces of citizen engagement through the short route of accountability (social accountability). Non-state actors like the civil society acted as a catalyst for these mechanisms like citizen report cards, citizen charters, community-based monitoring, Rogi Kalyan Samiti, social audits etc. To be fair, state provisions in India like the Right to Information (RTI) Act and the controversial Jan Lokpal Bill have also created newer spaces and instruments through which citizens can engage and scrutinise the state (Posani & Aiyer, 2009). Despite these newer spaces of accountability, their implementation has been sketchy, context specific and with mixed evidence on improvements in service delivery.

Therefore, although there is agreement that accountability in government is necessary, there is also a little consensus on which mechanisms should prevail at which levels. In addition, broad array of actors with multiple connections fill the accountability landscape. In some cases, these actors are both accountable to one set of actors while simultaneously exercising accountability over another set. For example, public providers, health ministries, finance ministries, parliamentary health committees, insurance fund agencies and hospital boards are often linked to multiple types of accountability among each other or a higher-up power. These connections create layered webs of accountability with varying degrees of autonomy and sources of control/oversight (Brinkerhoff, 2004).

To conclude in the words of Mark Bovens, accountability is often used in an overly broad sense, as a synonym for a variety of evaluative, but contested and contestable concepts, such as responsiveness, responsibility and effectiveness (Bovens, 2006). There is enough literature that argues the meanings of accountability in different contexts and settings as mentioned or how accountability is perceived by different actors both at conceptual and theoretical level.

2.4 Framework for Analysis

This study adopts the Institutional and Development Framework (IAD) proposed by Ostrom (2011), from the discipline of economics in analysing accountability relationships at the frontline of service delivery in a democratic state. The rationale of using this framework flows from the gaps in the frameworks used by other studies discussed earlier. However, the study does acknowledge that many alternative approaches are available and valid. The rationale of using the IAD framework is that the assumptions in this study (see 2.5.1) corresponds to the framework.

According to the basic assumptions of the IAD framework, politics of service delivery and policy making can be understood through the rules, codes of conduct and norms inherent in social structures, called institutions (Ostrom, 1990). Institutions play a significant role in our daily lives by influencing social, political and economic behaviour. Yet until recently, policy analysis has often ignored the role of institutions. In addition, a fact established by political science scholars is that, "the patterning of social life is not produced solely by the aggregation of individual and organisational behaviour but also by institutions that structure action" (Clemens & Cook, 1999). It is therefore crucial to bring in the framework of analysing institutions to study the accountability processes (Figure 2.5).

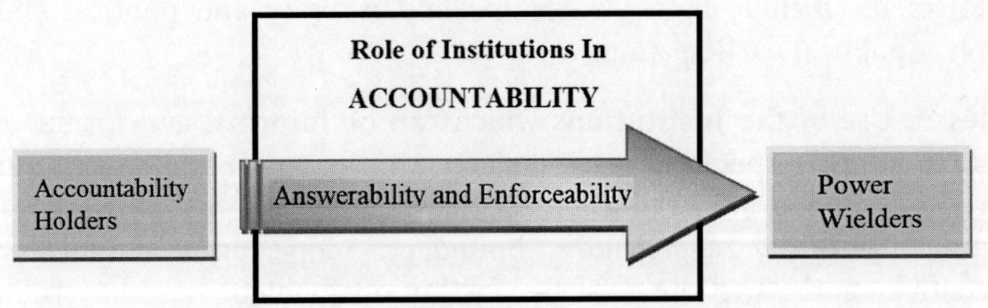

Figure 2.5: Institutions & Accountability

Source: Compiled from Ostrom 1990; Clemens & Cook, 1999.
Illustrations by Author

According to Ostrom, that policy work in various sectors can be improved if we include institutions in our analysis (Polski & Ostrom, 1999). When we accept that accountability is a practice of governance, it follows that the concept entails a relationship between the governing and the governed actor, a relationship characterised by roles and rules. Accordingly, the concept of accountability appoints roles to different actors, i.e. the accounting actor and the accountable actor. These roles are defined, maintained and regulated by a set of 'rules' inherent in the concept, i.e. the aspects of answerability and enforceability, respectively. These roles and rules delineate legitimate spaces of action for the actors involved in the relationship of accountability (Garn, 2010). Also, institutions exist wherever there are actor engaging with each other, like at frontline of service delivery at village level and one needs not only imagine it at the tertiary levels.

Using the IAD framework, I developed a conceptual framework for accountability relationships in Figure 2.6 & 2.7. The context of this study is public health service delivery which features in the **Policy or Action arena** in Figure 2.6. It includes behaviour of all the actors, individuals and groups who are routinely involved in the action arena. In public health service delivery, one can identify these actors and group them into categories - users/patients, user associations, providers in government and private sector, government administration from Ministry to PRIs, NGOs or professional associations or unions, local politicians etc. Three conditions influence behaviour of these actors in this Policy or Action arena, namely:

a. **Physical and Material Conditions** – These essentially include all the inputs for a policy area in terms of capital, labour, technical expertise, financial, infrastructure, distribution etc.

b. **Community attributes** or culture that involves demography, norms, values, beliefs, commonly held understanding, preference of the people in communities under focus. These community attributes also determine the 'Citizen Capability' (from Sen's Capability Approach, see Comim et al., 2008) in terms of social, political and economic endowments. Social endowments include education and caste, economic endowments include land ownership, employability and political endowments involves political participation.

a. **Rules-in-Use of the Institutions** which can be informal and formal and found at three levels – operating level, collective choice level and constitutional level. Institutions shape interaction and choice making among actors. These include position, authority, aggregation, boundary, scope, information and payoffs (incentives and sanctions). These institutions which are not visible (unlike organisations) in-turn determine the institutional capacity of the actors in the policy arena. Institutional capacity includes processes like monitoring, regulation, information sharing and planning. For instance, incentives and authority can determine how well information is collected, maintained and shared with actors for programme evaluation at the provider level.

All these three conditions influence actors in the policy arena, which together with citizen capability and institutional capacity creates patterns of interaction of which accountabilit is one of them, which is the focus of this study. The accountability relationships give rise to many kinds of institutional arrangements of accountability like the community-based monitoring, social audits, *jan sunwais*, and citizen report cards. Institutional capacities of various actors and agencies in public health service delivery also influence these arrangements.

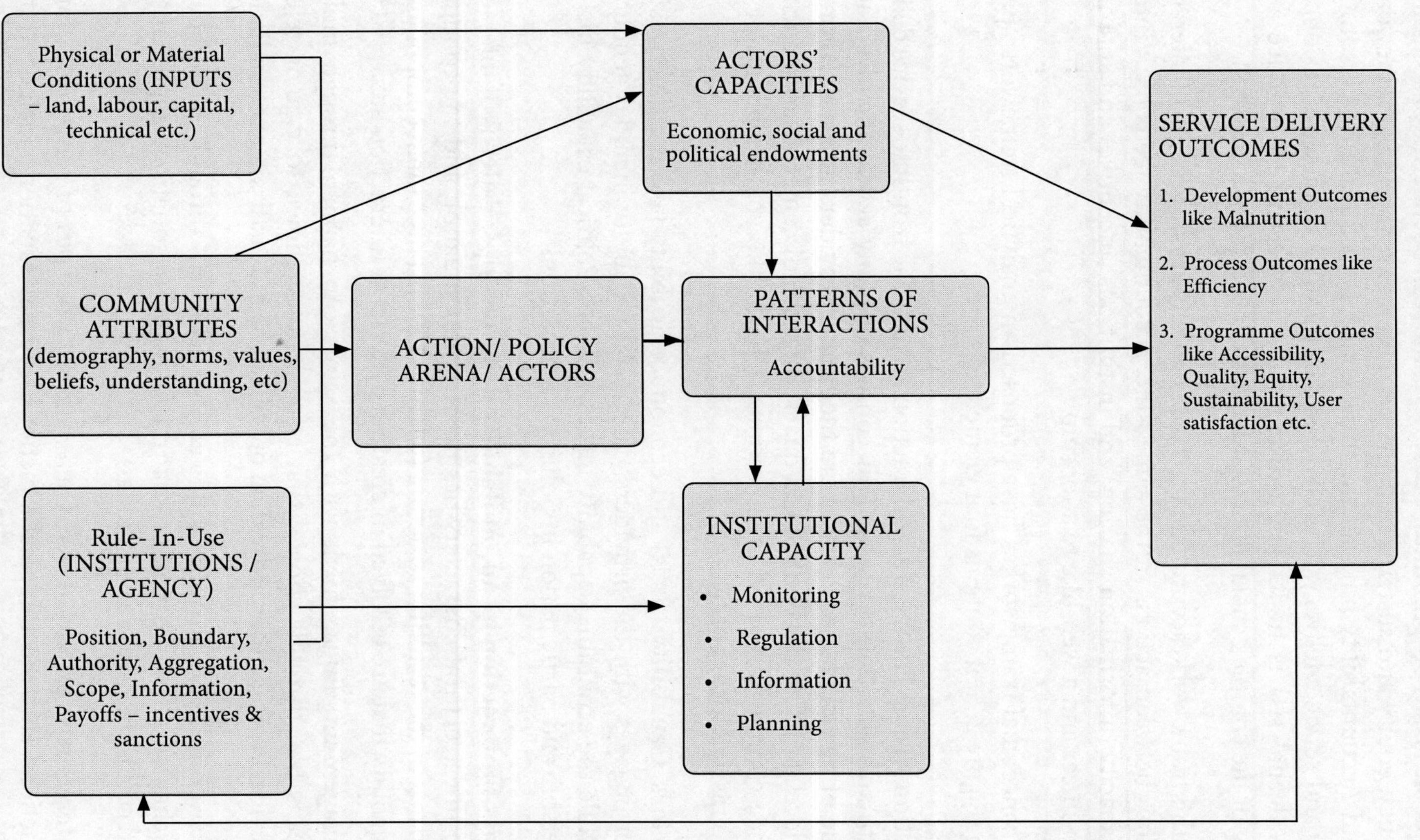

Figure 2.6: Conceptual Framework on Accountability in Service Delivery

Source: Compiled from Ostrom, 2011; The World Bank & IFPRI, 2010. Illustration by Author

Finally, accountability and its institutional arrangements influence **Service Delivery Outcomes** of public health programmes. These outcomes can be in terms of accessibility, quality, efficiency, equity and sustainability. As per Figure 2.7, the IAD Framework on Institutions and Accountability links all the three concepts of the study – institutions, accountability and service delivery. The advantage of the IAD framework (as opposed to the technical analysis) is in its multi-disciplinary perspective to produce a rich understanding of the complex social policy situations (Polski & Ostrom 1998).

As seen in this framework, accountability is conceptualised as a 'process' of interaction and relationships between actors. At the same time, accountability feeds back into the institutional capacity (information sharing) and institutions (incentives and authority), showing a non-linear and a web-like relationship.

From the conceptual framework, I have proposed an analytical framework specific to this study in Figure 2.7. It contains four elements:

1. **The Action Arena:** For the study, the action arena is the frontline service delivery of health and nutrition services. This consists of many actions involved at the frontline of service delivery. These are the health providers at the PHC or sub-center level, at village level like local quack, anganwadi center; users; panchayat members; community-based organisations (CBOs) like youth mandals or self-help groups and local politicians.
2. **The Actors' Capability:** social and economic capability largely influences how an actor engages with the providers. The social capability includes gender and caste while the economic capability includes assets. Political capability includes membership and participation in political organisation.
3. **Patterns of Interaction in Accountability Relationships:** Patterns of interaction refer to the structural characteristics of an action situation and the conduct of participants in the resulting structure (Ostrom 1998). Three main components of accountability that are involved in creating patterns of interaction are:
   a. **Engagement:** Engagement with the actors can happen through multiple means like through choice, that also includes choice to exit or reject a provider; voice, either individual or collective and lastly silent compliance.
   b. **Answerability:** answerability can be achieved through a number of mechanisms like information sharing, dialogue, negotiations, representation and confronting power relations.
   c. **Enforcement or Sanctions:** There can be two types of sanctions – formal sanctions and the informal sanctions. Formal sanctions include transfer order, suspensions, fines, complaints or third-party action like NGO action. Informal sanctions include rude behaviour, shame, embarrassment and fear.

4. **Service Delivery Outcomes:** finally, the delivery of services results in health outcomes like reduction in child under-nutrition, access and utilisation of services and user satisfaction.

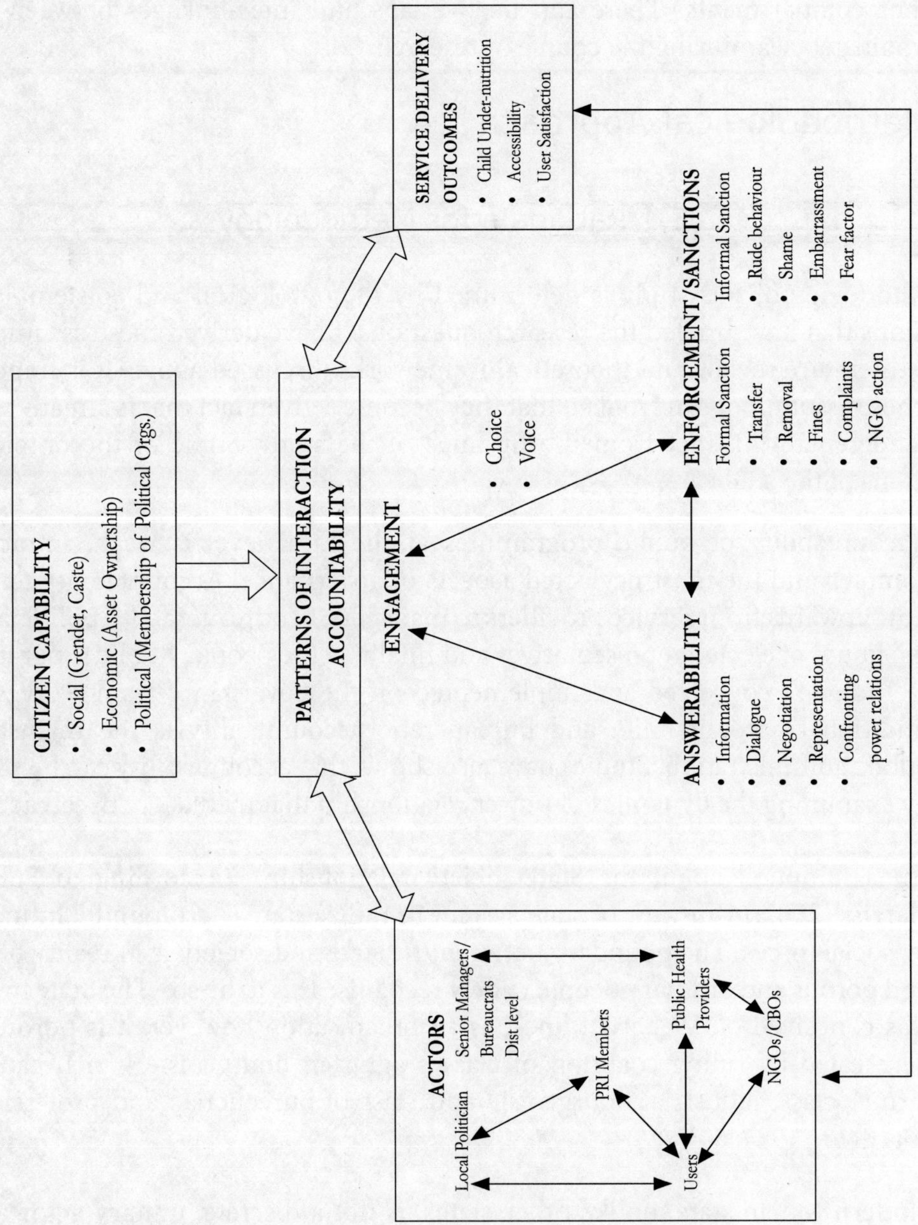

Figure 2.7: Analytical Framework used in the study

Source: Illustration by Author

With this theoretical and conceptual understanding on the linkages between institutions, accountability and public service delivery, a focus of the study discussed in the following section would delimit the study in its scope. The concepts and sub-concepts mentioned in these theoretical frameworks are not mutually exclusive, exhaustive or water-tight compartments. There can be overlaps and inter-linkages between them which would get clear during the course of research.

2.5 Methodological Approach

2.5.1 Rationale for Methodology

The methodology of this study is determined by the ontological and epistemological assumptions that have briefed the research questions. I have derived these assumptions from the literature review and theoretical frameworks discussed above. It is important to state these assumptions upfront so that they become a given fact that is already widely known and remain distinct from the findings of the study. Some of the ontological assumptions of the study are:

- Accountability of public programmes at the local level is weak, intractable, complex and the most neglected aspects of governance. Accountability tends to flow upwards from service providers to managers, to bureaucrats, to politicians, to the house of elected representatives and finally to the people. Public programmes in India are conceived and implemented on the governance framework where traditional accountability and bureaucratic accountability is the mainstay of public administration. Studies have also shown that accountability can be studied by examining the dynamics of power relationship that mediate between actors.

- An assumption about the State-society relationship - According to Fuller & Harriss (2001:14) review of state system in India, 'state is profoundly influenced by social forces. The boundary between the state and society is in reality blurred and porous and ordinary people widely recognise this to be so. 'The State in India was conceived on Weberian lines, as an organisation however, it is porous and permeated by ruling coalition of classes agrarian bourgeoisie – rich capitalist farmer class, industrial bourgeoisie and class of bureaucrats and professionals' (Bardhan, 1984: 64).

  Modern Indian state, unlike other states, is not a discrete, unitary actor acting impersonally above or outside the society. But '*sarkar*' appears on many levels and in many centers and its lower echelons are always staffed by people with whom social relationship can or could exist. The faceless bureaucrats do actually have faces. Therefore, the boundary between the state and society is not only unclear, it is also fluid and negotiable according to the social context and position.

The state does not consist of an 'actual organisation' separated from society. As the state expanded, a profound gap developed between the bureaucratic elite (which often corresponded well with the Weberian rationality) and the personnel at the lower levels, whose 'vernacular everyday discourses' were not structured around principles of formal rationality at all. An important reason for the modern Indian State's failure to implement its policies successfully is, therefore, the fact that it is 'overstretched' and its policies are finally implemented by those very low down in the bureaucracy and they are re-interpreted beyond recognition.

- Assumptions about collective action. There are institutional spaces for users to engage and participate in public health programmes like Village Health and Sanitation Committees (VHSCs) and Rogi Kalyan Samitis (RKSs). Despite these, the capacity to demand accountability is still weak in India. According to the latest evaluation of NRHM (IIPS, 2010), majority of PHCs and CHCs had registered RKSs and majority of panchayats had formed VHSCs in Maharashtra. Yet only 39% surveyed households had heard of VHSC and less than 1% had heard about RKS. According to Olson (1965) communities are not homogenous entities and even if they are, they would not come together owing to power relations among its members, despite a common interest, unless either incentive or coercion is present. In most cases of community participation, there is elite capture.

The main **epistemological** assumption of the study is that a researcher can study these relationships of accountability from Institutional and Development (IAD)[4] perspective rooted in its very own set of assumptions. These are:

- An institutional analyst must either estimate from survey measurements or make intelligent assumptions about preferences in order to construct a model of decision behaviour in the action arena (Polski & Ostrom 1998).

- Also, the IAD framework is meant to study policy analysis and design, which in the context of this study is public service delivery in general and child health and nutrition services in particular.

- The framework inherently incorporates knowledge and information gaps about how institutions affect the incentives of users in any public service, for instance on forest resources, which may result in substantial levels of deforestation in some locations while improving forest conditions in other locations. Therefore, two opposite contexts are again part of the framework's assumptions.

- The analysis can be based on empirical observations of past and present events, hypothetical forecasts and simulations, or a combination of both.

4 The IAD framework was suggested by Polski and Ostrom in 1998 after which Elinor Ostrom, an American political scientist, received a Nobel in Economics in 2009.

These assumptions will provide qualifications and justifications to the research design, methods and tools explained as follows.

2.5.2 Research Design

Research design provides 'a framework for the collection and analysis of data' [43]. Based on the theoretical assumptions and analytical framework, the research problem demands an **Exploratory Research**. The rationale for using this design is that there is low knowledge about accountability relationships between actors at the frontline of service delivery. In addition, there is a paucity of empirical studies on the issue as explained in the section on "Rationale for the Study" in Chapter 1.

I developed a research design where analytical concepts of the study were linked with its objectives and data collection tools (Table 2.1). I linked each of the study objectives to concepts, data collection tool and type of respondents. According to the analytical framework in Figure 2.7, since actors and processes of accountability are inextricably linked to outcomes, it is imperative to select sites based on its performance on health and nutrition outcomes. Service delivery outcome on health & nutrition is the only concept amongst others in the analytical framework that is measured and for which credible data is widely available. But before one reaches the actual study site, several choices are required to be made at every level of geographical division. For instance, from state to districts to blocks and finally end at villages. Therefore, to begin with, one needs to select a site based on this verifiable indicator. Two significant and frequently used indicators of outcomes in health and nutrition programme implementation are percentage of children weighed in an anganwadi center, denoting accessibility or utilisation of ICDS services to some extent and nutrition status of the children measured in terms of percentage of under-nourished children.

I selected two sites or cases from within Maharashtra that have registered poor and better health outcomes respectively, for instance on the rate of malnutrition which is a key indicator. I did this so that I can study the relationships of between the provider and user in both the scenarios. The study, however, does not attempt to explain reasons for these outcomes. The study will be limited to explaining what institutional processes exist in such contexts.

Also, according to the analytical framework, most accountability relationships between actors occur at the frontline of service delivery. Therefore, the most basic unit that encompass the study objectives in totality is a village. According to Bardhan (2009), accountability is also more direct at the local level, if the democratic processes work. There is more vigilance on issues where more local stake is involved, as the idea is that it is our money you are wasting or stealing. Electoral sanctions may be more effective at the local level, than at central level where multi-dimensionality of electoral issues dilutes responsbility.

Table 2.1: Methodological Linkages

Objectives	*Theoretical Concepts*	*Issues*	*Respondents*	*Tools*
1. To understand how accountability, as an element of good governance, plays a role in better or poor service delivery of public health programme at the frontline level. a. To identify relationships of accountability existing between various actors - providers, users, user groups, local politicians/PRI members and local NGOs, at the frontline of public health service delivery.	Institutional Capacity for ensuring Accountability i. Information Sharing ii. Monitoring & Evaluation	1. What are the various types of records maintained for monitoring and evaluation of the ICDS/NRHM programmes? 2. What is the frequency of updating these records? 3. To whom is this data/information send and how is it used - Is it send only to the hierarchy up or also to the people? 4. Have you heard about a jan sunwai (public hearing)? What happens there? If you have attended one, how was your experience? 5. How many RTIs do you receive in a week/month? What are the major concerns in the RTI? 6. How monitoring done – with data alone or physical inspection? 7. Is there any interaction and feedback at the Gram Sabha? What is your opinion on the same? 8. Are you confronted with people asking questions about the quality of services? 9. Are there any standards against which the monitoring is done like IPHS or citizen charters? 10. What is your role in RKS / VHSC? 11. What is the outcome of monitoring according to you? 12. What kind of incentives do you have or are given upon your performance evaluation?	• Providers Anganwadi worker (AWW) • Auxiliary Nurse Midwife (ANM) • Accredited Social Health Activist (ASHA) • Medical Officer (MO) of Primary Health Center (PHC)	In-depth Interview And Secondary data – Records or Minutes of meetings of Village Health and Sanitation Committee (VHSC) and Rogi Kalyan Samiti (RKS)
b. To understand how accountability relationships are enacted between frontline public providers and users in public health service delivery.	Nature of Engagement i. Choice (Exit) ii. Voice (collective) iii. Rude accountability (individual) iv. Silent compliance or inaction v. Co-governance	1. Why did they choose this provider? 2. Is there any voice in the way users engage with the providers if the services are poor? 3. How is this voice exercised and with what implications? 4. At individual levels are rude forms of accountability prevalent? 5. How and when is it exercised? Give examples. 6. Why do people silently comply and put up with poor services? 7. Is there any agency that helps people voice their concerns and demand accountability on their behalf? How is it done?	Users of the service – Head of the households and mothers of children below 6 years.	Semi-Structured Interview Schedule

Source: By Author

Table 2.1 Continued

Objectives	*Theoretical Concepts*	*Issues*	*Respondents*	*Tools*
b. To understand how accountability relationships are enacted between frontline public providers and users in public health service delivery.	Nature of Engagement i. Choice (Exit) ii. Voice (collective) iii. Rude accountability (individual) iv. Silent compliance or inaction v. Co-governance	1. Why did they choose this provider? 2. Is there any voice in the way users engage with the providers if the services are poor? 3. How is this voice exercised and with what implications? 4. At individual levels are rude forms of accountability prevalent? 5. How and when is it exercised? Give examples. 6. Why do people silently comply and put up with poor services? 7. Is there any agency that helps people voice their concerns and demand accountability on their behalf? How is it done?	Users of the service – Head of the households and mothers of children below 6 years.	Semi-Structured Interview Schedule
2. To analyze how users, especially the poor, demand or negotiate better services and entitlements through informal mechanisms when the formal mechanisms of accountability fail or exclude them? a. To identify and compare various institutionalised formal accountability mechanisms with informal forms of accountability. b. To examine whether informal forms of accountability have a comparative advantage over formal ones or vice versa.	Answerability i. Information sharing, dialogue and negotiation. ii. Representation (confronting power relations) Sanctions or Enforcement i. Formal negative sanctions – transfer, removal or dismiss, fines, complaints, NGO action ii. Informal negative sanctions – rude behaviour, shame, embarrassment, fear iii. Formal positive sanctions -recognition, rewards, promotions. iv. Informal positive sanctions -popularity, respect status	1. Are you aware about the institutional spaces meant for eliciting answerability in health services like VHSC and RKS in your village? 2. Do you think you as a user of a service your concerns are well represented? 3. Explain some instances in which you have confronted the provider for poor service and held dialogue with them? 4. Are you aware about mechanisms of answerability – elections, RTIs, jan sunwais, social audit, CBM? 5. Has any such exercise happened in your village? How do users participate in these and benefit from it? 6. In wake of poor quality / access /affordability of service, what kind of sanctions are levied on the providers? 7. What kinds of deficits in health services have attracted such sanctions?	• Users of the service – Head of the households and mothers of children below 6 years. • Frontline provider – ANM, AWW, ASHA, MO.	Semi Structured Interview Schedule Data on individual children – nutrition status from the anganwadi centres.
3. To revisit the idea of accountability and good governance in light of empirical findings.	Integration of all previous concepts –as a conclusion chapter.	None	None	None

Source: By Author

The study also demands to be based in rural India because as per contemporary trends, there is a significant increase in the utilisation of government health facilities in rural areas between 2004 and 2011. A study of five states has shown that over half of those who sought outpatient treatment (54%) and almost half (48%) of those who sought hospitalised care depended on public facilities (Nagaranjan, 2013). Only with certain level of utilisation of public services, can accountability processes be studied. Hence, guided by this rationale and the conceptual framework, the processes and relationships of accountability can be studied in an Indian village. A research design that can justify such a need is the **Comparative Case Study Research Design.**

Case studies are sites for the employment of both quantitative and qualitative research and associating them with qualitative research only, is not appropriate (Bryman, 2008). For this study, since the cases are chosen purposely on the grounds that it will allow for a better understanding of the objectives of the study, two villages chosen can be termed as **Critical Cases**. One of the standard criticisms of case study designs is that findings derived from it cannot be generalised. It is true to some extent as the external validity in a case study is restricted. However, those in favour of case studies argue that they aim to generate an intensive examination of a particular case, in relation to which they engage in theoretical analysis. The crucial question is not whether the findings can be generalised to a wider universe but how well the researcher generates theory out of the findings (ibid.). Thus, case studies can be associated with both theory generation and theory testing.

2.5.3 Context

Study context. Two national public health programmes - NRHM and ICDS are the context areas of the study. It is because both of these programmes converge on major child health outcomes; both having a component of community interface and both are predominantly rural in nature. National Rural Health Mission (NRHM) which has since 2014 been renamed as National Health Mission (NHM) is an important policy commitment of the Indian state together with other programmes like Integrated Child Development Services (ICDS), Rural Water Supply Programme and Total Sanitation Campaign (TSC).[5]

NRHM, which is one of the most significant public health policy initiatives, was rolled out as the country's biggest primary health programme. A comprehensive framework for accountability through community-based monitoring (CBM) is one of the important mandates of the NRHM. It proposes an intensive accountability framework through a three-pronged process of external surveys, stringent internal monitoring and

5 These flagship programmes fall under the 'Traditional Public Health' (as against the curative services of ambulatory and hospital care) which is further categorised into - 'Population Based Public Health Interventions' and 'Preventive and Promotive Public Health Interventions'.

an innovative approach of community-based monitoring of health services through community mobilisation initiatives like monthly "health and nutrition day", the VHSC and the RKS (Sinha 2008, Husain 2011). For the first time in India, the government introduced an intensive accountability framework for the Public health institutions in a generalised manner (Kakde, 2010). Thus, I choose NRHM as the programme for this study. There was evidence that health services had improved in places within Maharashtra where NRHM carried out CBM. However, I did not choose districts where CBM happened because such a process was not organic but was facilitated by one civil society organisation called SATHI-CEHAT in the state. Such an intervening factor can be a subject of independent research by itself. It also did not align with research questions of the study and hence was not considered.

The Integrated Child Health Services (ICDS) is another public health programme which is linked to outcomes of NRHM and where there is a wide gap between policy and implementation. Experts have demanded for improved convergences and accountability in the ICDS service delivery. For instance, one of the many policy recommendations in the ICDS includes selection of anganwadi workers by the gram panchayat, through a supervised process that involves the community to ensure improved accountability of the anganwadi worker towards the community. Lack of local accountability and poor governance are among other factors like poor capacities affecting the management such a large public programme.

Leakages, low motivation levels and poor community ownership are cited to be some of the problems that have plagued ICDS (Sinha, 2008). According to a study by Nandini Nayak and N C Saxena on ICDS in Bihar and Jharkhand, it shows that the effectiveness of ICDS is constantly being held up because children have no "voice" in the system owing to which there is no self-correction mechanism whereby implementation failures lead to outspoken protest and timely redressal. As a result, problems that could be solved easily are often left unaddressed like vacant posts of supervisors for months together leading to complete lack of supervision or prolonged disruption of food distribution in the anganwadis (Dreze, 2006). The Government of India has also institutionalised 'nutrition' in the local accountability framework through the Village Health Nutrition and Sanitation Committee (VHNSC). Therefore, ICDS was selected as another programme for the study.

Both the NRHM and the ICDS programmes have a historical trajectory in terms of its policies, programmes and structure of implementation that evolved over a period since their introduction. There is an over-flowing body of analysis on the flaws and critique of these programmes both at the level of policy and implementation. Attempting this analysis would not have added any value to the research problems of this study or to the body of knowledge on the subject in general. That body of literature falls in the domain of Health Systems Development and that is why I did not consider it for the study. Also, since both these programmes formed only a context of this research, I did not attempt any policy critique or historical analysis of these programmes. It meant that the study took the current policy, implementation processes, institutions within ICDS and NRHM like the institution of the Anganwadis, structure of PHCs or VHSC at village level as 'given' and 'out there', because that is the basis on which current public service delivery is structured. This, however, does not mean that I am not overtly concerned about the structural flaws of these programmes. In fact, this study is an attempt to add both theoretical and empirical knowledge to public service delivery in general and nutrition and health services in particular, with implications for improving policy design and its implementation.

Geographical or Spatial context. I choose the state of Maharashtra purposely as it suited the study objectives and its analytical framework. While Maharashtra on an average may be a developed state, it cannot escape the fact that this development is grossly skewed and has benefited a small minority of urban based middle classes and the richer peasantry in the sugar growing belt of the state (Mishra et al., 2008).

Large-scale disparities persist in Maharashtra, across rural-urban areas, within urban and rural areas, across classes, gender, and caste groups for access to basic public services and programmes and especially public health services. Historical analysis also reveals that these inequities in access to healthcare services have got worse over the last decade and a half, that is, post structural adjustment policies (ibid.). The gross inequities we see in access to public health services are very strongly associated with the role that the state plays in the health sector.

Limited data available across districts also shows wide variation in distribution of health infrastructure highlighting economic, social and regional disparities. Drought prone regions of Marathwada, North Maharashtra and Vidharbha are known to be the economically backward regions and lag in health outcomes as compared to rain-fed Konkan and Ratnagiri regions. These inequities are a part of many exogenous factors like agro-climatic conditions and overall structural inequities of caste, poverty and gender that we see elsewhere in the society. As mentioned earlier, a larger proportion of people both in rural and urban areas use public health services including communicable disease prevention, immunisation, family planning and contraceptive services, RCH services like antenatal care, pregnancy and delivery related care etc. However even for these services, the underprivileged sections suffer gross inequities in access because of a weak and unreachable public health system. When these underprivileged people are forced to seek care, then it is at a tremendous cost of indebtedness.

According to a recent study by an NGO in rural areas of five states - Assam, Jharkhand, Rajasthan, Tamil Nadu and Uttarakhand, across all economic classes, barring the highest class (over Rs 2,000 monthly per capita expenditure), a majority of people paid for hospitalisation charges by borrowing money (Nagaranjan, 2013). This only confirms that healthcare expense is one of the most common reasons for indebtedness.

According to the assumptions of the IAD framework used in the study, when we analyse outcomes, we are analysing the performance of a policy system. Hence, we need an objective standard or principle for comparison (Polski and Ostrom 1998). The first step would be to identify two districts within Maharashtra that differ in health outcomes.

Maharashtra has 35 districts, which are divided into six regions – Konkan, Pune, Nagpur, Nashik, Aurangabad and Amravati (Figure 2.8). A ranking of districts in Maharashtra in select health and development indicators can provide us a rationale for purposively selecting the study districts. Researchers have often used the Human Development Index (HDI) as a macro indicator to rank countries, states and districts based on key development policy outcomes.

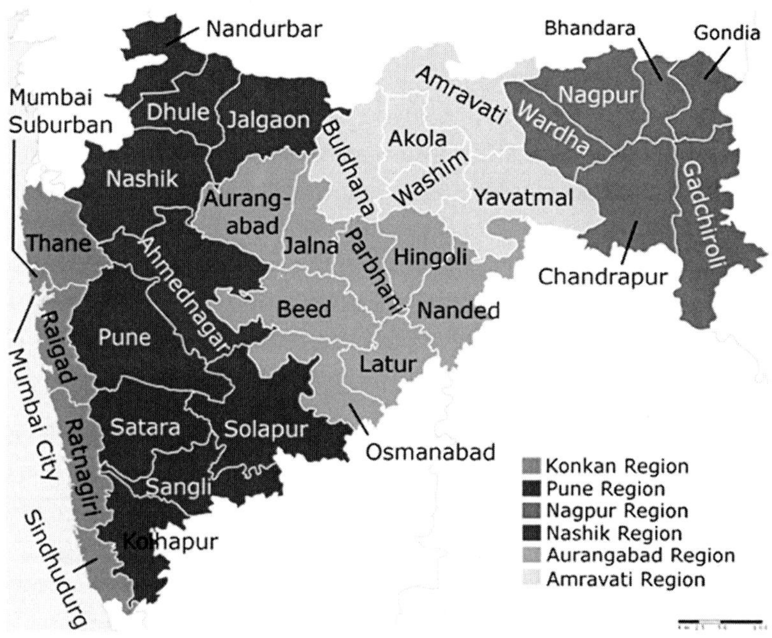

Figure 2.8: Districts and Regions of Maharashtra

Source: http://mapsof.net/map/political-map-maharashtra

Since one needs to start from the macro level of the State to go to micro level of a village, the HDI was the only valid indicator to begin with. Mishra & others had suggested an updated HDI for districts of Maharashtra by using four socio-economic indicators: per capita income for 2000-01 (at constant 1993-94 prices); infant mortality rate for 2001; literacy rate for 2001 and mean years of schooling for 1999-2000 (Table 2.4 Appendix I). These HDI values will not be comparable with that given in the Human Development Report Maharashtra, 2002 as the latter was based only on one indicator of per capita income (Mishra et al., 2008).

This revised HDI ranking included health and development indicators along with economic and educational hence, one can select a district with a superior HDI ranking and another with a low ranking out of 35 districts in Maharashtra. Accordingly, I selected Satara from Pune region, with a HDI rank of 2 out of 30 districts of Maharashtra; and

Osmanabad from Aurangabad region, with a HDI ranking of 29 for the study (see Table 2.4 Appendix I). As per another ranking by the IIPS on a composite index, Satara ranked 7th and Osmanabad ranked 27th out of 35 districts (Figure 2.9 Appendix I). Both the selected districts were in contrast on human development and health outcomes. Few other factors also supported my selection.

While there are districts which are worse off than Osmanabad and better than Satara, I choose these two because of some commonalities. For instance, both Satara and Osmanabad are predominantly rural in nature with miniscule tribal population. In addition, both these districts have been sites of sociological studies related to politics and health in the past, which can inform this study on historical backdrop, political dynamics and socio-cultural context of these districts.

For instance, Satara was a context of a political-anthropological study by Anthony T. Carter (1974) titled – 'Elite Politics in Rural India: Political Stratification and political alliances in Western Maharashtra'. This monograph was a political anthropological research done in Girvi village in Phaltan block of Satara district. In Osmanabad district too, there are two unpublished studies available, on women's reproductive health. One is by Kulkarni & Jaswal, 1999 and the other on social accountability by Kumar, 2006; 2007 conducted in Tuljapur block by the School of Rural Development of TISS based in Tuljapur.

2.5.4 Data Collection

After deciding the broad geographical locale of the study in districts of Satara and Osmanabad within Maharashtra, it was required to select blocks and villages. Health facilities like the PHCs, Sub-centres in all blocks or *talukas* of the two districts of Satara and Osmanabad, along with district headquarters are mapped in Figure 2.10 & Figure 2.11 respectively (see Appendix I). The study had to be conducted in villages as it was the smallest unit in rural setting that can demonstrate relationships of accountability between providers and users. Therefore, the unit of analysis for the study was a village. A **Multi-stage Area Sampling** method was adopted so that the study can identify blocks, clusters and finally villages where the study will be conducted (Table 2.2). At each level of selection, there was a rationale for choosing the location and hence every selection was purposive, guided by the analytical framework of the study. The selection of blocks within the study districts could not have been random but had to be based on some measurable indicators.

Government data on ICDS is widely available and accessible starting from state level, to the district, block and village level. Although one can always question the authenticity of this data as most often it is an underestimation, but this is the only credible source of data available. Therefore, it was logical to take two indicators from the ICDS management and information system (MIS) to choose the blocks. According to the ICDS MIS, two indicators that were directly applicable to the study were - percentage of beneficiaries receiving ICDS services from the eligible population and second, percentage of children malnourished (moderate and severe) of those weighed.

Table 2.2: Multi-Stage Area Sampling

Maharashtra (35 Districts)			*Criteria for selection*	*Type of Data – Secondary / Primary*
District ⇩	Satara	Osmanabad	Human Development Index (HDI)	Secondary Data - Ranking of Districts (CEHAT & IIPS) Table 2.4 & Figure 2.10 in Appendix I
Block ⇩	Koregaon (From 16 blocks)	Tuljapur (from 11 blocks)	Two service utilization indicators - percentage utilisation of ICDS and malnutrition rate among children under-6 years.	Secondary Data -ICDS MIS (Govt Website)Table 2.5 & 2.6 in Appendix I
ICDS Cluster ⇩	Wathar Kiroli (From 6 ICDS clusters)	Mangrol (From 8 ICDS clusters)	Percentage of malnutrition among children under 6 years	Secondary Data -Block level ICDS data from CDPO / Block Office Table 2.7 & 2.8 in Appendix I
Village ⇩	Surli (From a cluster of 12 villages)	Nanduri (From a cluster of 15 villages)	Distance from nearest PHC – up to 5 km and population size of approx. 2000.	Secondary Data -Village level data from ICDS Supervisor Table 2.9 & 2.10 in Appendix I
House-hold	All	All	Households with children under six years listed or not listed under anganwadi center	Primary data

The logic of choosing the first indicator was that accountability relationships can be studied only when there are sizeable percentage of beneficiaries availing and accessing the ICDS and the NRHM services in the village. Since Satara was selected as a district with a higher HDI rank, it was logical to select one block within this district where the utilisation of services was maximum while the percentage of malnourished children was negligible as per the ICDS MIS.

Essentially that block could act as a proxy for the whole district. Similarly, a block was to be selected from Osmanabad that would be one with a high utilisation of services and yet high rate of under-nutrition, similar to what the district rank in HDI signifies. This selection for once, does not mean that findings of this study can be generalised for the whole district. Selection also did not imply that there is no poor performing block in Satara district or a better performing block in Osmanabad district. The selection of the blocks was made to match the rationale of the selection of the districts.

From all 16 blocks in Osmanabad, Tuljapur had a highest utilisation of ICDS services (91.2%) while child under-nutrition was second highest at 14.2% after Osmanabad Urban at 16.7% (see Table 2.5 Appendix I). Osmanabad Urban was an urban block and hence it was not selected. In Satara, Koregaon block had high utilisation of ICDS services (76.5%), second to Patan block at 86.2% and a lowest percentage of under-nutrition (7.7%), out of all 11 blocks (see Table 2.6 Appendix I).

Accordingly, Koregaon block in Satara district and Tuljapur block in Osmanabad districts were chosen for the study. For selecting a village from each of the two blocks, another set of criteria was used as per the analytical framework. The first criterion of selecting the village was that it should be located within a radius of 5 km of a PHC. Such a condition ensures that community in that village are aware of government health services through a PHC and can access it. Usually a PHC has about 20-25 villages within 5 km radius. There was no point in selecting a village 20 km away from a PHC. The second criterion was that the chosen village should be a medium-sized village with a population of approximately 2000 people and one which would have its own *panchayat*. This was done because technically *panchayat* is a formal public institution run by public funds and which is accountable to its *gram sabha* or the entire village community. Therefore, accountability relationships in such a village could be identified and studied easily as compared to other villages that may not have its own panchayat and maybe sharing it with an adjacent village.

Also, since the study considered village as a unit of analysis in a case-study design, the size of the village had to fit into practical concerns of time and resources to collect maximum information and data from that geographical area. In addition, the population norm of 2000 people would mean that there will be at least two anganwadi centres running in the village. As per the Supreme Court guidelines on universalisation of the ICDS, one anganwadi centre is mandatory for every 1000 population. While selecting a village it was also ensured that the anganwadi centres should have been in operation since last five years and were not new. Such criteria would ensure that some rapport building between the ICDS staff and the community exists to be able to study it.

Fieldwork was initiated in February 2012 to obtain secondary data from the ICDS government offices of both the districts. Secondary data was required to objectively select block, cluster and finally a village. The data included list of blocks and information on select ICDS indicators in those blocks like number of children receiving supplementary nutrition or number of children moderately under-nourished. Subsequently, ICDS Block Offices in Koregaon (Satara) and Tuljapur (Osmanabad) were approached. The ICDS Block office is usually headed by a Child Development Project Officer (CDPO) while in the Health Department, it is the Taluka Medical Officer (TMO), who administers all PHCs and sub-centres in that block.

A formal letter from my supervisor and the university was given to the block officials of the ICDS and Health departments. The letter informed them about the study objectives, its policy and programme implications and requested their cooperation. In Osmanabad, ICDS Tuljapur Block office was located inside a small campus of public health department. For Satara, ICDS block office was located inside a panchayat samiti office building in Koregaon city. The next step was to select an ICDS cluster within each of the selected blocks (Table 2.2). In Satara, each block is divided into several ICDS clusters known as 'beats'. For instance, Koregaon block in Satara was divided into 6 beats – Tadvale, Ekambe, Koregaon, Rahimatpur, Arvi and Wathar Kiroli (see Table 2.7 Appendix I).

Similarly, Tuljapur block of Osmanabad district was divided into 8 projects – Salgara, Kakramba, Mangrol, Katgaon, Savargaon, Malumbra, Andur and Itkal (see Table 2.8 Appendix I). According to the child nutrition data provided by Koregaon CDPO, Wathar Kiroli beat had 99% utilisation of services (indicated by the indicator of percentage of children being brought to the anganwadi centres and weighed) while any form of malnutrition, including moderate and severe was 5.8%, lowest among six blocks. In Tuljapur block, Mangrol project had one of the highest utilisations of ICDS services at 97.5%, while malnutrition was also highest at 21.1%. Both Wathar Kiroli and Mangrol are large villages and were also the locations for the PHCs. Therefore, Wathar Kiroli PHC and Mangrol PHCs were chosen as the ICDS clusters.

After identifying the projects within the selected blocks and districts, the last step was to choose a village from a list of villages. Usually studies draw a random sample or a stratified sample forming 10% households from a cluster of many villages. However, for this study, since social, economic and political capabilities of households are part of the study, drawing a random sample can exclude very poor households, extremely rich or the politically powerful ones. Also, since this is a Case Study Research Design, the unit of analysis is a village. Such a research design eliminates the need for drawing a sample. Therefore, I included all households with children under age six in the study.

Households with children under six ensured that majority of the eligible population for ICDS & NRHM programme are included. This population comprised of women in the reproductive age group of 15-45 years; children below six years and adolescent girls. Selection of such households was possible from a list of all under-six children obtained from the Anganwadi that maintains record of births and deaths in a village. In addition, a door-to-door survey of all households was carried out to identify households with children under six. This method resembled a census and ensured that the study included even those households who may not access anganwadi services. Thus, according to the theory of methodology, the study did not draw a sample but comprised of a universe sample.

The selection of the villages followed a series of processes. Villages under each project or beat is organised with reference to a PHC that cover the population. The village level data and list are prepared by the ICDS Supervisor. The ICDS Supervisors in charge of the respective blocks provided the list of all the villages that came under the ambit of Wathar Kiroli PHC and Mangrol PHC respectively (see Table 2.9 and Table 2.10 Appendix I). As mentioned earlier, less than 5 km and a population of approximately 2000 people were the criteria to select the villages. For Wathar Kiroli PHC, there were 6 villages out of 12 that were within the distance of 5 - 7 km from it.

However, some villages were either exceedingly small in population size or too huge to be taken as the case. For instance, Kaloshi and Durgawadi were too small while Wathar, Targaon and Kiroli were too huge to be considered a case for this study. The only village that justified the criteria was Surli, which had a population of 2003 as per 2001 census and located 3.5 km from the Wathar Kiroli PHC. The main road outside the village had a local bus stand and the state transport buses ply with a good frequency ending in a depot in Wathar Kiroli village where the PHC was located.

Surli was located 40 km from Satara city; 20 km from Koregaon city and 280 km from Mumbai. Instead of commuting to-and-fro from the Satara city, I decided to stay in or near the study village. Vathar Kiroli Panchayat was one the villages where the panchayat implemented the World Bank aided water project and hence boasted of infrastructure facilities like water pumping station and a panchayat guest house. I completed the fieldwork in Surli village in 2 weeks in months of May-June 2012. I stayed at the Wathar Kiroli panchayat's guest room. *Gram sevaks* and visiting government officials used this guest house. Wathar Kiroli guest house was at 3 km from Surli village, so I either travelled in a local '*tam-tam*' (modified auto) or a state transport bus or walked at times.

For Mangrol PHC, out of 15 villages under its ambit, six villages were situated at 5 km from it. Of these, Sindhphal and Mangrol were huge villages with population of about 5000 people while the others like Kalegaon, Dhanegaon, Sardevadi and Bori were small villages with a population of less than 1000 people, as per 2001 census. Nanduri village although was located 7 km from Mangrol PHC and had a population of 1500 people, it was the closest village fitting into the study criteria and hence I selected it. The access of Nanduri village to Mangrol PHC was convenient as a newly built Tuljapur-Itkal road connected them and on which state transport buses plied. I completed fieldwork in Nanduri in two weeks in July-August 2012.

Osmanabad is 411 km away from Mumbai and is an overnight train journey. I was stationed at TISS School of Rural Development at Tuljapur which is about 22 km from Osmanabad city and Nanduri was further 25 km away from TISS campus and closer to the adjoining district of Solapur.

Tools and Techniques. The research design of the study follows Case Study Research design that involves intensive and in-depth study of a social unit in its totality by employing triangulation as suggested by Goode and Hatt (1952). According to Denzin & Lincoln (2005), there are four distinct types of triangulation – triangulation of theory, investigator, data and methods.

The study used triangulation of data using both qualitative and quantitative data collection tools. The assumption behind data triangulation is the recognition that no single type of data is complete (Jayaram, 2010). Acknowledging that no observations or interpretations are perfectly repeatable, triangulations also serve to clarify meaning by identifying diverse ways in which a case is being seen (Denzin & Lincoln, 2005). The tools for data collection follow the methodological linkages in Table 2.1, linking each of the study objectives with corresponding operational concepts, tentative questions to be asked, tools for data collection and prospective respondents.

The first and the third objective of the study demands employing in-depth interview schedule to collect data from frontline providers that included Anganwadi workers, ANMs, ASHAs, ICDS Supervisors and Medical officers from PHC. I choose in-depth interview as a tool because it required a one-on-one interaction with the researcher and the researched to generate data. I identified concepts, sub-concepts and themes on institutional processes and procedures used for ensuring accountability to create a common interview guide as a tool, again based on study objectives (Table 2.1). An interview guide was designed to be multi-lingual in nature using three languages of Marathi, Hindi and English to help me ask questions to the respondents and ensure they understood in a best possible manner.

In addition, the objective also requires collecting secondary data on formal institutional mechanisms like the minutes of the meetings of Village Health and Sanitation Committee (VHSC) and Rogi Kalyan Samiti (RKS). Only the Mangrol PHC Medical Officer shared the RKS data while Surli PHC MO did not refuse but kept delaying it and finally did not share. Moreover, RKS as an institution is at the level of PHC and not village, hence not included in the study.

An anganwadi worker of Surli shared its VHSC data in form of its income and expenditure statement. Nanduri village had its VHSC only on paper and was not functional. I took an informed consent from all the respondents after sharing the objective of the study. Since I could understand Marathi but not too conversant with it, so I asked the questions in Hindi while the respondents answered either in Marathi or Hindi or both. I recorded all the interviews on a digital recorder after taking permission from respondents. In all, I conducted 16 in-depth interviews from frontline providers (Table 2.3).

The second and third objective of the study required to collect data from the households on the nature of their engagement with the frontline providers and how they make claims in cases of poor services or failures in services delivery (Table 2.1). In a rural setting, a questionnaire is not an appropriate tool as respondents cannot fill it themselves. Hence survey interview schedule was best suited to elicit information from many households. As per anganwadis records, there were 450 households in Surli while Nanduri had 250. However, the study's sample included only those households that had children under six years. According to the lists procured, a total of 102 children were registered in Surli and Nanduri had 122 children registered in its anganwadis (Table 2.3).

Based on the analytical framework and study objectives, a set of tentative questions was initially prepared (Table 2.1) which was later developed into the Survey Interview Schedule. The schedule was again multi-lingual using Marathi, Hindi and English and designed into two parts. Part I had three distinct sections while part two had remaining two sections, all aligned with the second and third objective of the study.

Sections in part I included general background information of the household like family composition, asset ownership, housing and its social capability in terms of memberships in community organisations. Questions pertaining to these were divided into the following three sections:

a. Identification Particulars: This section included questions on the location of the household, its official address and description of landmarks near it so that I could relate its data with the house visited during the time of analysis.

b. Background Information & Personal Data: This section included questions on socio-economic and demographic profile of the household like the caste, family composition and occupation details of members, housing and ownership of assets.

c. Membership in community organisations and involvement in community activities: this section included questions related to awareness and participation in village level institutions like gram sabha, small saving group or mandals.

Part II comprised of the following two sections: -

d. Nature of engagement: the section had questions on the existing accessibility of health providers on maternal health and child nutrition services and how these services are perceived by the users.

e. Answerability: questions in this section were aimed at eliciting information on strategies users are using to claim services in case of poor quality or medical emergency.

The interview schedule was pre-tested in Surli village in the month of May 2012 just before the actual survey took place. The interview is meant to be administered to the head of the household for part I and jointly to the head of the household and the mother for part II of the schedule. The pilot interview took almost 1 hour and 45 minutes in one household. After the pilot, I realised to change the order of asking questions from the respondents. I administered part II of the schedule first, which entailed talking to the mother about the healthcare access for her children and perception of the providers, followed by asking questions in part I from the head of the household.

Table 2.3: Data Collection

Unit of Data →	*Household*	*Frontline Health Functionary*	*Child*	*Village*
Tool used →	Survey Interview Schedule	Semi-structured Interview	Anganwadi Records	Records from Anganwadi Centre or Gram Panchayat
Nanduri (Osmanabad)	69	7 Interviews • 2 AWWs • 1 ANM • 1 ICDS Supervisor • 1 Medical Officer, PHC • 1 ASHA worker • 1 Taluka Medical Officer	122	• Village Household Profile Survey ICDS • Village Community Map • Nanduri Gram Panchayat Income and Expenditure Annual Statement • Rogi Kalyan Samiti (RKS) Minutes of Meetings
Surli (Satara)	60	9 Interviews • 2 AWWs • 1 ANM • 1 ICDS Supervisor • 1 Medical Officer, PHC • 2 ASHA workers • 1 Local quack • 1 former sarpanch	102	• Village Household Profile Survey ICDS • Village Community Map • Village Health and Sanitation Committee (VHSC) Financial Statement • Surli Gram Panchayat Income and Expenditure Annual Statement
TOTAL	129	16	222	

After the pilot, I removed questions related to community-based monitoring or patient satisfaction surveys as these were technical terms which the community was not aware about. About 130 copies of the schedule were printed for the survey. A Focus Group Discussion (FGD) with mothers was also planned to collect data for this objective. An FGD guide was also prepared and pre-tested. During the pilot testing of the FGD tool, I realised that mothers hardly shared their views and did not speak much. The reason was that the central assumption of the FGD tool was not being met. It was that respondents need to be randomly chosen, strangers or unknown to each other to be able to express their views without inhibition and open to be influenced by other's opinions, either in agreement or disagreement while making a point. This condition was not being met in the study since mothers were residents of the same village, knew each other and hence hardly expressed their views in the discussion. Therefore, FGDs could not be used in this study.

Survey Implementation. Entry in a village for data collection is a sensitive process. I could understand Marathi but was not fluent in the language. Hence, I hired an interpreter who was an undergraduate student of TISS Tuljapur campus. He was a resident of Osmanabad district and fluent in Marathi, Hindi and English. The first village of my study was Surli. As a hack, I had read that entry to the village becomes easy once its children know about it! This study did involve children too, although indirectly. On entry into the village, I headed straight to the anganwadi centre to meet the anganwadi worker. I shared the purpose of my research and clarified that the research is not to evaluate them or aimed at finding fault with their work but will be used for purely academic purposes. In the meantime, anganwadi workers had also received information from their CDPO's office to extend cooperation for the study. I also met the Sarpanch and shared the purpose of the visit.

Despite having a list of names of children, identifying houses could have been a daunting and time-consuming task. It was because people do not number their houses in a village nor are there names of streets. Also, houses are dispersed across the village. I decided to involve a young boy or girl of the village itself who would volunteer and lead me to specific houses of children mentioned in the Anganwadi list. I adopted the same strategy in Nanduri village too and it clicked. This not only saved my time and effort but also helped me built rapport with the members of the household where the interview was to be conducted.

In Surli, there were 101 children registered with the two AWCs. Data was collected from 60 such households in Surli. Reasons for exclusion of some households are mentioned in Section 3.3.2. In addition to these, five houses were shut, or its respondents were unavailable after numerous follow up visits. In Nanduri, there were 122 children registered with the two anganwadis. Data was collected from 69 households in Nanduri while two households' members were unavailable despite repeated home visits. In all, 129 households were a part of the study with 839 members including 157 children. As a part of ethics in social science research, before the beginning of each interview, the following were shared with the respondents - the purpose of the research, researcher's intention on the use of the data, confidentiality of the identity of the respondents and their oral consent. Since most village residents were concerned about the outcome of this work, I told them that I plan to write a book about their village.

Data Entry, Data Cleaning and Analysis Plan. I entered primary data collected from 129 households through Survey Interview schedule into a computer programme to collate and analyse it. There were two choices before me – SPSS package and Microsoft Access. Going by the ease of entering data, MS Access was a better programme since one could create pages like one in the schedule and enter data, while it automatically creates a database is in the background.

As seen in Figure 2.12, the first page of the Survey Interview schedule shows data being entered for household number one. There were 11 pages in the schedule and hence I created 11 identical pages in MS Access, as seen in the top left ribbon of the screen shot window below. Owing to the visual ease and survey schedule matching with those in MS Access software, data entry for all 129 households was quick and with minimal errors.

The bottom left corner of the screen shows the current schedule number (one), being entered from 129 schedules in all.

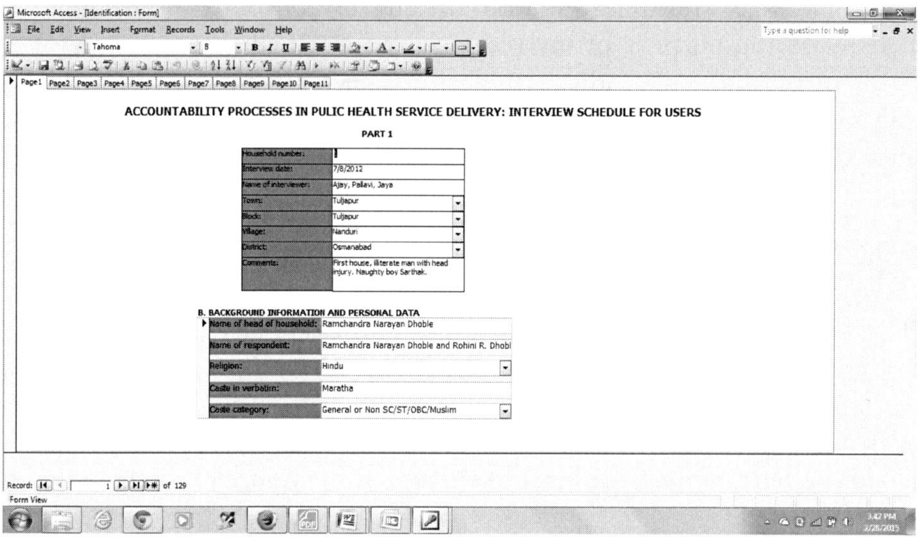

Figure 2.12 :Screenshot of First page of Household Survey Interview Schedule in MS Access (Data Entry)

ID	Household r	Sl no	Name	Relation to the head	Age	Age Cleaned	Sex	Literacy	Education	Education Cleaned	Occupation	Occupation Cleane
1	1	4	Sarthak Ramchandra Dhc	Unmarried child	4	4	Male	Child below 6 years	Pre-school Educatior	Pre School Educatio	Not applicable in case of childr	Not applicable
2	1	3	Ritesh Ramchandra Dhot	Unmarried child	6	6	Male	Literate only if schoc	Primary school upto :	Primary school	Not applicable in case of childr	Not applicable
3	1	2	Rohini Ramchandra Dhot	Spouse	22	22	Female	Literate only if schoc	High school upto 10tl	High School	Self employed in agriculture	Self employed in agricul
4	1	1	Ramchandra Narayan Dh	Head	28	28	Male	Illiterate	No education	No education	Self employed in agriculture	Self employed in agricul
57	10	4	Ramkrishna Tulsiram Jad	Grandchild	5	5	Male	Child below 6 years	Pre-school Educatior	Pre School Educatio	Not applicable in case of childr	Not applicable
58	10	5	Vasudha Tulsiram Jadhav	Grandchild	7	7	Female	Literate only if schoc	Primary school upto :	Primary school	Not applicable in case of childr	Not applicable
59	10	3	Archana Tulsiram Jadhav	Spouse of married ch	28	28	Female	Literate only if schoc	Middle school upto 7	Middle School	Housewife	Housewife
60	10	2	Tulsiram Madhukar Jadha	Married child	32	32	Male	High school and abc	Higher Secondary sc	Higher Secondary	Agriculture labour	Agriculture labour
61	10	1	Madhukar Bapurao Jadha	Head	64	64	Male	Literate only if schoc	Primary school upto :	Primary school	Service like Peon in Office	Services
638	10132	5	Boy Amol Bhosale	Grandchild	2 montl	0	Male	Child below 6 years	Child below school a	Child below school a	Not applicable in case of childr	Not applicable
639	10132	4	Vanita Amol Bhosale	Spouse of married ch	28	28	Female	High school and abc	High school upto 10tl	High School	Housewife	Housewife
640	10132	3	Amol Laxman Bhosale	Married child	31	31	Male	High school and abc	High school upto 10tl	High School	Self employed in agriculture	Self employed in agricul
641	10132	2	Sharda Laxman Bhosale	Spouse	55	55	Female	Literate only if schoc	Primary school upto :	Primary school	Self employed in agriculture	Self employed in agricul
642	10132	1	Laxman Ramchandra Bhc	Head	60	60	Male	Literate only if schoc	Primary school upto :	Primary school	Not applicable in case of elderl	Not applicable
643	10233	9	Jeevika Kishore Bhosale	Grandchild	6 montl	0	Female	Child below 6 years	Child below school a	Child below school a	Not applicable in case of childr	Not applicable
644	10233	6	Sumit Amit Bhosale	Grandchild	5	5	Male	Child below 6 years	Pre-school Educatior	Pre School Educatio	Not applicable in case of childr	Not applicable
645	10233	5	Damini Amit Bhosale	Grandchild	6	6	Female	Child below 6 years	Pre-school Educatior	Pre School Educatio	Not applicable in case of childr	Not applicable
646	10233	8	Sonali Kishore Bhosale	Spouse of married ch	21	21	Female	High school and abc	High school upto 10tl	High School	Housewife	Housewife
647	10233	4	Rupali Amit Bhosale	Spouse of married ch	23	23	Female	High school and abc	High school upto 10tl	High School	Housewife	Housewife
648	10233	7	Kishore Bapu Bhosale	Married child	28	28	Male	High school and abc	High school upto 10tl	High School	Self employed in agriculture	Self employed in agricul
649	10233	3	Amit Bapu Bhosale	Married child	30	30	Male	High school and abc	High school upto 10tl	High School	Self employed in agriculture	Self employed in agricul
650	10233	2	Shalini Bapu Bhosale	Spouse	45	45	Female	Literate only if schoc	Primary school upto :	Primary school	Housewife	Housewife
651	10233	1	Bapu Dada Bhosale	Head	55	55	Male	High school and abc	High school upto 10tl	High School	Self employed in agriculture	Self employed in agricul
652	10334	4	Pari Ramraje Bhosale	Unmarried child	1	1	Female	Child below 6 years	Child below school a	Child below school a	Not applicable in case of childr	Not applicable
653	10334	3	Samburaje Ramraje Bhos	Unmarried child	7	7	Male	Literate only if schoc	Primary school upto :	Primary school	Not applicable in case of childr	Not applicable
654	10334	2	Nandini Ramraje Bhosale	Spouse	25	25	Female	High school and abc	others like graduates	Graduates	Housewife	Housewife
655	10334	1	Ramraje baburao Bhosale	Head	30	30	Male	High school and abc	others like graduates	Graduates	Self employed in agriculture	Self employed in agricul
656	10435	5	Samriddhi Ajit Chavan	Grandchild	2 montl	0	Female	Child below 6 years	Child below school a	Child below school a	Not applicable in case of childr	Not applicable
657	10435	3	Ajit Arun Chavan	Married child	24	24	Male	High school and abc	Higher Secondary sc	Higher Secondary	Service like Bus Conductor	Services
658	10435	4	Sarika Ajit Chavan	Spouse of married ch	24	24	Female	High school and abc	others like post gradu	Post Graduates	Housewife	Housewife
659	10435	6	Sachin Arun Chavan	Unmarried child	24	24	Male	High school and abc	Others like post grad	Post Graduates	Not applicable in case of childr	Not applicable
660	10435	2	Laxmi Arun Chavan	Spouse	50	50	Female	Literate only if schoc	Middle school upto 7	Middle School	Housewife	Housewife
661	10435	1	Arun Shankar Chavan	Head	58	58	Male	High school and abc	High school upto 10tl	High School	service in a shop	Services

Record: 1 of 839

Datasheet View

Figure 2.13: Screenshot of Family Composition Database in MS Access

Once I had entered all data, the MS Access automatically created database for each of the tables present in a page. For instance, Figure 2.13 shows family composition database. One usually needs to clean the entered data as there can be typing or spelling errors or if

I have by mistake fed a verbatim non-categorised data. I created standardised categories for all close ended questions and converted numeric data like age into years especially in case of young children. I also factored spellings and 'no data entry' or 'not applicable' so that when analysis is run, the results are coherent and not spilled over to numerous invalid categories.

For data cleaning, I exported each of the databases created in MS Access to MS Excel since it offers high ease and flexibility to handle and process data. In Excel, for each database, I carried out the following steps - 'sorting' of columns on criterion to group entries together and then checking for errors or for adding standardised categories. I took care not to make changes in the original data but creating new columns for that indicator, for instance, 'Age Cleaned' or 'Education Cleaned'. After I had cleaned the data of errors in MS Excel, I pasted the databases again in MS Access since further analysis was to be carried out.

There were about 17 databases in all. Once I had cleaned the data, it was useful to link each database and its indicators with caste, asset category and village name (Figure 2.14) For instance, in the database on preference for providers, the caste, asset and village data was also integrated (see Figure 2.15).

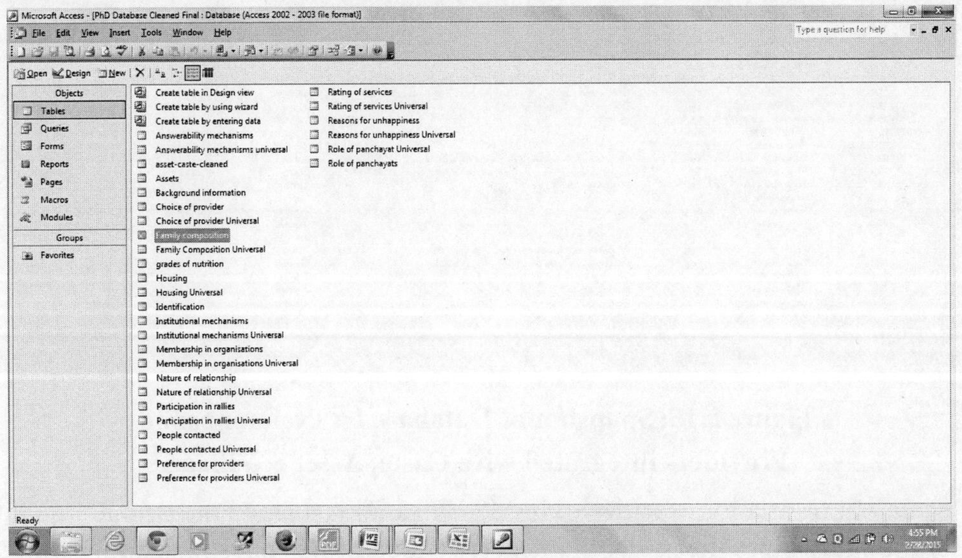

Figure 2.14: Screenshots of List of Databases for the Study

I did this so that during 'query' generation for making tables during analysis, all the indicators were upfront. After linking these, I created new databases with a suffix 'universal' in their title. Hence, 17 more databases were formed. After integration, the databases were ready for computation and running queries. Most queries were run on MS Access after which the results were pasted in MS Excel to create tables, to calculate percentages and to create graphs. I also exported some databases to SPSS so that creating tables and percentages was quick and easy. I had exercised caution while computing percentages within the category or across the category depending upon the logic of analysis in that table. I have retained open ended answers in the schedule and quoted as per the requirement of the analysis.

I first transcribed qualitative data generated from the in-depth interviews with providers from recordings to text. This text was a mix of Marathi and Hindi. I had to translate it into English before I could attempt any analysis. I hired a translator proficient in Marathi, English and Hindi. Since interviews were in conversational style, rooted in village context, therefore I retained its description while choosing the words and exercised caution not to rationalise any interpretations. The translator and I jointly translated interviews in English so that the nuisances of expressions, tone, person's context etc were factored in.

Microsoft Access - [Preference for providers Universal : Table]

ID	Household num	Provider	Do you access?	For what reason?	Comments	Reasons 1 Cleaned	Reas	Reaso	Village	Total asset v	Asset category	Caste category
1	1	Private hospital in town	Yes	For delivery and child birth.	Vikram Dabre a	Delivery	Chilc		Nanduri	1376080	A3	General or Non SC/ST/OB
2	1	Ayurvedic doctor	Yes	For treating the wounds in	Had taken him t	Chronic illness			Nanduri	1376080	A3	General or Non SC/ST/OB
3	1	Home remedy	Yes	Cold, cough etc		Cold cough			Nanduri	1376080	A3	General or Non SC/ST/OB
4	1	Local quack	Yes	He is like our family doctor	Dr. Bhansode vi	Family doctor for any			Nanduri	1376080	A3	General or Non SC/ST/OB
5	1	Rural Hospital	Yes	Husband had got a head ir	Civil hospital Os	Serious ailment			Nanduri	1376080	A3	General or Non SC/ST/OB
6	1	Anganwadi center	Yes	for nutrition and education					Nanduri	1376080	A3	General or Non SC/ST/OB
7	1	PHC	No	Not applicable	We do not trust				Nanduri	1376080	A3	General or Non SC/ST/OB
8	2	PHC	Yes	For delivery and also for im	I would rate it a:	Delivery	Imm		Nanduri	4527250	A4	General or Non SC/ST/OB
9	2	Local quack	Yes	For cold cough and fever	Swami doctor	Cold cough fever			Nanduri	4527250	A4	General or Non SC/ST/OB
10	2	Private hospital in town	Yes	For women sexual health	Yadav hospital :	Women issues			Nanduri	4527250	A4	General or Non SC/ST/OB
11	2	Anganwadi center	Yes	For child and self					Nanduri	4527250	A4	General or Non SC/ST/OB
12	2	Ayurvedic doctor	No						Nanduri	4527250	A4	General or Non SC/ST/OB
13	2	Home remedy	No						Nanduri	4527250	A4	General or Non SC/ST/OB
14	2	Rural Hospital	No						Nanduri	4527250	A4	General or Non SC/ST/OB
15	3	Private hospital in town	Yes	For Delivery	At a private hos	Delivery			Nanduri	562350	A2	General or Non SC/ST/OB
16	3	PHC	Yes	For delivery	One of the deliv	Delivery			Nanduri	562350	A2	General or Non SC/ST/OB
17	3	Local quack	Yes	He is a family doctor and v	Dr. Bhansode	Family doctor for any			Nanduri	562350	A2	General or Non SC/ST/OB
18	3	Anganwadi center	Yes	The child goes for leanring					Nanduri	562350	A2	General or Non SC/ST/OB
19	3	Ayurvedic doctor	No						Nanduri	562350	A2	General or Non SC/ST/OB
20	3	Home remedy	Yes						Nanduri	562350	A2	General or Non SC/ST/OB
21	3	Rural Hospital	No						Nanduri	562350	A2	General or Non SC/ST/OB
22	4	Private hospital in town	Yes	For delivery and women's r	Two of the boys	Delivery	Chilc		Nanduri	1765445	A3	General or Non SC/ST/OB
23	4	Rural Hospital	Yes	For Delivery	Civil hospital Os	Delivery			Nanduri	1765445	A3	General or Non SC/ST/OB
24	4	Anganwadi center	Yes	My children cannot go to a					Nanduri	1765445	A3	General or Non SC/ST/OB
25	4	Ayurvedic doctor	No						Nanduri	1765445	A3	General or Non SC/ST/OB
26	4	Home remedy	No						Nanduri	1765445	A3	General or Non SC/ST/OB
27	4	Local quack	No						Nanduri	1765445	A3	General or Non SC/ST/OB
28	4	PHC	Yes	For cold and cough					Nanduri	1765445	A3	General or Non SC/ST/OB
29	5	Private hospital in town	Yes	For delivery and childhood	Yadav Hospital	Delivery	Chilc		Nanduri	1159300	A3	SC
30	5	Rural Hospital	Yes	For getting HIV tests done		ANC			Nanduri	1159300	A3	SC
31	5	Ayurvedic doctor	Yes	Skin problem - a tumour oı	Solapur doctor	Chronic illness			Nanduri	1159300	A3	SC
32	5	Anganwadi center	Yes	for child and self					Nanduri	1159300	A3	SC
33	5	Home remedy	Yes	fever, cold					Nanduri	1159300	A3	SC

Record: 3 of 889

Datasheet View

Figure 2.15: Snapshot of Database on Preference for Providers integrated with Caste, Asset & Village

I typed out translations as a script in MS Word. This formed the primary qualitative data for the study. Since the in-depth interview schedule had questions under conceptual themes, this primary qualitative data was also organised under these themes, separately for both the study villages. While writing the chapters, such an organisation helped to analyse convergences and divergences within-case and across-case and use quotes when required. It was not possible to include the entire textual data as a part of annexure of this thesis; however, I have used conceptual richness or exact quotes from respondents wherever necessary in the analysis.

2.6 Issues of Validity and Reliability

Validity means if the tool or the instrument is measuring what it is intended to measure (Jayaram, 2009). Validity is also concerned with notions of truth, for it depends on the theoretical, methodological and ontological/epistemological position you adopt (Jayaram, 1989). As per the theoretical assumptions of this study, the reality is external to the actor and can be understood by means of observer categories and can be explained by means of relationships between these categories. It is also important to justify several types of validities of this study. Measurement validity for instance, is extremely significant especially for quantitative research that measures various social science concepts. Measurement validity means if a measure of a concept really represents the concepts they are supposed to be tapping, because if they do not, the study's findings will be questionable (Bryman, 2008). To attempt high measurement validity for the study, a link was established between study objectives, theoretical concepts, tentative questions, respondents and tools (Table 2.1). According to this table, the survey interview schedule was a valid tool to measure the concept that emerged out of second and third objectives of the study while in-depth interview was best suited to measure the concept that represented first objective. Most questions in the interview schedule could be coded, compared and measured. There are few open-ended questions which will be analysed qualitatively. Validity is also inversely related to the number of respondents if the aim of the study is to understand the meanings.

One of the epistemological critiques of the interview technique is the process of interviewing is a social interaction like any other in which the interview influences the interviewee's responses. Also, answers a respondent gives to questions, may well be a direct function of his or her interaction with the interviewer rather than anything else and that (as a result), these answers might not match his or her actual behaviour or attitudes (ibid.). To counter this critique, I added hypothetical questions in third person, on issues of perceptions so that the respondent need not answer about his or her experience but talk for others. Using this technique, a researcher can avoid personalising the question to the respondent directly and yet the answer received may actually convey what the respondent feels personally.

Reliability is concerned with the question of whether the results of the study are repeatable (Bryman, 2008). It is concerned with data and its replicability. For a technique of data collection to be reliable, it should produce results which are not affected by the process of collection. For a survey to be reliable, it must be reasonable to assume that each time the survey is repeated and applied to the same respondents, it will produce comparable results. Also, the more representative a sample of the population as a whole, the more reliable it is (ibid.). Since study involved a census which is not a sample and the process of data collection followed rules of social-science research, the reliability of the study can be said to be high.

2.7 Limitations of the Study

The most limiting aspect of the study was of language barrier. I was not conversant in Marathi since my mother-tongue is Hindi. I learnt conversational Marathi before the data collection commenced for the study. A prolonged stay for more than a decade in the city of Mumbai helped me to pick up basic language skills. Yet, linguistically Marathi in rural Maharashtra is different than the one spoken in Mumbai. Hence, during the pilot study, I decided to hire a male under-graduate student from social work in rural development to accompany me during fieldwork. I also hired a translator for transcribing recorded interviews. Therefore, any lack of nuanced understanding of social context of the respondents needs to be attributed to this limitation. Since the study was not based on interpretive methodological paradigm and its assumptions, this limitation could not adversely impact qualitative analysis attempted in the study.

Another aspect where I had faced an impediment was in designing the study's household survey. Many of its questions were not standardised unlike large scale national surveys, for example, the NSSO or the NFHS. Although I did attempt to refer to these large surveys for indicators especially on socio- demographic ones like types of housing, drinking water and educational profile. However, there were questions and indicators which were specific to the study like participation in local community organisations or access to providers other than public providers or awareness about formal instruments of accountability. Validity and reliability of such surveys is generally high but the same cannot be said about smaller surveys like the one designed specifically for a study.

Household data especially at the village level for the two case villages would not have been possible without the use of survey. Therefore, one cannot expect reliability of the survey instrument to be the same as that of large surveys. Many open-ended questions within the household survey and other types of data like village level documents and semi-structured interviews in a mixed method approach, helped limit the weakness of such a survey design.

The findings of the study are situation specific to the two cases and hence can only be generalised to similar context like the one in the study – a typical Indian village and not to the whole population in general. The study included a worst-case scenario in a poor HDI ranked district of Osmanabad and a best-case scenario in a better HDI ranked district of Satara. Findings could have been richer if the study also included and compared a better case in Osmanabad and a worst case in Surli and to have compared these four scenarios within the districts and across the districts. I acknowledge that such scenarios also exist, and I could have factored it. However, limited resources and time did not allow for such multiple comparisons.

Although there were 275 families in Nanduri and 428 families in Surli according to Anganwadi surveys (2012), but only 69 households from Nanduri and 60 households from Surli became part of the study. It was so because other than seven households which were locked or respondents unavailable, all households with children under-six years were included. Such a scenario was not pre-empted before data collection began. Hence, as per the study design, I used data from 129 households in all. This sample formed about 18% of the total households in both villages.

***

References

1. Ackerman, J. (2004). Co-governance for accountability: beyond "exit" and "voice." *World Development, 32*(3), 447–463.
2. Bank, T. W. (2004). *World Development Report 2004 Making Services Work for the Poor*. Washington D. C: The World Bank and Oxford University Press.
3. Bardhan, P. (2009). Governance Dilemmas in Service Delivery. In *Does Decentralization Enhance Service Delivery and Poverty Reduction.*
4. Bardhan, P. K. (1984). *Land, Labor, and Rural Poverty: Essays in Development Economics*. Columbia University Press.
5. Bovens, M. (2007). Analysing and Assessing Accountability: A Conceptual Framework1. *European Law Journal, 13*(4), 447–468.
6. Bovens, M. A. P. (2006). Analysing and Assessing Public Accountability. A Conceptual Framework. *European Governance Papers (EUROGOV), 100*, 1–37.
7. Brinkerhoff, D. W. (2004). Accountability and health systems: toward conceptual clarity and policy relevance. *Health Policy and Planning, 19*(6), 371–379.
8. Bryman, A. (2008). *Social research methods.* Oxford; New York: Oxford University Press.
9. Carter, A. T. (1974). *Elite politics in rural India*. Cambridge University Press.
10. Clemens, E. S., & Cook, J. M. (1999). Politics and institutionalism: Explaining durability and change. *Annual Review of Sociology*, 441–466.
11. Comim, F., Qizilbash, M., & Alkire, S. (2008). *The capability approach: concepts, measures and applications*. Cambridge University Press.
12. Cornwall, A. (2000). *Beneficiary, consumer, citizen: perspectives on participation for poverty reduction*. Swedish Internaitonal Development Cooperation Agency, Stockholm.
13. Denzin, N. K., & Lincoln, Y. S. (2005). *The SAGE Handbook of Qualitative Research*. SAGE.
14. Drèze, J. (2006). Universalisation with quality: ICDS in a rights perspective. *Economic and Political Weekly*, 3706–3715.
15. Fuller, C. J., & Bénéï, V. (2001). *The Everyday State and Society in Modern India*. C. Hurst & Co. Publishers.
16. Funnell, W. N., Cooper, K., & Lee, J. (2012). *Public sector accounting and accountability in Australia* (Second). Sydney: UNSW Press.

17. Garn, K. D. (2010). *Dynamics of Accountability in the Community Based Monitoring of Health Services Programme, Tamil Nadu, India*. Department of Public Health, University of Copenhagen, Copenhagen.

18. Gaventa, J. (2002). Exploring Citizenship, Participation and Accountability. *IDS Bulletin, 33*(2), 1–14. https://doi.org/10.1111/j.1759-5436.2002.tb00020.x

19. George, A. (2003). Using accountability to improve reproductive health care. *Reproductive Health Matters, 11*(21), 161–170.

20. George, A. (2009). 'By papers and pens, you can only do so much': views about accountability and human resource management from Indian government health administrators and workers. *The International Journal of Health Planning and Management, 24*(3), 205–224. https://doi.org/10.1002/hpm.986

21. Glynn, J. J., & Murphy, M. P. (1996). Public management: failing accountabilities and failing performance review. *International Journal of Public Sector Management, 9*(5/6), 125–137.

22. Goetz, A M, & Gaventa, J. (2001). Bringing Citizen Voice and Client Focus into Service Delivery. *IDS Bulletin, IDS Workin*.

23. Goetz, Anne Marie, & Jenkins, R. (2001). Hybrid forms of accountability: citizen engagement in institutions of public-sector oversight in India. *Public Management Review, 3*(3), 363–383.

24. Goode, W. J., & Hatt, P. K. (1952). *Methods in social research* (Vol. vii). New York, NY, US: McGraw-Hill.

25. Goyal, J. (2011). Social Audits in Outcome Budgeting: An experiment of accountability in Maharashtra. *Indian Journal of Social Work, 72*(4), 537–562.

26. Grant, R. W., & Keohane, R. O. (2005). Accountability and abuses of power in world politics. *American Political Science Review, 99*(01), 29–43.

27. Hodge, G. A., & Coghill, K. (2007). Accountability in the Privatized State. *Governance, 20*(4), 675–702. https://doi.org/10.1111/j.1468-0491.2007.00377.x

28. Hossain, N. (2010). Rude accountability: Informal pressures on frontline bureaucrats in Bangladesh. *Development and Change, 41*(5), 907–928.

29. Hughes, O. E. (2003). *Public management and administration: an introduction* (Third). New York: Palgrave.

30. Humphreys, P. C. (1998). *Improving public service delivery*. Dublin: Institute of Public Administration.

31. Husain, Z. (2011). Health of the National Rural Health Mission. *Economic & Political Weekly, 46*(4), 53.

32. Institute, T. W. B. and I. F. P. R. (2010). *Gender and Governance in Rural Services: Insights from India, Ghana, and Ethiopia*. World Bank Publications.

33. Jayaram, N. (1989). *Sociology: Methods and Theories. Adapted to Indian needs rom Tony Bilton et al "Introductory Sociology."* Macmillan India Limited.

34. Jayaram, N. (Ed.). (2009). Positivism. *MPhil/PhD Social Theory Course.* Tata Institue of Social Sciences.
35. Jayaram, N. (Ed.). (2010). M.Phil PhD Class Lecture on Triangulation. Tata Institue of Social Sciences.
36. Kakde, D. (2010). *Compiled Report of Community Based Monitoring of Health Services Under NRHM in Maharashtra.* Pune: Support for Advocacy and Training to Health Initiatives SATHI.
37. Kulkarni, A., & Jaswal, S. (1999). *An Exploratory Study on Women's Health in Rural Maharashtra.* School of Rural Development, Tuljapur: Tata Institute of Social Sciences.
38. Kumar, S. (2006). *Report on Piloting the Application of Social Accountability Tools in South Asia: Pilot of Community Score Card in Satara District.* School of Rural Development, Tuljapur: Tata Institute of Social Sciences.
39. Kumar, S. (2007). *Parallel Bodies & the Panchayati Raj Institutions: A Study of Village Based Special Committees in Three Districts of Maharashtrra.* School of Rural Development, Tuljapur: Tata Institute of Social Sciences.
40. Maharashtra-location-map.jpg (JPEG Image, 600 × 673 pixels) - Scaled (0%). (2014, August 26). Retrieved from http://www.mapsofindia.com/maps/maharashtra/maharashtra-location-map.jpg
41. McGarvey, N. (2001). Accountability in public administration: a multi-perspective framework of analysis. *Public Policy and Administration, 16*(2), 17–29.
42. Mishra, S., Duggal, R., Lingam, L., Pitre, A., Sardeshpande, N., & Shukla, A. (2008). A report on health inequities in Maharashtra. *SATHI, Pune, 411*, 29.
43. Mulgan, R. (2000). 'Accountability': An Ever-Expanding Concept? *Public Administration, 78*(3), 555–573.
44. Nagaranjan, R. (2013, February 13). Rural public health usage goes up, so does healthcare cost. *The Times Of India.*
45. O'donnell, G. (1999). Horizontal accountability and new poliarchies. *Lua Nova: Revista de Cultura e Política*, (44), 27–54.
46. Olson, M. (1965). *The logic of collective action: Public goods and the theory of group.* Harvard University Press Cambridge.
47. Organisation, W. H. (2010). *World Health Statistics.* Geneva: WHO.
48. Ostrom, E. (1990). *Governing the commons: The evolution of institutions for collective action.* Cambridge university press.
49. Ostrom, E. (2011). Background on the institutional analysis and development framework. *Policy Studies Journal, 39*(1), 7–27.
50. Ott, S. J., & Russell, E. W. (2013). *Introduction to Public Administration: A Book of Readings.*
51. Pollitt, C., & Bouckaert, G. (1995). *Quality improvement in European public services: concepts, cases and commentary.* Sage.

52. Polski, M. M., & Ostrom, E. (1998). An institutional framework for policy analysis and design.

53. Posani, B., & Aiyer, Y. C. N.-A. I. W. P. N. 2. (2009). State of Accountability: Evolution, Practice and Emerging Questions in Public Accountability in India. Center for Policy Research.

54. Potts, D. H. (2005). *Accountability and the right to the highest attainable standard of health*. Human rights Centre, University of Essex.

55. Roberts, N. C. (2002). Keeping public officials accountable through dialogue: Resolving the accountability paradox. *Public Administration Review*, *62*(6), 658–669.

56. Romzek, B. S. (2000). Dynamics of public sector accountability in an era of reform. *International Review of Administrative Sciences*, *66*(1), 21–44.

57. Romzek, B. S., & Dubnick, M. J. (1987). Accountability in the Public Sector: Lessons from the Challenger Tragedy. *Public Administration Review*, *47*(3), 227. https://doi.org/10.2307/975901

58. Roy, S. D. (2013, October 2). Apex medical council overrules state unit, faults two doctors. *The Times Of India*, p. 7.

59 Rubenstein, J. (2007). Accountability in an unequal world. *Journal of Politics*, *69*(3), 616–632.

60. Schedler, A. (1999). *The Self Restraining State: Power and Accountability in New Democracies*. Lynne Rienner Publishers.

61. Service Delivery. (2013, September 18). Retrieved from http://www.img.kerala.gov.in/index.php?option=com_content&view=article&id=596&Itemid=266

62. Sinha, D. (2008). Social Audit of Midday Meal Scheine in AP. *Economic and Political*

CHAPTER 3

Malnutrition and Local Institutions: Insights from the Two Cases

3.1 Introduction: Profiling of Cases

The premise of the theoretical framework of this monograph is that, at the village level, a web of institutions interacts with each other through processes that include accountability relationships and influence service delivery outcomes. Some of these institutional processes are position, boundary, authority, information, collectives, and payoffs in terms of incentives and sanctions. These are all man-made and operate at the local level to influence public services like Integrated Child Development Services (ICDS). The local institutions can only be understood within a specific context which is attempted in this chapter through profiling of the two villages – Surli and Nanduri.

According to the methodological assumptions and research design, the study follows a case study design with two villages as its cases. However, it is not an ethnography[1] of a village, but a study contextualized in a village setting. Therefore, this qualification needs to be kept in mind while describing and analysing the cases.

Fieldwork for this study was conducted from May 2012 till August 2012. The first trip was for a week to the Satara and Osmanabad districts and their respective villages Surli and Nanduri. These visits enabled the author to obtain permissions from the district administration necessary for the recruiting of local volunteers from the village to pilot test survey tools.

The actual fieldwork happened for a period of 2 weeks at each of the study villages. In all, the fieldwork happened for 180 days over a span of four months. Informed consent was gathered from all participants before interviewing them. Specifically, all respondents were

1 Ethnography, a primary method used in the discipline of anthropology, is a systematic approach to understanding the beliefs, rituals, patterns, and institutions that define a culture. 'Ethnography,' as used traditionally, labeled a research process where an anthropologist lived in a small community for a longer duration like 11 months to a year, to learn the details of their daily life (Allard and Anderson, 2005).

informed about the objectives of the study and that results would likely be published in research papers, a thesis or a book. They also consented that their personal data would be used only for furthering research.

Out of 35 districts of Maharashtra, Surli is in a district with high Human Development Index (HDI) rank of two while Nanduri is located in a district with a poor ranking of 29. This chapter begins with a discussion on the socio-economic and demographic profile of the sample, looking specifically at household composition, gender, sex ratio, caste, occupation, literacy, education, and economic class. Critical discussion on the politics of measuring child malnutrition[2] both at macro and micro levels and in comparison, to both case villages, follows this profiling. The chapter summarises key observations and questions long-held notions about the relationship between the supply of services like a well-functioning Anganwadi Center (AWC) or a Primary Health Centre (PHC) and users' access to these services.

3.1.1 Profile of Surli

The village of Surli is located in Wathar (Kiroli) cluster of the Koregaon block. The block is located in Satara district within Pune circle of Western Maharashtra region. Surli is 660 meters above the sea level and is located 20 km towards east from the district head-quarters in Satara and 235 km from Mumbai (Figure 2.10).

The nearby cities to Surli are Satara, Wai, Karad and Phaltan. Surli has three Anganwadi Centers (AWCs) and a Zila Parishad primary school with students up till grade four. While one of the AWCs buildings was constructed through a grant from the World Bank, another one runs also inside school classroom. The third AWC in Surli was located on the other side of the road and operates from a makeshift shed.

'Made with Sponsorship from the World Bank' (*jatakeye bank sahayit* in Marathi) was painted on the outer walls of one of the AWC (Figure 3.1). Having been to ICDS centres in other Indian states as well, this was an unusual text.

It is a known fact that the World Bank, being a multi-lateral agency, usually works directly with Central Governments of a country and does not directly sponsor or fund any community-based projects. When I asked the ICDS supervisor about this, her reply was rather intriguing.

The supervisor explained that the World Bank's brand acts as a serious endorsement to their work in the eyes of the community. Indirectly and unknowingly, she revealed that perhaps credibility of their own work, representing the State, remains undervalued.

2 Malnutrition is used to mean under-nutrition in this study. Although, both words are distinct, as malnutrition is derived from word malfunction; and includes both under-nutrition and over-nutrition. In this research, I have used the word malnutrition.

The local administration promotes international agencies in this manner to instil public confidence. Indirectly and unknowingly, she revealed that perhaps credibility of their own work, representing the State, remains under-valued. This response made me question why a community would doubt their services, especially if there were low incidences of malnutrition and high utilization of services, meaning that the AWCs were doing effective work in the village? Low incidence of malnutrition was also one of the assumptions on the basis of which Surli was chosen as a study village.

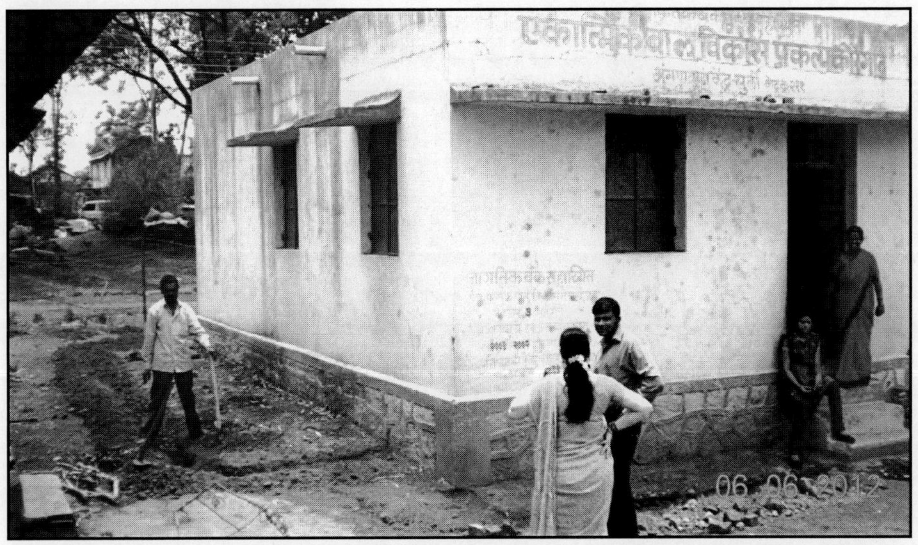

Figure 3.1: Anganwadi Centre in Premises of Village School, Surli

Source: From fieldwork, 2012. Note: ICDS Supervisor instructing a labourer to prepare a trench for the kitchen garden while the AWW looks on. AWWs & Helpers have colour coded uniforms – Magenta-coloured saris with black borders for AWW and Mustard-coloured saris with black border for Helper

Community Resource Mapping for Surli was jointly prepared at the Gram Panchayat's (GP) office, with inputs from the locals. When asked if participatory resource mapping exercises were done by the GP, its *gram sevak* (Panchayati Raj Institution's or PRI's facilitator) informed that they do not have the village map but PHC may have one. It was almost like evading the question. Like most village habitations, Surli's boundaries are defined by a state highway on its right side and an open sewerage (*nalah*) flowing on the north end (Figure 3.2). Community resources like cultivable land, main crops and social resources like community taps, village school, AWCs, panchayat office, village doctor, temples etc. are marked in the community map. Surli is no different than most Indian villages where scheduled caste (SC) households and those belonging to the Below Poverty Line (BPL) lay on the margins of the village and farthest away from its entry point from the road.

As per the government reporting requirements under ICDS, the AWCs have to fill a format called the three-monthly family survey (Figure 3.3 Appendix II). It is a household survey conducted by AWCs to provide a glimpse into the social profile of 'all' families residing in a village. The survey also lists numbers of all 'potential' or 'eligible' ICDS beneficiaries like number of children under age six, pregnant women, lactating mothers and adolescent girls.

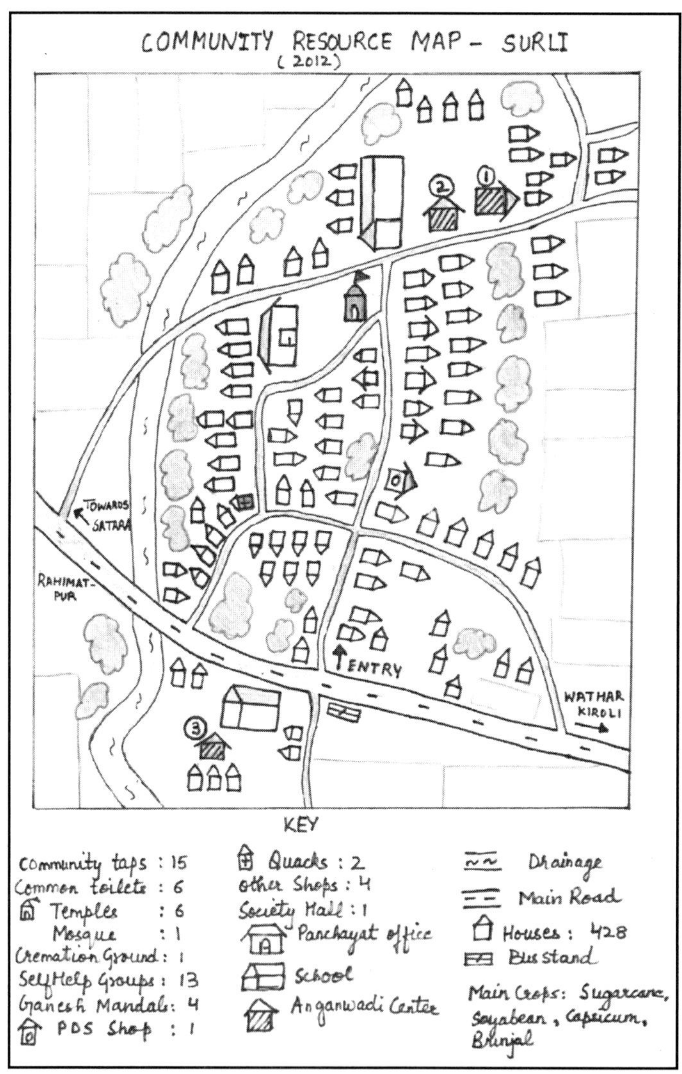

Figure 3.2 : Community Resource Map, Surli

Source: Illustration by Author

In Surli, this format was readily given by the AWW. Accordingly, in Surli, AWCs conducted this survey which was a part of the ICDS Management Information Systems or MIS (Figure 3.3). The information in AWC family survey pertains to April 2012 to June 2012.

Surli had 428 families in all, with a total population of 2003, of which 1043 were males and 960 were females. This means that for every 1000 males, there were 920 females in Surli. According to this data, 11.3% people (59 families) were below the poverty line[3] and 10.3% people (49 families) belonged to the SC category. In addition, the BPL and SC categories are not mutually exclusive. The village had no scheduled tribe (ST) family. This conformed to this block-level demography of having negligible presence of tribal communities. Also, Other Backward Class (OBC) as a category, was not recognised in the village survey.

Furthermore, the source included 35 pregnant women and lactating mothers; 188 women in the age group of 15-45 years; 131 children below the age of 6, and 90 adolescent girls aged 11 – 18 years. These formed the vulnerable population. These are also the potential and eligible beneficiaries of ICDS.

This data should not be mistaken for actual number of ICDS beneficiaries or study participants. This only indicates a universe for AWCs operations in a village. In both case studies, this information formed the first level understanding of the macro socio-demographic character of the villages.

3.1.2 Profile of Nanduri village

Nanduri is a village in Tuljapur taluka or block in Osmanabad district of Maharashtra. It falls in the Aurangabad division of the Marathwada region (see Figure 2.11). Nanduri is located 42 km towards south from district head-quarters, Osmanabad, 18 km from Tuljapur and 426 km from Mumbai. The nearby cities to Nanduri are Tuljapur, Solapur, Osmanabad and Umarga. The habitation area of the village is 10 acres while the surrounding area comprises of about 1000 acres of land, of which 500 acres is cultivable land while the remaining is grass land. Nanduri had two AWCs, a Zila Parishad (ZP) primary school and a secondary school run by a private trust. Both the AWCs were located in the premises of the ZP school. While one had its own building, the other was running in the school classroom in a makeshift arrangement since its building was under construction when the survey happened.

The community resources map of Nanduri was drawn based on cues from a hand-drawn map put up at the panchayat office. It was prepared through participation from the locals (Figure 3.4).

Like Surli, the boundaries of the village here are similarly defined by a highway on one end and a small tributary called *Harna* on the other. Nanduri's community resources include community toilets, a community hall, community taps, a primary school and AWCs. A large number of households were dependent on 11 community taps for

3 A family is considered Below Poverty Line (BPL) if combined income of all its members is equal to or less than Rs. Rs. 27,000 annually. A family comes in 'Others' category if its monthly income is Rs. 6000 or above.

domestic water requirements. The village had 10 community toilets, five each for men and women, constructed by the panchayat at one end of the village. The panchayat had also constructed shops and a community hall at the central location of the village, but most were yet to be occupied. Although Nanduri falls in the Marathwada region, which is known to be drought prone, interview revealed that the ample water infrastructure had been put in place. As the deputy sarpanch of the Nanduri GP shared,

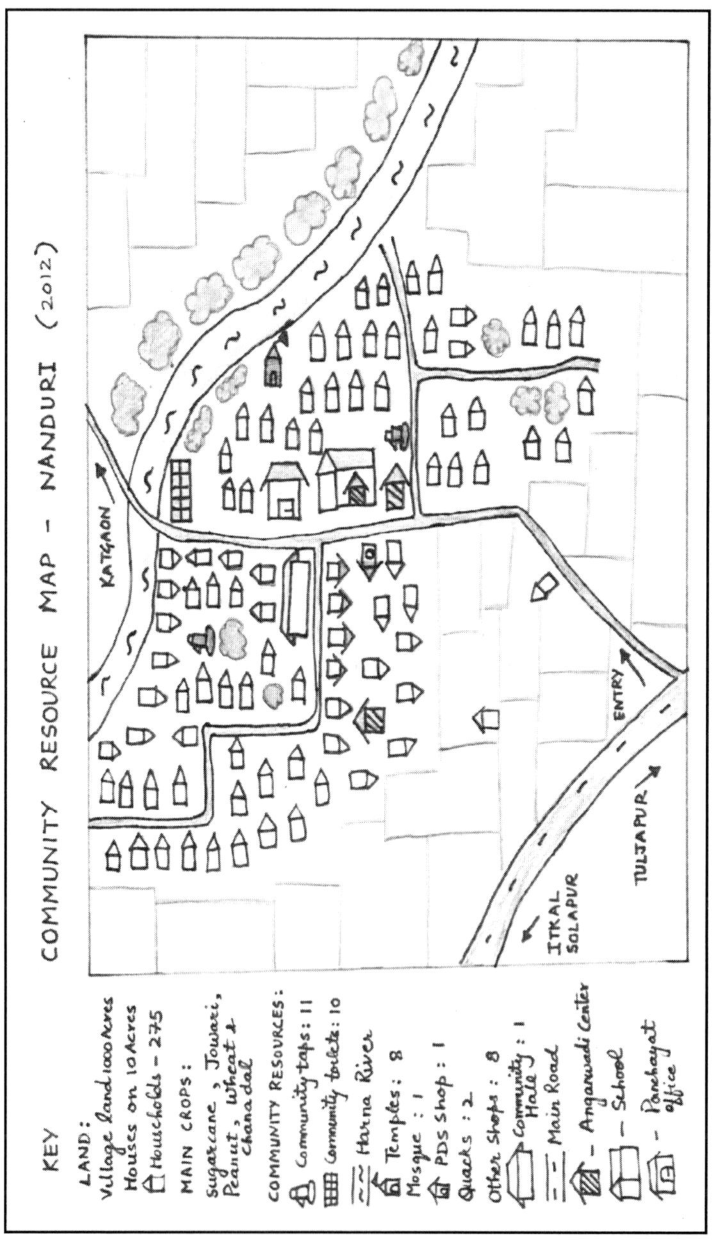

Figure 3.4: Community Resource Map, Nanduri

Source: Illustration by Author

"We have enough water, so much that the entire district does not have so much water as our village. The government had provided a 20 thousand litre tank, but we installed a sixty-thousand litre tank. A dispute is going on with the government as they have not reimbursed us the money for building an additional 40 thousand litre tank. Secondly, we had laid a water pipeline to a 3.5 km water source which is a well. Now in summer months, there is less water even in that well. To counter this, we got all water sources connected with each other. Now our water tanks are mostly full. So, there is no problem of water as such." – GP member, Nanduri

Interviews with other functionaries like the AWWs also revealed that availability of potable water was not a problem in Nanduri as there were eight water reservoirs or ponds in and around the village.

Incidentally, sugarcane was one of the major crops grown around Nanduri. The village demographic information was scattered since the quarterly family survey by AWCs did not happen in Nanduri. Instead, I gathered this information by combining segregated data from Nanduri panchayat office and the AWC registers (Figure 3.5 Appendix II). In December 2012, there were 275 families recorded in Nanduri with a total population of 1338, of which 682 were males and 656 were females. Sex ratio of the village was 961 females for every 1000 males, demonstrating the sex ratio of Nanduri was more equally distributed than that of Surli.

The SC population of the village was 14.7% (198 people) while the BPL population was 10.6% (143 people). There was a small presence of STs, comprising of only 3.5% of the population (47 people). Compared to Surli, Nanduri had a surprisingly higher percentage of the SC population and ST population, yet marginally lower percentage of families belonging to the BPL category. The total eligible ICDS beneficiary population of Nanduri as per AWC lists comprised of the following: 26 pregnant and lactating women, 135 children below the age of six, 299 women in the age group of 15 to 45 years and 28 adolescent girls in the age group of 11 to 18 years.

3.2 Profile of the Sample

The sample of the study consisted of all the households in the village that had a child below age six, as Chapter 2 details. While conducting the survey, the presence of a village youth volunteer in the survey team enabled inclusion of households that were not registered with the AWCs. At the same time, unidentified or ghost names procured from AWC lists were removed (see Table 3.11). A total of 129 households were part of the study, of which 60 were in Surli and 69 in Nanduri.

3.2.1 Condition of Housing and Toilets

The size of the household depicts the family type (Table 3.1). Surli had about 13.3% households who had nuclear families with four or less members. This was higher in

Nanduri at 24.6%. In rural areas, family size is causally linked to ownership of land holdings. This is true in case of Nanduri where a majority of the households who had 4 or less members, were either a family with landless labourers or belonged to SC/ST communities. In Surli, highest percentage of households were those with five to six members at 45%. Nanduri had an equal number of households with five to six members, while those with seven or more members constituted 37.7%.

Public service indicators like type of housing, water, toilets and electricity connection provide a glimpse on the socio-economic profile of the villages (Table 3.2). All houses in Surli were pucca houses, of which 8.4% were built either under the BPL or Indira Awas Yojna (IAY) scheme. In Nanduri, there were a sizeable number of *kaccha* houses (10%) and semi-*pucca* houses (11.6%). Of the pucca houses (78%) in Nanduri, about 14.4% were built under the BPL or IAY schemes. The higher presence of SC & ST households in Nanduri explains why more houses are built under these schemes. Surli also had the distinction of achieving 100% rural electrification. Almost all households (except one) had toilets within premises of home, while a large majority of the households (83.3%) had taps inside the house.

Table 3.1: Household Size of the Sample

Household Size	*Surli*		*Nanduri*		*Total*	
	Count	%	Count	%	Count	%
4 & less	8	13.3	17	24.6	25	19.4
5 to 6	27	45.0	26	37.7	53	41.1
7 & more	25	41.7	26	37.7	51	39.5
Total	60	100.0	69	100.0	129	100.0

In Nanduri, the picture was just the opposite. A majority of households in Nanduri (81.2%) did not have toilets within its premises. Also a majority of them (56.5%) rely on community taps as their source of water. There were also a handful of households (11.6%) with no electrical connectivity. This is reflected in overall community facilities in the village. Nanduri had 11 community taps and 10 community toilets. The households in Nanduri without tap connection in their houses, obtained water from community taps and then stored for domestic use. It was found during the survey that community toilets built by the Panchayat laid unused. This is a common observation when such physical assets are often constructed, but not utilised. Qualitative data during the interviews reveal that most people without toilets in their houses (including women) go to the fields instead of using community toilets. When asked about the poor usage of the community toilets, a male office bearer of the Nanduri gram panchayat shared,

> *"We [have] got so many toilets made for the village, separately for men and women. Toilets have overhead water tank, tap, light[ing] everything. We cannot*

forcibly take the women there and ask them to use it. During the monsoon, near the river, the grass grows tall, they put a stone or wood plank and then do it in open. This is the problem every year. We have taken numerous steps. Unko aadat pad gaui hai, nahi karte, aap kitna bhi suvidha de do.' (No matter how many facilities you give them they will not use it because they are habituated in their ways)." – GP member, Nanduri

When I asked possible reasons for the trend and if economic constraints were one of the main reasons, he replied, "It is not the question of money here. Those who have money, they can construct toilets in their house. But they also do not make [them]. They have gotten used- to doing it outside".

Table 3.2: Status of Public Services for Sample Households

Public Service Indicator	***Category***	***Surli***		***Nanduri***		***Total***	
		Count	%	Count	%	Count	%
Type of House*	Kaccha	0	0.0	7	10.1	7	5.4
	Pucca	60	100.0	54	78.3	114	88.4
	Semi Pucca	0	0.0	8	11.6	8	6.2
	Total	60	100.0	69	100.0	129	100.0
Government Built Housing	BPL (Below Poverty Line)	1	1.7	3	4.3	4	3.1
	IAY (Indira Aawas Yojana)	4	6.7	7	10.1	11	8.5
	None	55	91.7	59	85.5	114	88.4
	Total	60	100	69	100	129	100.0
Electricity	No	0	0	8	11.59	8	6.2
	Yes	60	100	61	88.41	121	93.8
	Total	60	100	69	100	129	100.0
Toilet within premises	No	1	1.7	56	81.2	57	44.2
	Yes	59	98.3	13	18.8	72	55.8
	Total	60	100	69	100	129	100.0
Source of drinking water at home	Bore well & tap	5	8.3	0	0	5	3.9
	Community tap	5	8.3	39	56.5	44	34.1
	Tap within home premises	50	83.3	30	43.5	80	62.0
	Total	60	100	69	100	129	100.0

*Type of House classification is as per NSS Survey

With the absence or no exposure of these mechanisms in Nanduri, more than 80% of the poor and lower middle asset quintiles did not have toilets in their homes. Surprisingly, more than 70% households in upper middle and rich quintile also did not have toilets in their houses. of all the asset classes, the highest percentage of households that had toilets within premises of home were the middle asset quintile (33.3%).

Data from the survey indicates that income may not be the reason for lack of toilets in houses in Nanduri. Asset quintile[4] of households in both the villages was cross tabulated with presence of toilets within household premises (Table 3.3). In Surli, most households, irrespective of income class, had toilets in their houses. Reasons for this include incentivising central government schemes like Total Sanitation Campaign[5] in which the district administration aggressively promotes open-defecation-free villages. Surli had won *Nirmal Gram Puruskar*, an award for open-defecation-free village and also *tanta-mukt* (conflict free) village. These incentives or awards ensured that most houses had toilets and had no country-liquor shops in the village. Liquor shops in villages is assumed to be one of the reasons behind domestic and community conflict and a risk to local self-governance (PRIs). Therefore, the State incentivises with awards to villages to be conflict-free and hence better governed.

Table 3.3: Asset Quintile and Presence of Toilets in Household Premises

Village	*Toilet within premises*	*No*		*Yes*		*Total*	
	Asset Quintiles	Count	%	Count	%	Count	%
Surli	Poor	0	0.0	8	100.0	8	100.0
	Lower Middle	1	12.5	11	91.7	12	100.0
	Middle	0	0.0	16	100.0	16	100.0
	Upper Middle	0	0.0	12	100.0	12	100.0
	Rich	0	0.0	12	100.0	12	100.0
	Total	1	12.5	59	98.3	60	100.0
Nanduri	Poor	14	82.4	3	17.6	17	100.0
	Lower Middle	15	93.8	1	6.3	16	100.0
	Middle	6	66.7	3	33.3	9	100.0
	Upper Middle	10	71.4	4	28.6	14	100.0
	Rich	11	84.6	2	15.4	13	100.0
	Total	56	81.2	13	18.8	69	100.0

Note: Poor quintile has household asset value falling in range of Rs. 20,000 to Rs.5,32,050; lower middle as Rs.5,32,050 to Rs.10,18,915; middle as Rs. 10,18,915 to Rs. 14,06,300; upper middle as Rs. 14,06,300 to Rs. 28,42,600 and rich as Rs. 28,42,600 to Rs. 3,09,40,850.

This observation resonates with mainstream discourse on rural sanitation that defecating in open is often linked to 'mindset' and 'culture'. It is also evident from Swachh Bharat Mission's (previously Total Sanitation Campaign) advertisement featuring actor Vidya Balan. The campaign's punch line, "*Jahan soch, wahan sauchalaya*" (where there is a mindset, there will be a toilet) suggest this most clearly.

4 The development of asset quintiles is mentioned in Section 2.2.

5 Total Sanitation Campaign (TSC) was introduced in 1999 by Indian Government to accelerate sanitation coverage throughout the country, particularly in rural areas (Irigoyen, 2017).

The assumption of this campaign is that even economically well-off households do not construct toilets within house premises because of reasons that pertain to mindset or culture. Sociologically, this phenomenon is often explained through the concepts of purity and pollution of the Hindu caste system and Brahmanism[6]. Insights from households' interviews with women respondents reveal another facet to this issue. During one of the interviews in a seemingly well-off household, I continuously probed as to why the head of the household did not construct toilet in the house premises. She responded, *"They* (male members of the family) *will do it, but I do not want to have a toilet in the house at the first place"*. Taken aback, I asked for her reasons behind this. She replied,

> *"First of all, it is me who is responsible for filling water in the house from the common tap. In addition to the existing responsibility of household chores and child-care, the responsibility of cleaning the toilet would also fall on me. So, it is fine when everybody in the house goes out to relieve themselves, at least, I am saved of additional work." – A woman in Nanduri*

Interviews with other women who stayed in households without toilets evinced similar responses. Clearly, women had a choice to get it built in the house but she chose not to have it, unlike the protagonist of Bollywood film "Toilet, Ek Prem Katha" (Toilet, a Love Story) who overcame many barriers to get one in her marital house.

Not having toilets relates to caste, gender inequalities and patriarchy other than cultural and poverty, an observation which this data confirms. Of the total 13 households that had toilets within the house premises in Nanduri, seven were from the general category and six were from SC, OBC and Muslims combined. Interestingly, all the three Muslim households in Nanduri had toilet in their houses. The rest were two households from SC families and one from OBC. Of the seven households that belonged to a general category, a majority (five households) were from a poor to middle asset quintile.

Field data reveals that the presence of a toilet is likely to be found in a SC/OBC/ Muslim household than a general category Hindu household. This points to the role played by patriarchy and caste in perpetuating gender inequalities in the decision of having a toilet in home. Since this is not a sociological analysis of a village nor an objective of the study, but only its context, reasons or explanations are not attempted. In Satara, presence of toilets in most households were a result of institutional factors of Surli village being part of the Total Sanitation Campaign. In Satara, gender inequalities were ironed out by effective implementation of sanitation campaign.

---

6 Traditional norms of purity and pollution are crucial in determining sanitation practices in India including use (or lack) of toilets. Hindu norms of pollution and purity have many dimensions that centre on connotations of dirt and pollution, purity and cleanliness, physical spaces as pure or impure, and the human body as a site of purity and impurity (Mohanty and Dwivedi, 2019; Coffey and Spears, 2017).

At the village level, community toilets also include toilets at anganwadi centers and schools. While Surli AWCs had functional toilets in its AWCs, this was not the case in Nanduri (Figure 3.6). Nanduri AWC had a toilet but it remained locked and children were seen to be taken out in a queue, made to release in the open compound of the ZP school. There was no embarrassment or shame associated with this. None of the parents present in the school objected to this practice, despite my presence, implying that this was a way of life. When functionaries were asked about the non-functional toilet in the AWC in Nanduri, one of them shared,

> *"Toilet construction was not done properly. The hole is bigger and not meant for children. At times, children have even fallen into it. One has to keep paying attention all the time. At times one of us is not there, then how will one manage? So we make all children make a queue and do [it] in open. Toilet's drainage is also not proper as the effluent would spill out on the road just outside the school entrance; it used to stink and inconvenience people. So ZP people came and closed it."* – *AWW, Nanduri*

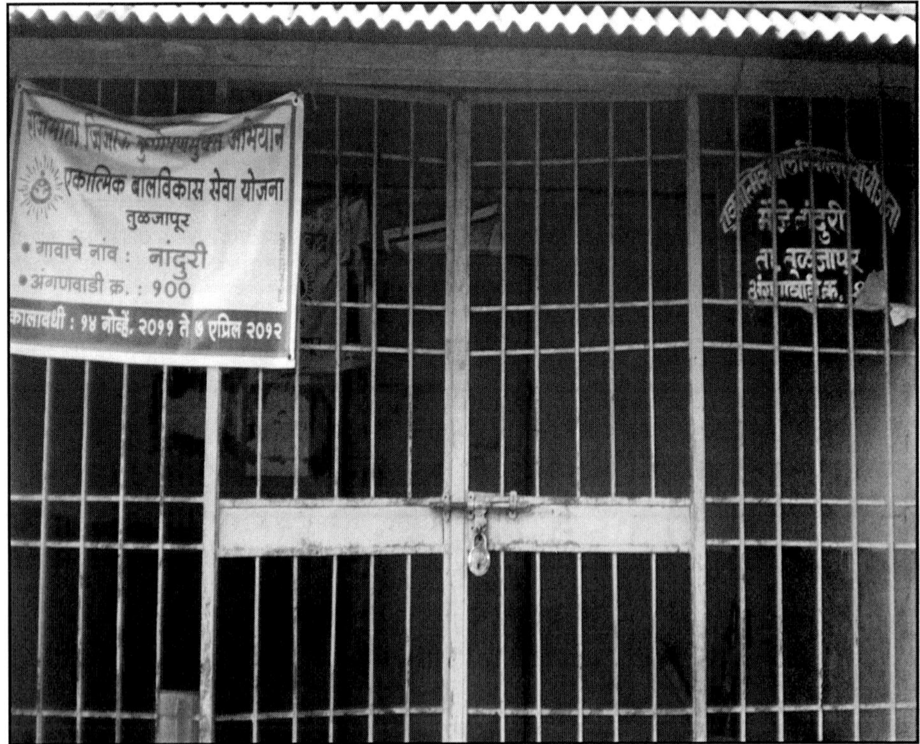

Figure 3.6: Anganwadi Centre in Premises of Village School, Nanduri

Source: From fieldwork. Note: Picture shows anganwadi helper bringing children in the open for urinating. The AWC building has a toilet but it remains unused and locked.

When I posed the same question to senior functionaries of the ICDS in Nanduri, they acknowledged that this was indeed the issue and that they were thinking about solutions. Such a trend is not new for the output-focused monitoring of the current NPM framework that places emphasis on physical deliverables that is construction of toilets, rather than user outcomes, like sanitation.

Despite large public money being spent on toilet construction in general India, toilet 'use' is still not guaranteed and is low. Toilets are linked with general sanitation which is known to influence child health and nutrition outcomes. It would also be interesting to see the relationship between child malnutrition and presence or absence of toilets in Surli and Nanduri. The section 3.4 on child nutrition attempts this analysis.

3.2.2 Socio Demographic Profile of the Sample

The socio-economic profile of respondents gives a glimpse on gender, social group, asset quintile and religion (Table 3.4). On gender distribution, Surli had a higher percentage of males (52.4%) than females (47.6%) while it is opposite in Nanduri, with a higher percentage of females (53.2%) than males (46.8%). This observation is linked to the fact that district Satara was known for its skewed sex ratio till 2011. Experts cite female foeticide and infanticide as a common reason, which is exacerbated by presence of diagnostic health-care infrastructure in more developed district like Satara[7].

Gender. Satara district is notoriously known for a prevalent gender biased tradition, where parents name their third or fourth-born daughter as '*nakoshi*' which means unwanted in Marathi, in a belief that their next child will be a boy. Till 2010, Satara was one of the districts with poor child sex ratio in Maharashtra. Child sex ratio (0-6 age group) in Satara was 880 females per 1000 males in 2009-2010. Action taken by the district health department revealed that more than 11 doctors from the district were involved in more than 100 cases of female foeticide (Patil, 2013).

In 2011, child sex ratio in Satara stood at 881 per 1000 males, although this was an improvement since 2001, as seen in Table 3.5 (Census of India, 2011; Sakal Times, 2011).[8] Surli lies in Koregoan block of Satara. The block had a mushrooming of private doctors within a radius of 5-10 km. In fact, in 2012, during the Maharashtra

---

7 It is a common observation that there is a high co-relation between sex-selective abortions (female foeticides) and presence of diagnostic facilities being available and accessible in that region. In 1994, Pre-natal Diagnostic Techniques (Regulation and Prevention of Misuse) Act came into force to prevent sex-selective abortions.

8 It is a well-established law of nature that males exceed females at the time of birth. It is believed that generally 943-953 female births take place for every 1000 male births, which implies that there is a deficiency of 50 females per 1000 males in every birth cohort. Many demographers believe that left on its own, this is an unalterable constant (Census of India, 2011).

government's drive to crackdown on illegal or unregistered sonography centres conducting sex determination tests, one doctor's clinic nearby Surli village was raided and shut down. It is the same time while this research was on.

Table 3.4: Select Socio-economic Indicators of Sample Households

Socio Economic Indicators	*Category*	*Surli*		*Nanduri*		*Total*	
		Count	%	Count	%	Count	%
Gender	Female	188	47.6	236	53.2	424	50.5
	Male	207	52.4	208	46.8	415	49.5
	Total	395	100	444	100	839	100
Social Group	General	36	60.0	52	75.4	88	68.2
	OBC	21	35.0	8	11.6	29	22.5
	SC	3	5.0	9	13.0	12	9.3
	Total	60	100.0	69	100.0	129	100.0
Asset Quintiles	Poor (Rs. 20,000 to Rs. 5,32,050)	9	15.0	17	24.6	26	20.2
	Lower Middle (Rs 5,32,050 to Rs. 10,18,915)	10	16.7	16	23.2	26	20.2
	Middle (Rs. 10,18,915 to Rs. 14,06,300)	17	28.3	9	13.0	26	20.2
	Upper Middle (Rs. 14,06,300 to Rs. 28,42,600)	12	20.0	14	20.3	26	20.2
	Rich (Rs. 28,42,600 to Rs. 3,09,40,850)	12	20.0	13	18.8	25	19.4
	Total	60	100.0	69	100.0	129	100.0
Religion	Hindu	57	95.0	66	95.7	123	95.3
	Buddhist	1	1.7	0	0.0	1	0.8
	Muslim	2	3.3	3	4.3	5	3.9
	Total	60	100.0	69	100.0	129	100.0

Note on Asset Quintiles: Each household's consolidated asset values were calculated after adding and converting all their assets into rupee value using standardised rates prevailing in 2012. All households' asset values were then arranged in a descending order. Most poor and most rich households were clearly grouped into quintiles marked by their asset values and asset ownership like land ownership and type of house. Other three quintiles could also be identified from the descending order using the same method. Source: Field level data compiled from household survey (2012)

There are other studies which indicate similar findings, in which sex ratio unfavourable to girls was a feature peculiar of a more developed district like Satara. In a study of 24 villages, women self-help groups in villages of the better developed districts of Maharashtra even gave loans to access sex selection technologies (De et al., 2012). The same study also revealed that sex selection was said to be practiced by the relatively affluent and upper castes.

Sex ratio of total population in Satara revealed a peculiar trend where there were 986 females per 1000 males in 2011 (Table 3.5). Sex ratio statistic is not the same and is different from child sex ratio. Child sex ratio (number of females per 1000 males in the age group of 0-6 years) can indicate exact gender inequalities. In case of Satara, sex ratio seems to be higher than average. But this should not be interpreted as less discrimination since child sex ratio remains highly unfavourable for girls. Experts have attributed such a discrepancy to women living without spouses because of higher mortality among men due to alcoholism, occupational injuries, and tuberculosis (ibid.).

Table 3.5: Comparison of Sex Ratio in Study Districts

State / District	*Sex ratio of total Population*		*Sex ratio of 0-6 age*	
	2001	2011	2001	2011
Maharashtra	922	925	913	883
Satara	995	986	878	881
Osmanabad	932	920	894	853

Source: Compiled from Census of India 2011 (Census of India, 2011b)

Although a poorly ranked HDI district, child sex ratio in Osmanabad was much better than Satara in 2001 at 894 per 1000 males. However, it deteriorated in a decade and by 2011, it decreased to 853 (Table 3.5). It is a well-established fact that less developed districts have low accessibility to sex-selective diagnostic technologies. With growth of urbanisation and privatisation of medical services, even in less developed districts like Osmanabad, child sex ratio dropped drastically by 41 points by year 2011.

In context of total population, Osmanabad is one among the six districts of Maharashtra including the infamous case of a doctor couple in Beed[9], where sex ratio is low (920 per 1000 males), in the range of 900 to 925 in 2011 (Rizwanullah, 2012). Other districts in this category are Pune (910), Beed (912), Aurangabad (917), Jalgaon (922) and Latur (924).

The age profile of the population of the two villages provides an interesting glimpse on the demographic patterns of the two villages (Table 3.6). The percentage of population in the age group of 0-6 years was the highest among all other age groups in both Surli (22.7%) and Nanduri (27.9%). It also shows that of the total population, children below six years were higher in Nanduri than in Surli. Nanduri also had higher percentage of girls (14.4%) than boys (13.5%) in the age group of 0-6 years while in Surli the percentage of girls was much lower (8.7%) than boys (14%). Also, the social composition of Nanduri had a higher percentage of SCs and STs as compared to Surli. Presence of ST is a factor that is known to have a positive impact on the sex ratio that favours girls.

9 Beed doctor couple surrendered in 2012 on charges of conducting illegal abortion on an eight month pregnant woman who had died during the operation. The couple has also been accused of carrying out sex determination tests and feeding female foetuses to dogs. The doctor couple got sentenced to 10 years of rigorous imprisonment in 2019.

Table 3.6: Age Profile of Households' Members according to Gender

Age Profile	*Gender*	*Surli*		*Nanduri*		*Total*	
		Count	%	Count	%	Count	%
0-6 years	Female	34	8.7	64	14.4	98	11.7
	Male	55	14.0	60	13.5	115	13.8
	Total	89	22.7	124	27.9	213	25.5
7-18 years	Female	14	3.6	36	8.1	50	6.0
	Male	17	4.3	16	3.6	33	3.9
	Total	31	7.9	52	11.7	83	9.9
19-29 years	Female	59	15.1	64	14.4	123	14.7
	Male	33	8.4	40	9.0	73	8.7
	Total	94	24.0	104	23.4	198	23.7
30-39 years	Female	22	5.6	17	3.8	39	4.7
	Male	46	11.7	44	9.9	90	10.8
	Total	68	17.3	61	13.7	129	15.4
40-49 years	Female	10	2.6	13	2.9	23	2.8
	Male	8	2.0	8	1.8	16	1.9
	Total	18	4.6	21	4.7	39	4.7
50-59 years	Female	28	7.1	17	3.8	45	5.4
	Male	15	3.8	9	2.0	24	2.9
	Total	43	11.0	26	5.9	69	8.3
60 years & above	Female	20	5.1	25	5.6	45	5.4
	Male	29	7.4	31	7.0	60	7.2
	Total	49	12.5	56	12.6	105	12.6
Grand Total		392	100.0	444	100.0	836	100.0

A similar trend is also confirmed by another age group category of 7-18 years. Nanduri had a substantially higher percentage of girls (8.1%) in the age group of 7-18 years as compared to boys (3.6%). The gender gap continues in the age group of 7-18 years with percentage of females was found to be lower (3.6%) than that of males (4.3%) in Surli. The age group of 19-29 years is the only age group where the percentage of females is substantially higher (15.1%) than males (8.4%) in Surli. The observation is true for Nanduri too. This is so because 19-29 years age group witness majority of marriages among females who migrate from one village to another. Migration owing to marriage is a well-established reason for this trend.

Caste, Occupation & Asset ownership. There was a distinct difference in social composition between Surli and Nanduri. While Surli had a higher percentage of OBCs, percentage of SCs was higher in Nanduri. Such composition directly implies higher economic status of households in Surli than in Nanduri. It is so because OBCs as a group is economically better off than SCs and is politically more empowered. Incidentally, many of Maharashtra's chief ministers have been from Satara region. In terms of religious composition, majority of the households in the survey (95%) in both the villages were Hindus, with a miniscule presence of Muslims and Buddhists. Surli had 65% households belonging to general (non-SC/ST/OBC) category; 35% OBCs and 5% SC. Households from OBC category in Surli were the following castes - Parit, Navhi, Gurav, Jangam, Wadar, Sonar and Dhangar.[10] The SC families reported their castes as Mahar, Navbodh, and Mang. The castes in general category included Maratha and Bhat. The social composition of Nanduri was different in terms of higher presence of SC households and lower OBCs as compared to Surli. General category in Nanduri was 75.4%; SCs at 13.0% and OBCs at 11.6%. General category castes in Nanduri included Maratha and Lingayat. The OBC castes in Nanduri were Koli, Teli and Dhangar while SCs castes were Mahar and Chambar.

The occupational profile of the sample was captured by asking the head of the household about the primary occupation of all family members. The primary occupation of respondents in Nanduri and Surli according to age and gender is shown in Table 3.7 and Table 3.8. There was no occupation reported in the age group of under-15 years old in both the villages. It could be true that there was no child labour in these villages. One also cannot rule out the possibility of under-reporting by the head of the household, nor was it possible to cross check this information during the survey.

As a primary occupation, respondents who reported self-employed in agriculture (working on family owned farms) formed the highest percentage of the total population. This was in both villages although Nanduri reported a higher number than in Surli. In Nanduri, it was found that as the age group increased, more numbers were engaged in self-employed agriculture, which was the highest in the age group of 56-65 years (52.6%) (Table 3.7). In this age group, a higher percentage of males (68.2%) reported this activity while highest percentage of females (33.3%) who reported to be self-employed in agriculture were in the age group of 46-55 years.

Surli (22.7%) and Nanduri (27.9%). It also shows that of the total population, children below six years were higher in Nanduri than in Surli. Nanduri also had higher percentage of girls (14.4%) than boys (13.5%) in the age group of 0-6 years while in Surli the percentage of girls was much lower (8.7%) than boys (14%). Also, the social composition of Nanduri had a higher percentage of SCs and STs as compared to Surli. Presence of ST is a factor that is known to have a positive impact on the sex ratio that favours girls.

10 One of the questions asked in the household interview schedule during the survey was 'caste in verbatim'.

Table 3.7: Primary Occupation of Sample Households' Members in Nanduri (n=444)

Category	*Sub category*	*> 15 yrs*	*16-25 yrs*	*26-35 yrs*	*36-45 yrs*	*46-55 yrs*	*56-65 yrs*	*66 & above*
		%	%	%	%	%	%	%
Agriculture labour	Female	0.00	10.7	6.2	27.3	11.1	12.5	0.0
	Male	0.00	16.7	21.4	6.3	28.6	27.3	18.2
	Total	0.00	12.5	15.9	14.8	16.0	21.1	9.1
Animal Husbandry	Female	0.0	0.0	0.00	9.1	0.0	0.0	0.0
	Male	0.0	0.0	0.0	6.3	0.0	0.0	0.0
	Total	0.0	0.0	0.0	7.4	0.0	0.0	0.0
Housewife	Female	0.0	76.8	75.0	27.3	50.0	56.3	54.5
	Male	0.0	0.0	0.0	0.0	0.0	0.0	0.0
	Total	0.0	53.8	27.3	11.1	36.0	23.7	27.3
Manufacturing*	Female	0.0	0.0	0.00	0.0	0.0	0.0	0.0
	Male	0.0	0.0	0.0	6.3	14.3	0.0	0.0
	Total	0.0	0.0	0.0	3.7	4.0	0.0	0.0
Non Agricultural Labour**	Female	0.0	0.0	3.1	0.0	0.0	0.0	0.0
	Male	0.0	0.0	3.6	0.0	0.0	0.0	0.0
	Total	0.0	0.0	3.4	0.0	0.0	0.0	0.0
Not Applicable***	Female	100.0	7.1	0.0	9.1	5.6	0.0	45.5
	Male	100.0	16.7	0.0	0.0	0.0	0.0	27.3
	Total	100.0	10.0	0.0	3.7	4.0	0.0	36.4
Self-employed in Agriculture	Female	0.0	3.6	6.2	27.3	33.3	31.3	0.0
	Male	0.0	37.5	42.9	62.5	42.9	68.2	54.5
	Total	0.0	13.8	29.5	48.1	36.0	52.6	27.3
Self-employed other than Agriculture****	Female	0.0	0.0	0.0	0.0	0.0	0.0	0.0
	Male	0.0	4.2	7.1	0.0	0.0	0.0	0.0
	Total	0.0	1.3	4.5	0.0	0.0	0.0	0.0
Services*****	Female	0.0	1.8	9.3	0.0	0.0	0.0	0.0
	Male	0.0	25.0	25.0	18.8	14.3	4.5	0.0
	Total	0.0	8.8	19.3	11.1	4.0	2.6	0.0
TOTAL	Female	100.0	100.0	100.0	100.0	100.0	100.0	100.0
	Male	100.0	100.0	100.0	100.0	100.0	100.0	100.0
	Total	100.0	100.0	100.0	100.0	100.0	100.0	100.0

Note: *Manufacturing category includes employment in dairy, oil mill, sugar mill. **Non-agriculture labour includes painter, construction and goldsmith. ***Not applicable category includes disabled, handicapped, retired or old people and children. ****Self-employed other than agriculture includes ration shop, barber, beauty salon, ironing, dyer and washer, electric shop, civil contractor, tailor, stationery shop, milk booth and shuttering shop. *****Services category includes government services (clerk in municipality/gram panchayat/postal department, AWC worker, school teacher/principal, gram sevak, ASHA worker, police constable, bus conductor and armed forces), driver (of car, JCB, jeep, auto, tempo, truck), commission agent, nurse, peon, priest, employee in private company.

Table 3.8: Primary Occupation of Sample Households' Members in Surli (n=395)

Category	*Sub category*	*> 15 yrs* %	*16-25 yrs* %	*26-35 yrs* %	*36-45 yrs* %	*46-55 yrs* %	*56-65 yrs* %	*66 & above* %
Agriculture labour	Female	0.00	0.0	2.9	10.0	10.0	0.0	0.0
	Male	0.00	0.0	10.9	0.0	0.0	3.8	0.0
	Total	0.00	0.0	8.1	4.3	7.9	2.6	0.0
Housewife	Female	0.0	95.5	88.6	70.0	72.4	92.3	55.6
	Male	0.0	0.0	0.0	0.0	0.0	0.0	0.0
	Total	0.0	72.4	31.3	30.4	55.3	30.8	25.0
Manufacturing*	Female	0.0	0.0	0.0	0.0	0.0	0.0	0.0
	Male	0.0	7.1	3.1	0.0	0.0	0.0	0.0
	Total	0.0	1.7	2.0	0.0	0.0	0.0	0.0
Non Agricultural Labour **	Female	0.0	0.0	0.0	0.0	0.0	0.0	0.0
	Male	0.0	0.0	6.3	0.0	33.3	3.8	0.0
	Total	0.0	0.0	4.0	0.0	7.9	2.6	0.0
Not Applicable***	Female	100.0	4.5	0.0	0.0	0.0	0.0	44.4
	Male	100.0	50.0	0.0	0.0	0.0	7.7	27.3
	Total	100.0	15.5	0.0	0.0	0.0	5.1	35.0
Self-employed in Agriculture	Female	0.0	0.0	2.9	10.0	13.8	7.7	0.0
	Male	0.0	14.3	37.5	61.5	66.7	61.5	63.6
	Total	0.0	3.4	25.3	39.1	26.3	43.6	35.0
Self-employed other than Agriculture****	Female	0.0	0.0	0.0	0.0	0.0	0.0	0.0
	Male	0.0	7.1	20.3	0.0	0.0	3.8	0.0
	Total	0.0	1.7	13.1	0.0	0.0	2.6	0.0
Services *****	Female	0.0	0.0	5.7	10.0	3.4	0.0	0.0
	Male	0.0	21.4	21.9	38.5	0.0	19.2	9.1
	Total	0.0	5.2	16.2	26.1	2.6	12.8	5.0
TOTAL	Female	100.0	100.0	100.0	100.0	100.0	100.0	100.0
	Male	100.0	100.0	100.0	100.0	100.0	100.0	100.0
	Total	100.0	100.0	100.0	100.0	100.0	100.0	100.0

Note: *Manufacturing category includes employment in dairy, oil mill, sugar mill. **Non-agriculture labour includes painter, construction and goldsmith. ***Not applicable category includes disabled, handicapped, retired or old people and children. ****Self-employed other than agriculture includes ration shop, barber, beauty salon, ironing, dyer and washer, electric shop, civil contractor, tailor, stationery shop, milk booth and shuttering shop. *****Services category includes government services (clerk in municipality/gram panchayat/postal department, AWC worker, school teacher/principal, gram sevak, ASHA worker, police constable, bus conductor and armed forces), driver (of car, JCB, jeep, auto, tempo, truck), commission agent, nurse, peon, priest, employee in private company. commission agent, nurse, peon, priest, employee in private company.

In Surli, the trend was similar, where a higher percentage of respondents who reported their primary occupation to be self-employed in agriculture increased with age (Table 3.8). Highest percentage of total population (43.6%) self-employed in agriculture was from the 56-65 year age group, followed by 39.1% in 36-45 years age group. A lower percentage of females reported to be self-employed in agriculture in Surli (13.8%), in the age group 46-55 years as compared to those in Nanduri.

The second largest category was of agriculture labour, percentage of which was again higher in Nanduri than in Surli. In Nanduri, percentage of people involved in agriculture labour again increased with age category. Agriculture labour was highest in age group of 56-65 years (21.1%), followed by 46-55 years (16%). Of this, women comprised a small proportion but was higher in Nanduri as compared to Surli. About 27.3% females in age group of 36-45 years were agriculture labourers. In Surli too, women who reported their primary occupation as agriculture labourers were mostly those aged 36 and older.

A higher percentage of males in Surli in the age group of 46-55 year were non-agriculture labourers (7.9%), mainly from the construction sector, as compared to those in Nanduri. Service was the third largest category of primary occupation, with a higher percentage of people reporting it in Surli as compared to Nanduri. In Surli, all age groups had a substantial percentage of people reporting to be in services that included government jobs, drivers, nurse, priests, clerks etc. The highest however, was in the 36-45 years category (26.1%), followed by the 26-35 years category (16.2%). In Nanduri, 19.3% people in age group of 26-35 years reported to be in services where the share of women was higher than those in Surli in the same age group.

A sizeable percentage of women in all age groups starting from 16-25 years reported to be housewives, that is, not gainfully employed outside the house. This however was higher in Surli as compared to those in Nanduri. Also, about 7.9% males in age group 46-55 years in Surli were non-agriculture labourers, which was higher than those in Nanduri. Manufacturing was reported largely in Nanduri in the age group of 36-45 years (6.3%) and 46-55 years (14.3%), and mainly by males. Of the remaining primary occupations, a higher percentage of people aged 26-35 years in Surli reported to be self-employed in professions other than agriculture (13.1%), as compared to those in Nanduri (4.5%). This category included occupations like running a ration shop or others like barbers, dyers and washers, and electricians.

Income is not a dependable indicator in assessing the economic class of the households. This is especially so in a rural setting. Consumption expenditure is often used as a proxy indicator in many large surveys like NSSO to assess economic class. However, this is not an econometric study. With a smaller sample size, a less complex method in form of household asset ownership was used. The assets of rural households were divided into eight categories – type and number buildings, livestock, farm equipment, vehicles including farming related, electrical appliances, household wooden furniture, other household items and finally land holding. Each of these categories had a comprehensive and exhaustive list of items listed under them, along with their numbers or quantities and current approximate prices (in Rupees). The cost of the house or shop was asked directly from the respondents and that was taken at face value. Land costs in the region however, were ascertained from the land records of the panchayat depending on the type of land (cultivable, dry or fallow). The standard costs for other assets were ascertained as per the current prevailing market rates (see Table 3.14 Appendix II). Once each item had its value, all asset values were summed up to get one consolidate value of asset ownership per household.

Table 3.9: Asset Quintiles as per Socio-religious groups

Village	*Asset Quintiles**	*General* %	*Muslim* %	*OBC* %	*SC* %	*Total* %
Surli	Poor	8.8	100.0	14.3	33.3	15.0
	Lower Middle	8.8	0.0	23.8	66.7	16.7
	Middle	23.5	0.0	42.9	0.0	28.3
	Upper Middle	32.4	0.0	4.8	0.0	20.0
	Rich	26.5	0.0	14.3	0.0	20.0
	Total	100.0	100.0	100.0	100.0	100.0
Nanduri	Poor	16.3	66.7	25.0	55.6	24.6
	Lower Middle	22.4	0.0	50.0	11.1	23.2
	Middle	14.3	33.3	12.5	11.1	13.0
	Upper Middle	22.4	0.0	12.5	11.1	20.3
	Rich	24.5	0.0	0.0	11.1	18.8
	Total	100.0	100.0	100.0	100.0	100.0

Note: Surli (n=60); Nanduri (n=69) * As per Notes of Table 3.4

Once all 129 households in the survey had a consolidate asset value, five quintiles were generated after putting all the values in descending order. Asset values lying between Rs. 20,000 to Rs. 5,32,050 were named as poor; Rs. 5,32,050 to Rs. 10,18,915 as lower middle; Rs. 10,18,915 to Rs. 14,06,300 as middle; Rs. 14,06,300 to Rs. 28,42,600 as upper middle and finally Rs. 28,42,600 to Rs. 3,09,40,850 as rich (see notes Table 3.4). Comparing the two villages, Nanduri had a higher percentage of households belonging to poor quintile (24.6%) as well as lower middle quintile (23.7%) as compared to 15.0% and 16.7% respectively in Surli (Table 3.9).

Of all the asset categories, middle class was the highest among all other classes at 28.3% in Surli while the same was 13% in Nanduri. The upper middle quintile was almost the same in both villages at 20%, and rich quintile was marginally higher in Surli (20%) than in Nanduri (18.8%).

Households from all socio-religious category belongs to each of the asset quintile (Table 3.9), which is intuitive. Since the numbers of households in categories like SC and Muslim were small, percentages were calculated within each category and not across categories. In Surli, the economic status of Muslim and SC households was worse than those of the general category or OBCs. Almost 100% households of Muslim and SC in Surli either belonged to poor or lower middle asset quintiles. Within the general category, a majority of households (58.9%) belonged to the upper middle and rich asset quintile, followed by the middle asset quintile (23.5%). Those in the poor and lower middle asset quintile were 8.8% each. For OBCs, the majority of households fell in the middle asset quintile (42.9%). This is followed by the lower middle (23.8%) quintile, while 19% households belonged to rich or upper middle asset quintile. About 14.3% of OBC households were poor in Surli.

In Nanduri, there was a higher percentage of households from all socio-religious categories who belonged to poor asset quintile, as compared to Surli. A majority of Muslim, SC, OBC, and even general category households belonged to the poor or lower middle asset quintile. The rich and upper middle households in Nanduri were 46.9% in all, which is lower than those in Surli. About 11.1% households of SCs also belong to upper middle asset quintile. Clearly, households in Surli were economically better off than those in Nanduri.

Education. Education is considered to be one of the main social determinants of rural development and gender empowerment. Status of both literacy and school education was collected in the household survey (Table 3.10). The percentage of those who are illiterate and those who can sign their names only (literate without school education) is more than three times in Nanduri (25.4%) as compared to Surli (8.3%).

Of this, the majority were women, with 15.9% in Nanduri and 6.7% in Surli. Of the total population, Nanduri had a higher percentage of children below age six (24.8%), compared with that of Surli (21.8%). Accordingly, the percentage of children who are in pre-primary level is higher in Nanduri (13.1%) than in Surli (11.2%). Of this, an equal percentage of girls and boys were enrolled in pre-primary in Nanduri (6.6%) while the percentage of females was half (3.4%) than males (7.7%) in Surli. Almost an equal percentage of people passed primary and middle school (till class IX) in Surli (33.5%) and Nanduri (33.9%). Surprisingly, the percentage of females attaining primary and middle school here was higher in both Surli (18.6%) and Nanduri (19.7%) as compared to men (14%) in both villages.

One distinct observation from the data on school education shows that Surli had a higher percentage of graduates or postgraduates (8.6%) than in Nanduri (4.7%). Surli also had a higher percentage of those who passed higher secondary or class XII (14.3%) than in Nanduri (6.6%). Among these, the percentage of females was lower than males, with both the villages aligning with a generalised, predictable trend. The percentage of people (of any age group) who had passed high school (class X) was higher in Surli (25.2%) than Nanduri (20.0%). Of these, the percentage of men was higher than women in Surli but equal in Nanduri.

Table 3.10: Literacy (age 7 & above) and School Education (age 3 & above) for Sample Households

Socio Economic Indicator	*Category*	*Sub category*	*Surli*		*Nanduri*		*Total*	
			Count	%	Count	%	Count	%
Literacy	Illiterate	Female	19	6.1	45	13.5	64	9.9
		Male	4	1.3	24	7.8	28	4.3
		Total	23	7.4	69	20.6	92	14.3
	Literate without schooling (sign only)	Female	2	0.6	8	2.4	10	1.5
		Male	1	0.3	8	2.4	9	1.4
		Total	3	0.9	16	4.8	19	2.9
	Literate (schooling between class 1 to 5)	Female	61	19.7	81	24.2	142	22.0
		Male	52	16.8	56	16.8	108	16.8
		Total	113	36.6	137	41.0	250	38.9
	Middle school and above	Female	74	23.9	46	13.8	120	18.6
		Male	96	31.1	66	19.8	162	25.2
		Total	170	55.0	112	33.5	282	43.8
	Grand Total		309	100.0	334	100.0	643	100.0
Education	Graduates & Postgraduates	Female	15	4.3	5	1.3	20	2.7
		Male	15	4.3	13	3.4	28	3.8
		Total	30	8.6	18	4.7	48	6.6
	Higher Secondary (12th)	Female	19	5.4	8	2.1	27	3.7
		Male	31	8.9	17	4.5	48	6.6
		Total	50	14.3	25	6.6	75	10.3
	High School (10th)	Female	38	10.9	38	10.0	76	10.4
		Male	50	14.3	38	10.0	88	12.0
		Total	88	25.2	76	20.0	164	22.5
	Primary & Middle school (Up to 9th)	Female	65	18.6	75	19.7	140	19.2
		Male	52	14.9	54	14.2	106	14.5
		Total	117	33.5	129	33.9	246	33.7
	Pre School Education (age 3- 6 years)	Female	12	3.4	25	6.5	37	5.1
		Male	27	7.7	25	6.6	52	7.1
		Total	39	11.2	50	13.1	89	12.2
	No Education	Female	20	5.7	50	13.1	70	9.6
		Male	5	1.4	32	8.4	37	5.0
		Total	25	7.1	82	21.6	107	14.7
	Grand Total		**349**	**100.0**	**380**	**100.0**	**729**	**100.0**

Assessment of this village-level data shows that Nanduri had a fewer percentage of those continuing higher secondary, graduate, or post graduate education than those in Surli. At the same time, a higher or an equal percentage of females attained high school as compared to males in Nanduri. Conversely, Surli females lagged behind males at this level. data also show less gender disparity in educational attainment in Nanduri, as compared to Surli. This observation also aligns with skewed child sex ratio favouring boys, in Satara. It would now be interesting to see the status of child malnutrition in two case villages with such distinct socio-economic-demographic features.

3.3 Status of Regional and Local Child Nutrition

Validity of government data on child malnutrition remains a contentious issue. Malnutrition is often said to be under-reported in the state ICDS MIS, while national surveys like NFHS or those by civil society and local NGOs have often reported higher numbers. For instance, while the ICDS is ideally placed to provide this data, the discrepancy seen between ICDS rates of malnutrition and the National Family Health Survey (NFHS) data is 1:17 (De et al., 2012). This means that for every single child reported to be under-nourished by ICDS data, there are 17 more reported by NFHS.

However, at the onset, the study took a district with a better HDI rank and another with a poor HDI rank. Even if one assumes that there are anomalies in reporting child malnutrition data at the village level, these anomalies will be present in both the villages and hence would not interfere in comparison. Also, the focus of the study is not to 'measure' the quantum of malnutrition in terms of extent, since the differential is a given, and part of the study design. Therefore, collecting primary data on child malnutrition in both study villages (by weighing of each child) would not have added value or justified the objectives of this study. Hence, these were not carried out.

Secondly, the reason for using government data is that it forms the basis on which current child health and nutrition programmes like ICDS and NRHM are delivered. Here, it is the institutional design which is the focus of the study. At the village level, there are hardly any incentives or disincentives for workers to misreport statistics, an observation also made by few independent ethnographic studies. Gupta (2001) argues that although there were few mechanisms to double-check the records kept by Anganwadi Workers, there was little reason to be suspicious of the figures that had been entered in the registers. The following section provides a glimpse of the status of child malnutrition at both micro (village) level and macro level (cluster, block and district) from government data segregated at various levels, starting from AWCs at village level; block level; CDPO's office at district level and ICDS Commissionerate at state level.

3.3.1 Macro level: From government data

Surli was one among the 14 villages that were a part of the Wathar Kiroli beat, also called cluster. Surli village was chosen as per the population criteria of the study as it only fitted population criteria and distance from the PHC. Since malnutrition issue had gained judicial and media attention at the time of study, coupled with extensive monitoring under the ICDS, data was available at all levels of administration, starting from district, block, cluster and village. According to village-level data procured from the Supervisor of Wathar Kiroli cluster, about 129 children under-six were weighed in Surli (see Table 2.9 Appendix I).

In the cluster, the average percentage of children who were moderately malnourished was 5.3%. Surli had 7.8% children under-six with moderately malnutrition, higher than the average in the cluster. The data shows 86% of Surli's children as normal weight. This meant that almost 14% of children in Surli had some form of malnutrition, a number which is considered high according to regional standards. Also, government data shows that about 98% children in Surli were brought to the AWC and weighed. In the same cluster, villages like Targaon had 3% of children who were moderately under-nourished, lower than Surli while Sathewadi had higher a percentage of children under-nourished at 14%. This data shows that even in a high HDI district like Satara with low child malnutrition, the percentage of malnutrition among children can vary from extremely low to high at the level of a village.

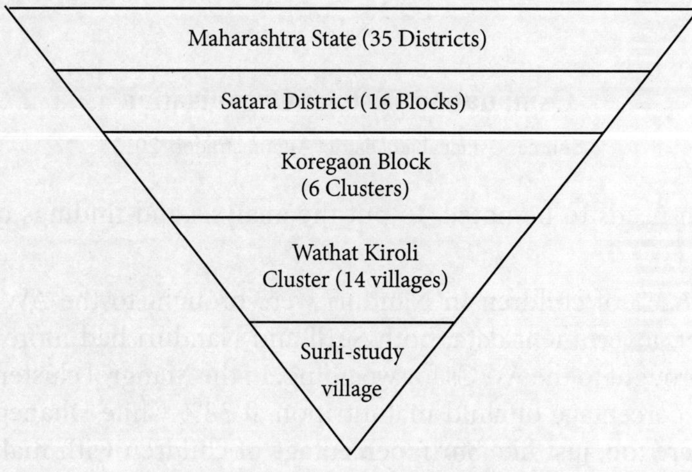

Satara District Organisation

Source: Satara District Administration, 2012

From village and cluster, if one moves up to the block, the law of averages nullifies any extreme variations in percentage of malnutrition. Cluster level data provided by the Block CDPO's office at Koregaon, shows that out of six beats, Wathar Kiroli beat had 99% of its children being brought to the AWCs and weighed, while any form of malnutrition, including moderate and severe was lowest among six beats, at 5.8% (see Table 2.7 Appendix I). Tadwale beat had the highest percentage of under-nourished children at 10.6%. Moving up from cluster to block levels, the Koregaon block was one among 16 blocks in Satara district which had lowest percentage of any form of child malnutrition (7.7%) and high utilisation (76.5%) of ICDS services (see Table 2.6 Appendix I). If one is to compare the state of child malnutrition between Surli and Koregaon, there is not much difference. Therefore, as per government records, Surli represented a site with lowest level of child malnutrition in the district.

Nanduri was chosen among 15 villages under the Mangrol cluster after applying the same criteria of population and distance from the PHC (see Table 2.10 Appendix I). Village level data procured from ICDS Supervisor revealed that any form of malnutrition among children, on an average, was 14.2% in Nanduri. This percentage was almost on par with the level of malnutrition in Surli, which is a higher HDI rank district.

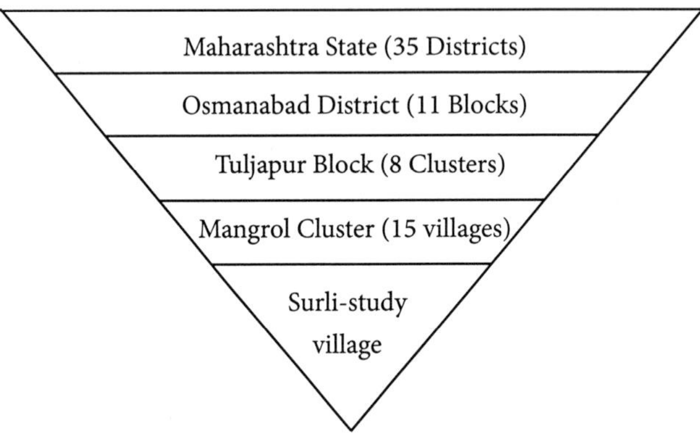

Osmanabad District Organisation

Source: Osmanabad District Administration, 2012

This observation needs to be noted, to put the analysis and findings of the study in a perspective.

Similarly, 96.3% of children in Nanduri were brought to the AWC for weighing. Therefore, as per government data, both Surli and Nanduri had more than 95% of its children being brought to the AWCs for weighing. In the Mangrol cluster, Kamtha village had the highest percentage of child malnutrition at 38% while Dhanegaon village had lowest at 5%. Here too, just like Surli, percentage of children with malnutrition varied and was low in some villages despite being in a poor HDI rank district.

Moving from village to cluster level, Mangrol cluster was one among eight projects in the Tuljapur block which had one of the highest utilisation of ICDS services at 97.5% (indicated by the percentage of children brought to the AWCs for weighing), while any form of malnutrition was also highest at 21.1% (see Table 2.10 Appendix I). The Tuljapur block in turn, was one among 11 blocks that had highest rate of child malnutrition at 14.2% and also had a high utilisation of ICDS services at 91.2% (see Table 2.5 Appendix I). Therefore, according to government data, Nanduri represented a site with highest level of child malnutrition in a poor HDI rank district of Osmanabad. Both the study villages Surli and Nanduri represented their respective districts of Satara and Osmanabad on the status of child malnutrition.

One can draw two conclusive observations from this preliminary macro level comparison between the two cases. First, government data hide much more than they reveal. The ICDS data is generated out of an extensive and strict MIS adhered to by the whole top-down bureaucratic and administrative machinery of the government, right from each AWC, to the village, cluster level, block, and finally the district levels. It is the only extensive source on functioning of ICDS that I could rely upon. In fact, there are numerous papers and studies that have documented the overpowering role of record keeping and reporting by frontline functionaries in ICDS (Gupta, 2001; Dreze, 2006; Sinha, 2006). Under the NPM framework of bureaucratic accountability, quantitative data assumes a key role in programme evaluation and policy making.

The problem is not with managerialism per se, but with its institutional design where actors are always bound by the inter-play of multiple institutional processes like hierarchies, incentives, rents, patronage and sanctions. There is always an incentive to under-report the negatives (which is hard to curb) and over-report the positives. From here, several questions arise. What can managerial accountability achieve if the data it generates cannot represent the status on ground? What are the positive impacts of managerial accountability on improving public programmes? These questions are not new but asking these questions in this context is important.

Secondly, child malnutrition is a pervasive issue, prevalent even in Surli located in Wathar Kiroli cluster and Koregaon block which reported the best record on child nutrition in a high HDI ranked district. Satara had high per capita income as compared to other districts where educational, literacy, and health indicators were also encouraging. Yet, it had almost similar high percentage of children malnourished as compared to Nanduri, which was located in the Mangrol cluster of the Tuljapur block. One also now needs to see village-level data on child nutrition outcomes to verify these findings.

3.3.2 Micro level: Anganwadi records

Anganwadi center is a crucial public institution that delivers child health, nutrition, and early childhood education services at the village level. As mentioned earlier, just like ICDS, data collated by government department are often contested and questionable. The data at the bottom most level of AWC at the village level cannot be any better. Experts believe that AWC data is often fudged as it is maintained for the sake of administrative monitoring. However, it is a type of secondary data which need not be totally dismissed and can be utilised with certain qualifications. For instance, I matched names of children with their father's names to tally with actual households surveyed for this study. This ensured verification of each child in the village. Ghost names of children (who do not exist) on AWC registers, is a widespread practice in ICDS programme, and such a check ensured selection of genuine cases only.

Politics of Measurement. Fudging was common in reporting 'grades of malnutrition' in anganwadi records. Once all 129 households this is so because, it is the 'grades' which gets reported for MIS and not the weights of children. There are hardly any incentives for weights of children to be fiddled as these are not computed or reported in this form.

Weights are often converted into Grades of Malnutrition and then reported as Grade I, II, III or IV malnutrition. Therefore, I discarded the grade data from the AWC records since this data had shown miniscule children under-nourished in Nanduri while Surli records show near zero malnutrition.

And, I retained children's weights recorded at AWCs and assigned fresh grades to the weights using internationally recognised WHO Child Growth Monitoring Standards, 2006 (see Table 3.12, Table 3.13 and Table 3.14 of Appendix II). It was found that the measurement of child malnutrition is an issue of politics, steered by national policies and influence of international aid agencies. Such politics unfolds in the following section. The AWCs included in the study used two indicators to measure malnutrition.

First is the weight-for-age indicator (WFA), currently used across the country. This is also termed as an indicator of under-weight, especially in National Family Health (NFHS) surveys. The WFA indicator has been used to measure child malnutrition in both ICDS for many decades. It classifies malnutrition in four categories - Grade 1 (Normal or ideal weight); Grade 2 (Slight malnutrition, equal to or greater than minus 2 SD or Standard Deviation); Grade 3 (Moderate malnutrition, equal to or greater than -3SD to less than -2SD) and Grade 4 (Severe malnutrition, less than -3SD) (NIPCCD, 2010). Before 2011, this indicator was used to identify children in Grade III and IV malnutrition, as those needing exceptional care and supplementary feeding. The data available with the AWCs used WFA metrics and hence was considered for the study.

The second indicator used by AWCs is weight-for-length/height (WFLH) to identify children with SAM (Severe Acute Malnutrition) also called wasting and MAM (Moderate Acute Malnutrition). In 2010, the Government of India adapted this new measurement according to criteria specified by the WHO and had begun its implementation as well. The argument given against WFA, is that WFLH is followed globally, instead of WFA measurement (Rajmata Mission, 2010). One needs to question international policy making bodies on why 'height' suddenly became a key statistic to determine malnutrition and they recommended usage of measurement like height-for-age (HFA or stunting) and WFLH (wasting)? Answers to these questions is a subject of study by in itself, however it is important to raise such questions here.

The children identified with SAM/MAM are cared for at the Village Child Development Centers (VCDC)[11] for nutritional rehabilitation, while those needing additional medical attention are either admitted to Child Development Center (CDC) at

11 VCDC is run at the existing AWC in the village and AWWs are given training for the same. Children are admitted for a maximum of 30 days and are given a special diet 6-7 times in a day. NRHM provided the funding for VCDCs from its 'RCH- Child Health' budget. It has a provision of Rs.32 per child per day, including the cost of the special diet, medicines/tonics and even incentives to AWW (Rs. 8 per child per day). Rajmata Jijau Mission took the responsibility of training all the AWWs in Maharashtra. VCDC operates 30 days a month from 8 am to 6 pm with two hours break in between. The spending on VCDCs was about Rs.10 crore in 2012-13 (Source: Rajmata Mission, 2010).

the PHCs or Nutritional Rehabilitation Centers (NRC) at district hospitals. Maharashtra's aggressive programme Rajmata Jijau Mission is claimed to be behind the decline in child stunting (height-for-age), between the periods of 2005-06 to 2012 (Hari & Jose, 2015). The mission's website mentions, 'There is difference in both these standards, such that there is 'no guarantee' that <-3SD children (severely underweight) as per WHO standards can be classified as SAM (wasting)' (Rajmata Mission, 2010). This means that a huge proportion of children in the state, despite being severely under-weight, may not qualify for the SAM/MAM category and hence are excluded from special feeding programmes of the state. There also is evidence of this trend in the official statistics (Figure 3.7).

If one compares percentage of children underweight (32.1%) with the percentage of children with wasting (19.3%) as per NFHS V, there is an enormous difference of 12.8%. It means that 28% of underweight children can be easily taken off the beneficiary list, if 'wasting' becomes the accepted indicator of malnutrition instead of under-weight.

There is also a difference of 6.3%, between children under-weight (21.8%) and those wasted (15.5%) as per the State's government Comprehensive Nutrition Survey Maharashtra 2012 Report. Therefore, with the introduction of SAM/MAM, the number of children to be identified for special complementary feeding in VCDC, drastically reduced.

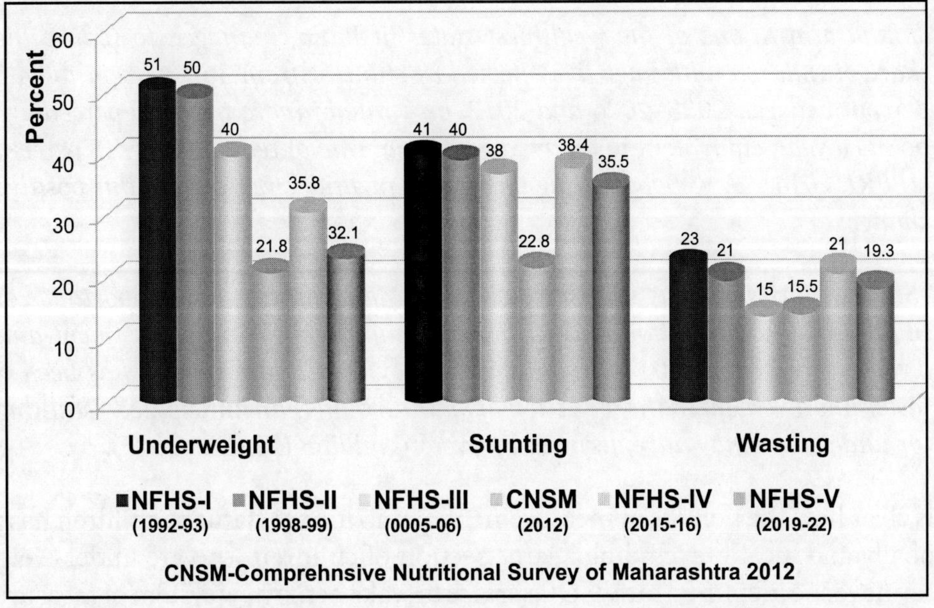

Figure 3.7: Child Malnutrition Indicators as per National Family & Health Surveys (NFHS) & Comprehensive Nutrition Survey of Maharashtra (CNSM)

Note: NFHS data represents children under-six while CNSM included children aged two and below. Under-weight includes Grades II, III & IV (mild, moderate & severe) malnutrition.

Source: NRHM

Reduction in malnutrition happened only in statistics but not on the ground. The report also cited that the drastic lowering of stunting cases in Maharashtra was because of the mission's efforts. On needs to note that the CNSM report included only children under two for its survey while NFHS was based on survey of children under-six. The CNSM report would obviously result in lesser numbers. Also, the report failed to explain that if one agrees that the mission's efforts paid off to reduce stunting, why did it have a negligible impact on reducing the number of under-weight children?

The answer lies in the politics of statistics and measurement. If the state can show lower numbers of malnourished children, through any statistic, it would need less investments and financial allocations towards it. The implementation machinery too will be more than contented with fewer numbers, than to protest against the new system. In addition, monetary incentives built-in this process will silence most functionaries. Child rights activists have cried foul over 2015 Union Budget cuts since previous year, calling it 'entirely bizarre'. Budget cuts were to the tune of 54.19% for ICDS and 21.63% for NRHM Reproductive and Child Health Flexi Pool (Chowdhury, 2015). For Budget cuts in FY 22 see section 5.6, pg 212

Despite such anomalies in nutrition measurements, the Global Nutrition Report touted the reduction in stunting in Maharashtra as a success story.[12] The report in its section titled, "How did Maharashtra cut child stunting?" mentions,

> *"Maharashtra, one of the wealthiest states in India, managed to reduce the share of children under age five affected by stunting from 36.5 percent to 24.0 percent between 2005–2006 and 2012, or a rate of more than 2.0 percentage points a year, equivalent to an average annual rate of reduction of 5.8 percent (IFPRI, 2014)." A webpage citing this report mentions reasons for this positive change,*
>
> *"Success stories such as stunting decline in Maharashtra show importance of multi-sector coordination and sustained commitment from government and civil society. As per 2013-2014 Rapid Survey on Children, there has been a faster improvement in the reduction of malnutrition than anticipated - stunting for under-fives may have declined by over 10 million (Mishra, 2015)."*

It is clear how the politics of measurement of nutritional status of children has played out globally and locally, excluding a large section of children who are under-weight but who may never be identified for VCDC service in wake of the new system of measurement. Stunting is also a tough statistic to compute in the context of a village where data on

12 The Global Nutrition Report was launched by International Food Policy Research Institute in November 2014. The report tracked worldwide progress for 193 UN countries in improving nutrition status. The report aims to contribute to country-led efforts to strengthen accountability and accelerate the reduction of malnutrition (Mishra, 2015).

length of a baby or height of a toddler are rarely complete at the anganwadi centers across Maharashtra. I could not include height/length data of children for this study too, as it was practically non-existent. A glimpse of village level data in the following section would help identify existing gaps and challenges in government monitoring of child nutrition at local level. Therefore, before assessing the child nutrition status, the first task was to assess the number of children in each of the study villages.

Table 3.11: Type and Source of Data for Under-six Children in Study Villages

Types of village level data	*Number of children in Surli*				*Number of children in Nanduri*			
	AWC HH Survey	Supervisor's Data	AWC Muster	Study Survey	AWC HH Survey	Supervisor's Data	AWC Muster	Study Survey
No. of children aged 6 & below	131	132	101	89	135	141	122	121
Children's names not tallying with household verification (ghost names)			38				28	
Households' respondents unavailable				5				2
Children not registered with anganwadi but part of study survey				26				27
Children with available weight data				63				94
Total children with available data	157							

Source: Collated from various village level data, 2012. Note: HH - household

Information Asymmetry. The number of children in a village, a basic and easily verifiable statistic, was surprisingly a primary issue of contestation and a source of corruption. There were 101 children under-six registered in Surli and 122 in Nanduri as per the lists of children procured from attendance registers of the AWCs in two case villages. This data was taken from one of the 22 registers which the AWCs maintain. Some of these registers are named as pre-primary attendance register, nutritional food supply distribution register, weight grading register, growth charts and immunisation register etc. This list also meant that children who do not come to AWC for any services will not be reflected in these registers. This number had to be verified with another source. There is the three-monthly family survey conducted by the AWCs to update birth/death & migration records known as AWC Household Survey. This survey pegged the number of children at 131 and 135 in Surli and Nanduri respectively, which is higher than the numbers in the AWC records (Table 3.11).

Comparing the percentage of children attending AWC using AWC muster and AWC household survey, it shows that a higher percentage of children in Surli (22.9%), as compared to children in Nanduri (9.6%), opted out of ICDS services. Many of these children were attending nearby private English-medium playschools. These children were identified and made part of the study. However, their weight-for-age data did not exist.

The number of children was also verified from a third source - data procured from the ICDS Supervisor. According to this list, the number of children in both villages was not much different from AWC surveys, at 132 in Surli and 141 in Nanduri. The minor difference between the two data can be attributed to children being added (owing to new births) if there was a gap of few months between these surveys. The fourth source was a primary survey I did through a door-to-door listing of households with children under-six years. This was done to check AWC lists and most importantly, to include those children who may not be registered with the AWCs.

Except five households in Surli and two in Nanduri who did not participate in this survey owing to unavailability of its members, the study included 'all' households in the village that had children under 6 years. According to study survey, there were 89 children in Surli and 121 in Nanduri. It was clearly a smaller number than that reflected in the three other sources mentioned above.

As the survey proceeded, I realised that there were ghost names of children & their families in the list given by the AWCs that simply did not exist in that village (Table 3.11). There were 38 such names of children in Surli and 28 in Nanduri which were simply fictitious. These ghost names were confirmed not only by village youth volunteer but also by local village folk. When confronted with the AWC workers on the ghost names, they pretended not to be aware and tried to duck the issue. I could not pursue the case in as an activist as that could have created friction in the community. However, the issue was brought up with anganwadi supervisors. The supervisors shared their sanctioning practices if such a case is proven and even promised to look into the matter (See Section 5.5.3).

Ghost names on AWC's muster roll has been a widespread practice indicating corruption practices at the bottom-most and frontline level of service delivery, the reasons for the same are discussed in Chapter IV. This cannot be termed as merely an accountability gap. There are multiple checks and balances prevalent in both ICDS and NRHM programmes to curb such malpractices. For instance, decentralised gram panchayat functioning; high managerial accountability in terms of strict reporting; organised MIS (Management & Information System), all these mechanisms are present to identify and curb these corrupt practices. However, malpractices only seem to increase despite these top-down accountability mechanisms. It is therefore important to view the trend from the perspective of institutional processes like authority, position, information etc. that shape relationships between actors at the frontline of service delivery.

Effectively, I collected data of 223 children in all, but the complete weight for age data was available only for 157 children - 63 in Surli and 94 in Nanduri. Records pertaining to age, weight and height of a substantial number of children did not exist as they were either not registered with the AWCs or were ghost names. The AWCs keep the records of eligible children pertaining to weight from first month onwards; the grade of malnutrition like Grade I, II, III or IV and also length or height from first month onwards. The two case villages had two AWCs each and hence data of children was collected from four AWCs.

A format was created with details like full name of child, their father's name, date of birth, weight, grade of malnutrition, and height from first month onwards till current age of the child. Entry for each child registered with the AWC was filled in this format. For instance, if a child was five years old at the time of survey, her weight for age, grade of malnutrition, and height for age was entered from first month up to 60th month (or 5 years).

As per the anganwadi records, most children weight was graded as 'normal' while a miniscule few were in grade I and II. It was quite unusual, given the extent of malnutrition prevalent in Osmanabad. I then decided to do away with AWC grades and instead used the WHO child growth monitoring standards to ascertain grade at each month for each child (see Table3.12 and Table 3.13 Appendix II).

The weight data procured from the AWCs was in Marathi. It was translated to English with the help of a translator and translated data was entered in an excel sheet after removing the ghost names. Also, those children who were not registered with the AWC were removed since their weights were not recorded in the first place. The unique household number that was given to each household during the study survey was then matched with each child's household data in Microsoft Access software. By doing this, I was able to link children's weight for age data with their household and family characteristics, like asset quintile, caste, educational status of mother etc. at the first level. Second, I could also co-relate child nutrition status with the responses of the head of the household gathered from household interviews. While entering this data, it was found that height data was grossly incomplete. Therefore 'height' could not be a consistent measure to ascertain nutritional status of children. Hence, height data was not included in the analysis.

3.3.3 Change in Malnutrition

Weight of a child by in itself cannot ascertain which grade of malnutrition the child falls. In Anganwadi centres, a child's weight is recorded every month. The same weight record is also used by the government monitoring of malnutrition. Weight data by itself cannot ascertain severity of malnutrition unless it is benchmarked against a standard. The standard used is called the WHO Child Growth Monitoring Standards, 2006.

Actual data on weights and grades of all children in the study can be seen in Table 3.14 in Annexure II. I used WHO standards to convert children's weights into grades of malnutrition (See Table 3.12 and Table 3.13, Appendix II). Weight data procured from the AWCs, I did not use 'grades' of malnutrition as these were either incomplete or faulty and did not match with WHO standards. I manually ascertained the grade for every month for each child using existing weight data and gave a score as per WHO standards.

In order to see the change in grades of malnutrition, the number of children in various grades were analysed between two time periods, at first month soon after birth and at six-month of age, for both the villages (Figure 3.8).

Although incidence of child malnutrition is high among children aged two in Maharashtra, malnutrition usually sets-in before the age of two (Hari & Jose, 2015). It is also the reason that Maharashtra's Rajmata Jijau Mission was conceived in 2005 with a focus on children under-two years. UNICEF too brought out a first of its kind report called the Comprehensive Nutrition Survey in Maharashtra (CNSM) in 2012, with an exclusive focus on children aged two and below. Therefore, the study's analysis, that follows, considered time periods under-two as justified indicators to access malnutrition.

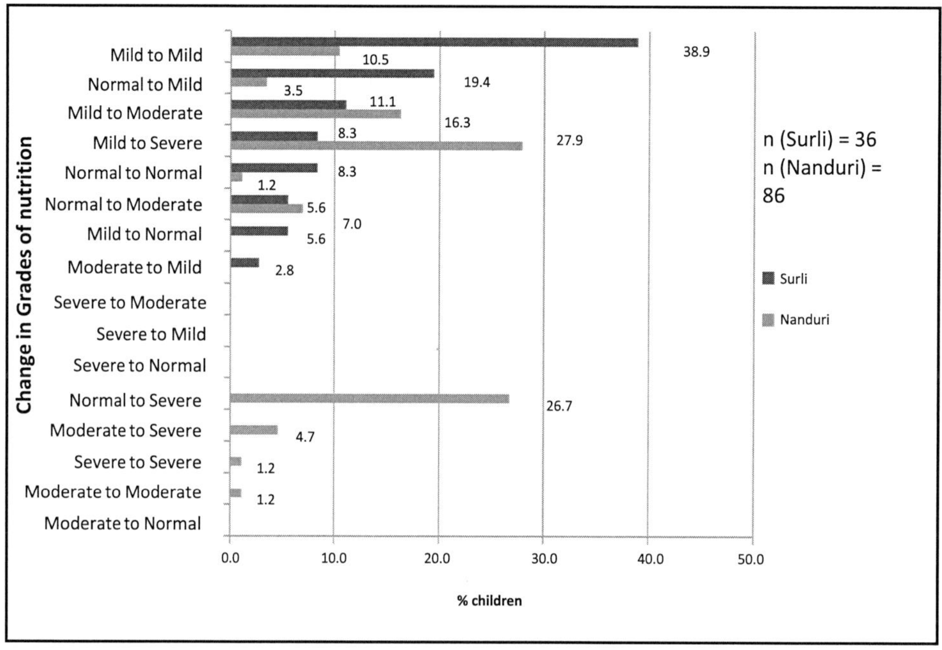

Figure 3.8: Change in Grade of Child Nutrition from First Month to Sixth Month

Source: Field level data compiled from AWC records and household survey (2012)

There were data for end points like one year, two years and so on till 60 months (five years). However the two end points – the first month after birth, and the time after six months had highest number of observations (n). It is also important to note that cross-tabulation was the only analysis possible with this kind of data which had nutrition grades (a nominal variable) of children at different age groups and at different time periods. The total number of children or observations (n) in Figure 3.8 is 122 - 36 from Surli and 86 from Nanduri. I included data of 122 children out of 157 because the remaining children were above six months. According to Figure 3.8, Nanduri had a high percentage of children who were normal at first month after birth but either became severely under-nourished (26.7%) or moderately under-nourished (7%) in six months while only 1.2% remained normal in that time period.

This shows that a substantial percentage of children in Nanduri were normal weight (26.7%) in the first month but deteriorated to severe malnutrition within six months. Children that were mildly undernourished in the first month slipped to either severe malnutrition (27.9%), became moderately malnourished (16.3%) or became mildly malnourished (10.5%) by the time they turned six. There was not a single child in Nanduri who improved in nutritional status towards normalcy within the first six months of birth. The progression of children in terms of nutritional status was much grimmer than the fixed statistic projected in government records and when compared to Surli. In addition, over 50% of children in Nanduri were severely malnourished by the time they turned six. Clearly, child malnutrition in Nanduri was under-reported as per district government records and was found to be higher and changed dramatically towards severe forms.

For Surli, the situation was not so grim. Here, about 19.4% of children who were normal weight in first month slipped to mild malnutrition after six months (Figure 3.8). Also, 8.3% of children in Surli who were normal in first month after birth remained in the normal weight category even after six months - indicating that higher percentages of children in Surli were normal in first month as compared to Nanduri. On the other hand, Surli being in a region and district that had lowest rate of malnutrition, a majority of children who had mild malnutrition in first month, either remained in mild category (38.9%); became moderately malnourished (11.1%) or even became severely malnourished (8.3%) after six months. This data reveals that a majority of children in Surli too had some form of malnutrition by the time they are six months. The only difference here is that most were in mild or moderate malnutrition unlike in Nanduri where most children deteriorated to severe malnutrition. Now here lies the answer to a question I posed in the beginning of this chapter – as to the reasons why the anganwadi center had poor credibility in the eyes of the community in Surli.

Therefore, this evidence supports a fact that children in better HDI ranked district have a better start and they also do not drastically slip to severe forms of malnutrition within first six months as compared to the children in a poor HDI ranked district.

It is clear that a majority of children in both Surli and Nanduri had some form of malnutrition at the time of birth, which deteriorated in the subsequent six months. Yet, the ICDS government statistics in both the villages reported more than 85% of children as normal in nutritional status. This is a cornerstone of NPM framework and managerial accountability that lays emphasis on record keeping and quantitative data monitoring. This is despite the fact that the situation on the ground can be just the opposite.

Crucially, this shows the benefit of using the village-level AWC data. Although the credibility and quality of AWC data is low, it provides a near-reality picture of the status of child malnutrition in both the villages that was counter-intuitive to the official version in government records. In order to access trends in change in the grade of child nutrition, another set of time period were factored to compare the two villages - six months and one year (Figure 3.9).

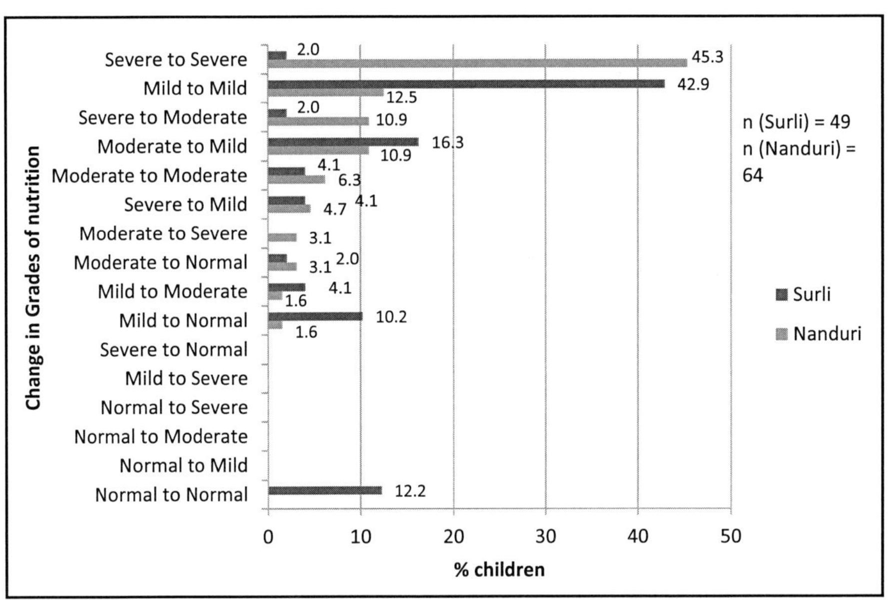

Figure 3.9: Change in Grade of Child Nutrition between Sixth Month and One Year

Source: Field level data compiled from AWC records and household survey (2012)

Between the time period of sixth month and one year, the situation in Surli somewhat improved or remained same. Conversely, the situation in Nanduri did not see much improvement. About 45.3% of children aged six months remained severely under-nourished in Nanduri, even after one year (Figure 3.9). In Surli too, about 42.9% children who were in mild category at six months remained in the category after one year. In terms of improvement, 16.3% and 10.2% children in Surli shifted from moderate malnutrition to mild and from mild malnutrition to normal. In Nanduri, this improvement was lower as compared to Surli with 10.9% children shifting from moderate malnutrition to mild and 4.7% from severe to mild malnutrition.

In both villages, there was a small percentage of children who deteriorated or remained under-nourished. In Surli, 4.1% slipped from mild to moderate, and in Nanduri 3.1% worsened from moderate to severe malnutrition. Therefore, in terms of rate of change in nutrition, children in Surli were nutritionally better off than those in Nanduri as their age progressed. The study did not factor in breastfeeding practices, which is known to play a role in child nutrition especially till six months to one year of a child's age. Hence this analysis is only meant to understand the nutrition status and its change among children in both study villages. However, it is also imperative to understand the socio-economic groups of children in various nutritional categories.

3.3.4 Asset Quintile and Malnutrition

Linkages between poverty and malnutrition are well documented. At the macro level, there is an inverse relationship between economic class and child malnutrition – higher the economic class, lower the rate of child malnutrition. Also, recent evidence shows that relative inequality in child malnutrition seems to be larger among wealth groups than social groups (Hari & Jose, 2015). Correlation tests like Phi & Cramer's V, Anova and Chi-Square was done to show possible correlation between households' consolidated asset value (a ratio variable) and nutrition grades (an ordinal variable), at a one-time period – for instance, at 18 months.

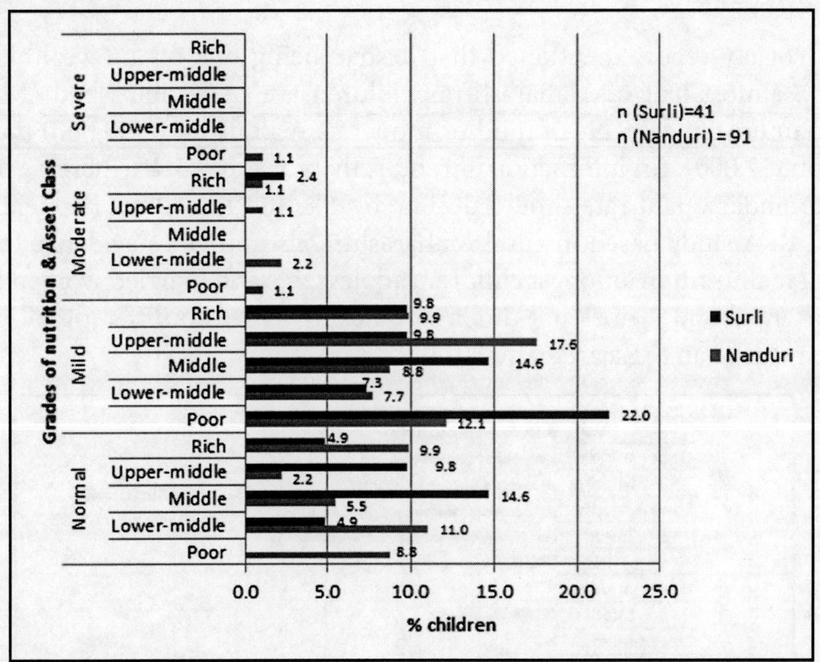

Figure 3.10: Grades of Nutrition among Children at Birth as per Asset Quintile

Source: Field level data compiled from AWC records and household survey (2012)

The tests values of 0.549 for Chi-square and 0.649 for Anova shows that this data does not support to carry out these tests. Gama test of correlation between households' asset quintile (an ordinal variable) and nutrition grade (an ordinal variable) at 18 months age was also carried out. The resultant value of -0.124 again revealed a negative or inverse relationship but not significant. Hence, only cross tabs between these variables were attempted for analysis in this section. Data from the study village also show that all asset categories, even the rich and upper middle had children with some form of malnutrition. The percentage of children under various grades of malnutrition, under each asset class, at birth and at one year, are compared in Figure 3.10 & Figure 3.11.

Of the children who were mildly under-nourished in the first month after birth, a majority of them (22%) were from poor asset quintile of Surli. In contrast, this was followed by 17.5% children from upper middle asset quintile in Nanduri and 14.6% children from middle asset quintile in Surli who had mild malnutrition in their first month. Surprisingly, about 9.8% of children who were mildly malnourished in first month were from the rich asset quintile, equally so in both villages. Of the percentage of children who were normal in the first month, a higher percentage were from the middle, upper middle, and rich asset quintiles in Surli, while in Nanduri, they were from lower middle and poor asset quintiles. For children who were moderately under-nourished in first month, 2.4% were from the rich asset quintile in Surli while 2.2% belonged to lower middle asset quintile in Nanduri. A similar observation has been reported in other independent studies.

A civil society report mentioned that despite being one of the wealthiest states in the country, almost half of Maharashtra's children are undernourished (Mishra et al., 2008). Also, more children die of mild or moderate malnutrition (33,000) than of severe malnutrition (12,000). An international trend is that for every 3-4% increase in per capita income, the underweight rate should decline by 1%. But this is not happening in India (Pawar, 2014). A study based in rural Maharashtra also provides evidence to this trend, that "overall malnutrition amongst children, adolescents and married women in the study area is substantial and it does not differ significantly between different socio-economic groups" (Parasuraman & Rajaretnam, 2011).

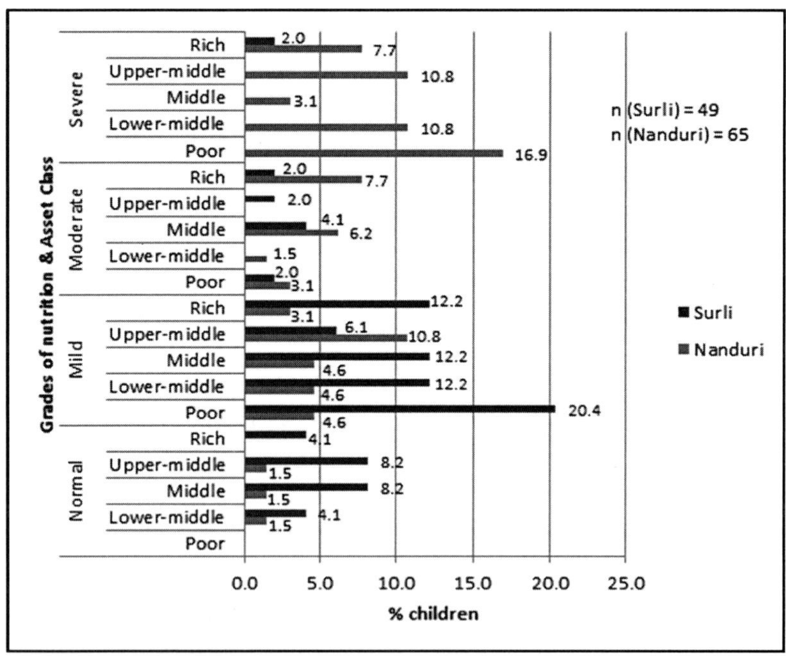

Figure 3.11: Grades of Nutrition among Children at One Year as per Asset Quintile

Source: Field level data compiled from AWC records and household survey (2012)

This data revealed that, at time of birth, malnutrition is not so significantly different among various asset quintiles, but more pronounced among the poor. There is a general consensus that there are factors other than social and economic that is responsible for child malnutrition, namely health and nutritional status of the mother, status of breastfeeding, medical interventions during pregnancy and after delivery, food security, water, and sanitation, etc. However, these factors are applicable to women from all asset categories, especially those from poor and lower middle class who are more vulnerable. And yet rich, upper middle and middle asset quintiles in both villages also had a substantial percentage of children who were mild malnourished. By the time children turn one year, the risk of malnutrition increases especially if weaning and solid food introduction is not appropriate. Figure 3.11 show that after one year, there was a distinct difference as well as a similarity in status of malnutrition among children of both villages.

The difference was that in Nanduri, there was a higher percentage of children in the severe malnutrition category, while the majority in Surli were either in the mild or normal category. The similarity was that these respective majorities had children belonging to all asset quintiles. The majority of children severely nourished in Nanduri belonged to all asset quintiles including the upper middle (10.8) and the rich (7.7%), but this was more pronounced for the poor (16.9%) and lower middle (10.8%) asset quintiles. In Surli too, a majority of children who were mildly under-nourished, were from all asset quintiles. Therefore, the nutritional status of children in Surli was better from that of children in Nanduri and it also improved over time. It shows that status of malnutrition does not vary significantly with asset quintiles but was starkly different in the two villages.

3.3.5 Social Category and Malnutrition

Literature has often cited strong linkages between social class and child malnutrition. Similar analysis was attempted here. Figure 3.12 shows cross-tab between percentage of children in various grades of nutrition and their socio-religious category, reported by the head of the household to which they belong. In both study villages, although percentage of Muslims & SCs was small, yet being a case study design, this analysis on social categories was attempted.

There were four socio-religious categories in both villages – General, Muslim, SC and OBC. The general group included all households except the SC, Muslims, or OBCs. In Surli, all children from Muslim households, 61.9% from the OBC category, and a marginally higher percentage (63.1%) from the general category were mildly under-nourished. In Nanduri, about 87.5% children from SC households, with similar percentages from OBC, Muslim and general, were in category of mild malnutrition (Figure 3.12). In the normal nutrition category, a higher percentage of children were from Nanduri than Surli. About 50% children from Muslim households; 42% from general category; 25% from OBC, and 12.5% from SC in Nanduri were normal in nutritional status at birth. However, Nanduri also had a higher percentage of children from OBC households (25%) in the moderate malnutrition category as compared to those in Surli. These observations point towards the fact that there was a substantial percentage of new-born children who were mildly undernourished in all social categories but this was more pronounced in SCs and Muslim. The change of status of malnutrition becomes visible if age of children is increased to 18 months or one-and-half years (Figure 3.13).

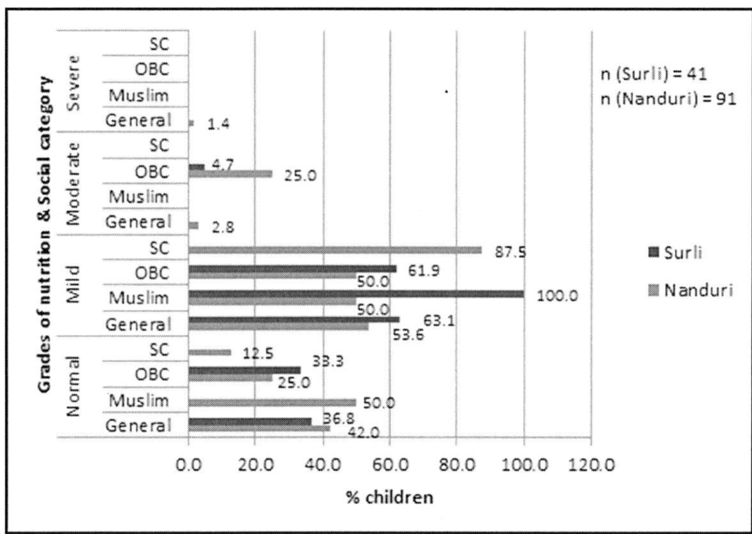

Figure 3.12: Grades of Nutrition among Children at Birth as per Socio-religious Category

Source: Field level data compiled from AWC records and household survey (2012)

For instance, children from OBC households who were mildly undernourished were 63.1% at birth, but at 18 months, this percentage came down to 56%. In Nanduri, the opposite happened where its children from normal category of all social groups deteriorated to mild, moderate, or even severe forms of malnutrition. In Nanduri, 50% of the children from OBC households and 40% from OBC households slipped to severe and moderate undernutrition, respectively.

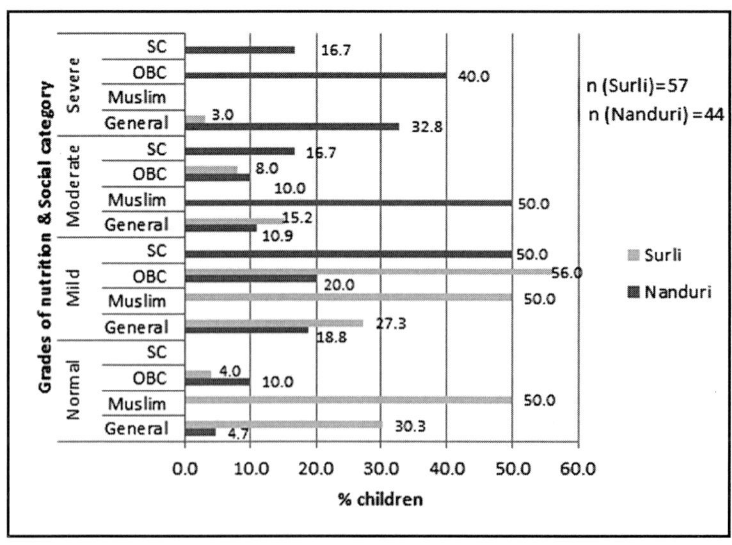

Figure 3.13: Grades of Nutrition among Children Aged 18 months as per Socio-religious Category

Source: Field level data compiled from AWC records and household survey (2012)

Furthermore, 50% children from SC households and 50% from Muslim households slipped to moderate and mild malnutrition, respectively. A substantial percentage of children from general category, constituting 32.8%, and 16.7% from SCs became severely under-nourished after 18 months in Nanduri. This data shows, in addition to economic factors (asset quintiles), child malnutrition did not vary significantly among caste but varied significantly between the two case villages.

3.4 Discussion and Conclusion

There are three main conclusions that can be drawn from these findings. First, as expected, a higher percentage of children were normal weight in first month after birth in Surli and that they did not deteriorate to severe forms of malnutrition. In addition, even if children in Surli did slip to some form of malnutrition, the situation had improved after 18 months. In Nanduri, soon after birth, many children drastically slipped to severe forms of malnutrition and over a period of time there were not much improvement but deterioration.

Second, child malnutrition was also seen among the affluent rich, upper middle and middle asset quintiles, although it was more pronounced among the poor. Data in the study also shows that child malnutrition did not vary significantly among asset quintiles or even among caste 'within' the villages but varied distinctly *between* the two villages.

Lastly, data also revealed that presence or absence of toilets in the premises of households as well as those in the AWCs seem to have little influence on rates of child malnutrition under aged two. Surli had 98.3% households with toilets in house premises together with functional toilet inside its AWC yet had a substantial percentage of children with some form of malnutrition at birth and at one year. Nanduri had more than 80% households without a toilet and also a substantial percentage of children were normal in first month after birth. Many experts believe that the mere presence of toilets may not guarantee their use by the households. This consequently explains its limited influence in tacking the issue of malnutrition.

This finding is also backed by a recent study that explored the relationship between sanitation and child health. A Study on Total Sanitation Campaign (TSC) in 80 villages of Madhya Pradesh show that TSC did increase the household level availability of sanitation facilities and to a lesser extent reduced open defecation. These improvements, however, were insufficient to improve child health outcomes (diarrhoea, parasite infections, anaemia and growth) (Patil et al., 2014; Asian Scientist Magazine, 2014). Findings from The Global Nutrition Report 2014 continue to zero down on sanitation as one of the most crucial and underlying determinants of malnutrition (Mishra, 2015). These findings, however, should not undermine the challenge of achieving large scale sanitation for public health.

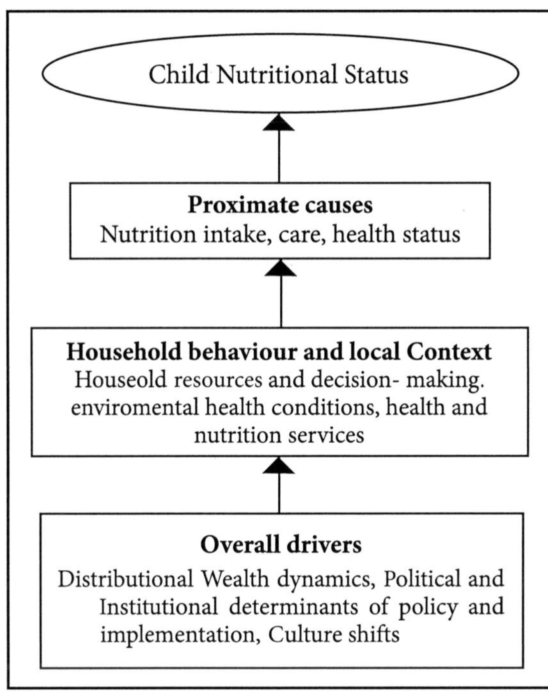

Figure 3.14: Factors Influencing Child Nutrition

Source: Walton, 2009

This study's observations on child malnutrition seem to question the mainstream logic that stunting, wasting, and underweight prevalence reduces as economic status or increased food security increases. Prasad (2010) in his article asks one of the basic question - is poverty alone causing malnutrition among Indian children. Citing NFHS-3 data using 'wealth index', Prasad cites that 19.7% children from richest households and 33.6% children from moderately rich households in India, are malnourished as well. Therefore, there is a disjuncture of nutrition with macro contextual development, economic class, and caste in the study villages. This is explained by Walton's paper showing an interplay of three causal factors that ensure good child nutrition outcomes (Figure 3.14). At the immediate level, the causal or proximate causes include nutritional intake, care, and status of mother. The second group of factors are household behaviour and the local context. Finally, the third factor are overall drivers like distributional wealth, culture, policy and institutional determinants (Walton, 2009).

According to Walton (2009), there is a break-down of causal chain determinants of child malnutrition. Here, a disjunction exists between prosperity and malnutrition. For instance, the behaviour of mothers (even those better off or educated) may be inconsistent with recommended practices. Rising wealth may have modest effect on food spending; while 80% may have access to AWC. Most however do not use it or despite access to safe drinking water only one third treat water to make it potable etc.

At the macro level too, there have been studies to support a disassociation between economic growth and child malnutrition. A study on association between economic growth and early childhood malnutrition, using 121 demographic and health surveys from 36 low-income and medium-income countries, provides evidence that there was "very small to null association seen between increase in per-head GDP and reductions in early childhood malnutrition" (Vollmer et al., 2014).

Another lead author of an India-specific study, Subramanian, argued that more than two-fifths of India's children are underweight and nearly half are stunted. This has not changed much since the early 1990s (Baragona, 2014). The study concluded that "the study failed to provide consistent evidence that economic growth leads to reduction in childhood malnutrition in India" (Subramanyam et al., 2011).

Evidence in this chapter for the village level (micro) clearly reveal that the AWC in Surli was well endowed with good infrastructure with its own building, water supply, toilet, etc. In addition, it was also a well-functional anganwadi that had children coming in and having hot cooked meals. It also conducted regular immunisation, weighing of the children, and distributed THR. Yet, Surli had almost equal proportion of its children under-two, like Nanduri, with some form of malnutrition at the time of birth. But, children in Surli did not slip to severe forms as they did in Nanduri. In fact, there were improvements in nutritional status over a period of time in Surli. The situation in Nanduri was poor to begin with and it further deteriorated. Also, these children who had moderate to severe forms of malnutrition in Nanduri included those from the upper-middle, rich asset quintile, and even those from the general category.

This finding reinforces the basic premise of this thesis that institutional factors, other than economic, social & developmental ones, influence child malnutrition outcomes. Malnutrition is not a dimension of current or future inequalities but is also causally related to unequal institutional structures (Walton, 2009). The question arises, what are those local institutional processes that can be attributed for the trend of child malnutrition witnessed in both study villages? The answer to these questions unfolds in the proceeding chapter on the nature of engagement between providers and users.

***

References

1. Allard, F., & Anderson, E. (2015). Ethnography - an overview. Retrieved 24 June 2020, from https://www.sciencedirect.com/topics/neuroscience/ethnography.
2. *Asian Scientist Magazine*. (2014, September 4). The mixed results of India's Total Sanitation Campaign. Retrieved September 10, 2014 from http://www.asianscientist.com.
3. Baragona, S. (2014, March 26). Rising wealth not enough to raise child health. *Voice of America*. Retrieved March 28, 2014 from http://www.voanews.com.

4. Census of India. (2011). *Chapter 5: Sex composition of Population (Provisional data)* (pp. 37–48). Census of India. Retrieved on February 11, 2014 from http://censusindia.gov.in.

5. Chowdhury, S. R. (2015, March 12). Children most neglected in the 2015-16 Union Budget: child rights organisations. Retrieved on March 18, 2015 from http://timesofindia.indiatimes.com.

6. Coffey, D., & Spears, D. (2017). Purity and pollution stand in the way of using loos. Retrieved 24 June 2020, from https://www.nationalheraldindia.com/book-extract/concepts-of-purity-and-pollution-come-in-the-way-of-using-loos

7. De, A., Sathyamala, C., Saxena, K. B., Kurian, N. J., & Priya, R. (2012). Public Report on Health. *Economic and Political Weekly*. 47(21), 43-54.

8. Dreze, J. (2006). Universalisation with quality: ICDS in a rights perspective. *Economic and Political Weekly*, *41*(34), 3706–3715.

9. Gupta, A. (2001). Governing population: the integrated child development services program in India. In Hansen, T. B., & Stepputat, F. (Eds.) *States of imagination: ethnographic explorations of the postcolonial state* (pp. 109-136). USA: Duke University Press.

10. Hari, K. S., & Jose, S. (2015). Progress in reducing child under nutrition. *Economic and Political Weekly*, *50*(3), 23–26.

11. IFPRI or International Food Policy Research Institute. (2014). Global Nutrition Report 2014: Actions and Accountability to Accelerate the World's Progress on Nutrition. Washington, DC.

12. Irigoyen, Claudia. (2017, August 25). India's Total Sanitation Campaign. Centre for Public Impact. https://www.centreforpublicimpact.org/case-study/total-sanitation-campaign-india.

13. Mishra, A. (2015, February 5). India is facing multiple burdens of malnutrition, says Global Nutrition Report. Business Today. Retrieved on February 12, 2015 from http://businesstoday.intoday.in.

14. Mishra, S., Duggal, R., Lingam, L., Pitre, A., Sardeshpande, N., & Shukla, A. (2008). *A report on health inequities in Maharashtra* (pp. 29). Retrieved on September 27, 2013 from http://works.bepress.com.

15. Mohanty, R., & Dwivedi, A. (2019). To What Extent does Culture Determine the Usage of Toilets by Urban Poor in India? | Centre for Policy Research. Retrieved 24 June 2020, from https://www.cprindia.org/news/8198.

16. Parasuraman, S., & Rajaretnam, T. (2011). Agriculture, food security and nutrition in Vidarbha: a household level analysis. *Economic and Political Weekly*, *46*(19), 42–50.

17. Patil, S. R., Arnold, B. F., Salvatore, A. L., Briceno, B., Ganguly, S., Colford, J. M., Jr, & Gertler, P. J. (2014). The Effect of India's total sanitation campaign on defecation behaviors and child health in rural Madhya Pradesh: a cluster randomized controlled trial. *PLoS Med*, *11*(8), e1001709.

18. Patil, V. (2013, April 12). Once among worst districts, Satara's sex ratio shows major rise. *Sakal Times.* Retrieved on July 15, 2014 from http://www.sakaaltimes.com.

19. Pawar, Y. (2014, March 16). Governments Rs 300-crore plan to tackle malnutrition in Maharashtra a waste of money: study. *Daily News & Analysis*. Retrieved on March 17, 2014 from http://www.dnaindia.com.

20. Prasad, C. Bhan. (2010, October 17). Why rich Indians are malnourished too. *Times of India*. Mumbai edition.

21. Rajmata Jijau Mother - Child Health and Nutrition Mission. (2010). Village Child Development Centers: The Concept. Retrieved on November 22, 2015 from http://nutritionmissionmah.gov.in.

22. Rizwanullah, S. (2012, June 19). Female feticide case: Beed doctor couple travelled 5 states to evade arrest. The Times of India. Retrieved on July 17, 2014 from http://timesofindia.indiatimes.com.

23. Sakal Times. (2011, June 3). Sex ratio improves in three districts. Retrieved on November 2, 2014 from http://www.sakaaltimes.com.

24. Sinha, S. (2006). Infant survival: A political challenge. *Economic and Political Weekly*, *41*(34), 3657–3660.

25. Subramanyam, M. A., Kawachi, I., Berkman, L. F., & Subramanian, S. V. (2011). Is economic growth associated with reduction in child under nutrition in India? *PLoS Med*, *8*(3), e1000424.

26. Vollmer, S., Harttgen, K., Subramanyam, M. A., Finlay, J., Klasen, S., & Subramanian, S. V. (2014). Association between economic growth and early childhood under nutrition: evidence from 121 demographic and health surveys from 36 low-income and middle-income countries. *The Lancet Global Health*, *2*(4), e225–e234.

27. Walton, M. (2009). The political economy of India's malnutrition puzzle. *IDS Bulletin*, *40*(4), 16–24.

CHAPTER 4

Providers and Users: Nature of Engagement

4.1 Introduction

In the context of public health services delivered by the state, accountability relationships exist between the provider and the user even if the user does not use the service. These accountability relationships operate within institutions of service delivery like the Integrated Child Development Services (ICDS) and erstwhile the National Rural Health Mission (NRHM). These programmes in turn are delivered through frontline organisations like Primary Health Centers (PHC), Anganwadi Center (AWC), private providers including formal and informal political system within the Panchayati Raj Institutions (PRIs).

These institutions affect 'choice' of the users in preferring one provider over other and these choices in turn influence performance of these service delivery systems (Global Development Network, 2009). Therefore, it is crucial to understand what choices users make to access women and child health services in different context, the reasons behind those choices, and finally how are these choices defining relationship between users and providers in context of a democracy like India and the rhetoric of accountability.

As per the conceptual framework of the study, accountability relationships manifest through interaction between the user and the provider and can be understood through the three components that constitute understanding accountability - engagement, answerability and sanctions (see Figure 2.7). This chapter deals with understanding the 'nature of engagement' between users and providers in terms of choice in access, level of trust and households' rating of services. The chapter aims to unpack the first objective of the study, which is to identify relationships of accountability existing between various actors at the frontline of public health service delivery and how these accountability relationships are enacted between various actors. Such an exercise is of particular interest in context of the two cases to see how the context impacts the nature of engagement.

The way respondents choose to access a health provider is the first step in understanding the extent of their engagement. Such choices can be the cause and also the result of the present nature of health and nutrition services. This interface is explored in this chapter. The common frontline health providers in rural India, mainly the anganwadi center (AWC), Primary Health Center (PHC) & sub-center, private doctor and local quack are the first point of contact of the population for primary health service delivery. Of these, anganwadi center and PHC are the institutional providers for maternal and child health services which forms the largest component of primary health care in rural India. In case of early childhood care and education (ECCE), ICDS is one of the main providers although there is a growing private sector of pre-schools, nurseries, and child day care centers in rural areas.

Mainstream literature points to a fact that a majority of rural population, including the poor choose private health providers over public health services. Problems of accessibility, lack of infrastructure, and personnel in public health system as a reason for people to choose private health. According to Kumar (2007), all indicators reveal lower reach and access to health services and care in rural areas than in urban areas. For instance, data from NFHS-III revealed that only 26 per cent of children with diarrhoea were given oral rehydration salt (ORS) and barely two-thirds (64 per cent) of children suffering from acute respiratory infection or fever were taken to a health facility (ibid.). Much of the analysis in the literature attributes such low access to poor supply side of public health services. NFHS data for instance, in itself, cannot explain if such low access is a problem of the poor demand, poor supply, or interplay of both (ibid.).

This chapter attempts to unpack not only why households choose to access a provider but also why they choose to reject others. It attempts to explain the reasons for those choices through understanding the nature of engagement between users and providers. Thus, the chapter aims to provide enough evidence to accept or reject the mainstream literature's argument of poor access of public health services among the rural poor.

The chapter is organised into four main sections. The first section provides an overview of policy and programme mandate of both ICDS and NRHM and the areas they converge towards maternal and child health outcomes. This is followed by an analysis of household's choice of various providers to access maternal and child health services. To unearth the reasons for such choices, the following section gives a glimpse of how households rate providers and the reasons for the same. Finally, the last section describes the resultant nature of relationship between the providers and the users that have a direct bearing in shaping accountability relationships between them. This leads to an understanding of the reasons behind households' choices in accessing frontline providers.

The chapter concludes by summing up significant findings in consonance with the study objectives.

4.2 Entitled Services

4.2.1 Current practice

Under ICDS[1], the AWC offer a package of services in an integrated manner converging with the PHC services. The range of health services available, their target group, and service provider are mentioned in Table 4.1.

Table 4.1: Package of Services Provided by Anganwadi centres under ICDS scheme

Services	*Target Group*	*Service Provided by*
Supplementary Nutrition	Children below 6 years including under-nourished children; Pregnant women & Lactating mothers, Adolescent girls	Anganwadi Worker and Anganwadi Helper
Immunization*	Children below 6 years; Pregnant & Lactating Mother	ANM/MO
Health Check-up*	Children below 6 years; Pregnant & Lactating Mother	ANM/MO/AWW
Referral Services*	Children below 6 years; Pregnant & Lactating Mother	AWW/ANM/MO
Pre-School Education	Children 3-6 years	AWW
Nutrition & Health Education*	Women (15-45 years)	AWW/ANM/MO

Note: * Services are delivered through public health infrastructure under the Ministry of Health & Family Welfare.
Source: http://wcd.nic.in/icds, 2012.

ICDS is by far the biggest community-based nutrition supplementation programme in India. If Right to Food is also integrated in the programme, it will become one of the largest rights-based, community-based comprehensive nutrition programmes of the world. However, currently household level food security is not guaranteed under ICDS which is often critiqued by experts as one of its weakest points. One of the major components of ICDS is the supplementary nutrition programme (SNP), which is delivered in two modes as per the type of beneficiary. Four target groups namely, young children aged 6 months to 3 years; children with any form of malnutrition below age 6; pregnant or lactating mothers and adolescent girls are given Take-Home-Rations (THR) (see Figure 4.1).

1 The ICDS is estimated to be the world's largest integrated early childhood program, with over 40,000 centres established nationwide. The program covers over 4.8 million expectant and nursing mothers and over 23 million children under the age of six. Of these children, more than half participate in early learning activities. The network consists of 3907 projects, covering nearly 70 per cent of the country's community development blocks and 260 urban slum pockets (Awofeso & Rammohan, 2011)

The THR was envisaged as a nutritious[2] pre-mix that can be cooked into a hot snack, convenient to the developmental needs of young children, mothers, and adolescent girls in the comfort of their homes. THR in study villages includes packaged savoury and sweet pre-mixes like *upma* (savoury semolina), *sheera* (sweet cracked wheat), *sattu* (gram flour) and *upeeth* (a flour mix) that require few minutes of cooking time to turn into hot snacks. The THR is primarily cereal and pulse mix, flavoured with condiments and spices and artificially fortified with nutrients. It is distributed to the beneficiaries once or twice a month for which they do not have to come to the centre on an everyday basis.

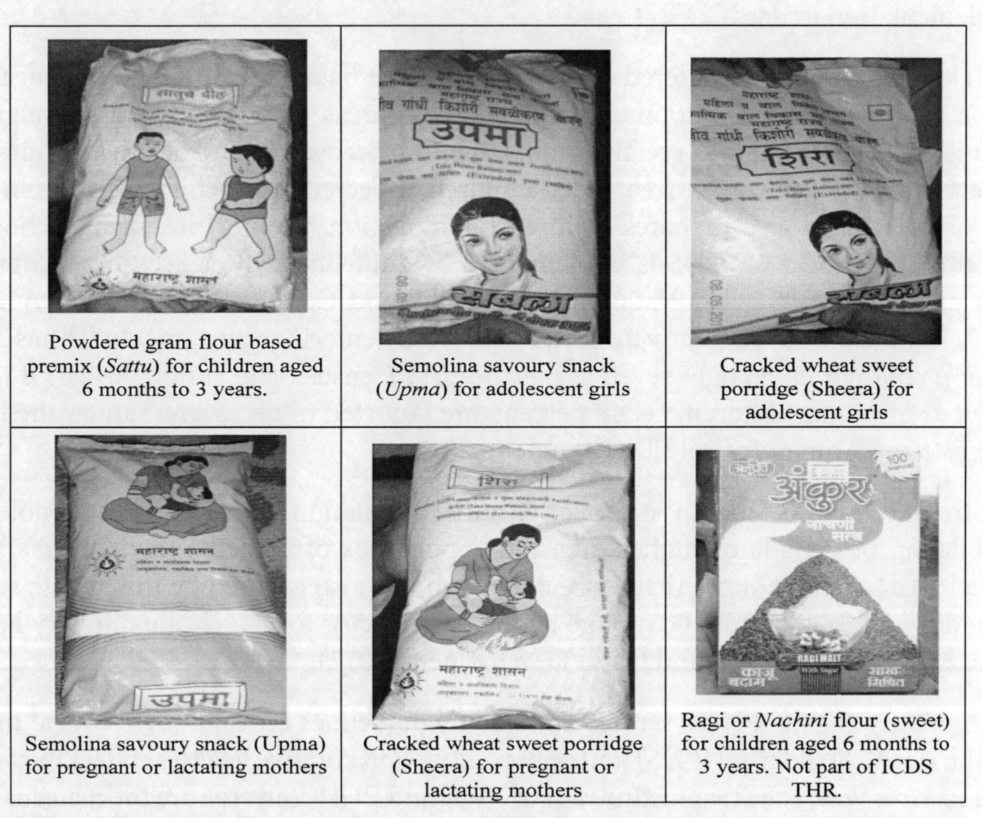

Powdered gram flour based premix (*Sattu*) for children aged 6 months to 3 years.

Semolina savoury snack (*Upma*) for adolescent girls

Cracked wheat sweet porridge (Sheera) for adolescent girls

Semolina savoury snack (Upma) for pregnant or lactating mothers

Cracked wheat sweet porridge (Sheera) for pregnant or lactating mothers

Ragi or *Nachini* flour (sweet) for children aged 6 months to 3 years. Not part of ICDS THR.

Figure 4.1: ICDS Take Home Ration (THR) & Weaning Foods in Maharashtra

Source: Author's fieldwork in Satara and Osmanabad, 2012.

2 Nutritious foods for children under six, comprise of 5 categories of foods – a. fruits and vegetables; b. pulses and sprouts; c. millets and cereals; d. nuts and oilseeds; e. dried fruits and jaggery. These foods that are largely plant based are also regional, seasonal, local and low cost, rich in macro and micro-nutrients. However in ICDS, the emphasis has largely been on cereal-pulse mixes or millet-based mixes only, which has often been critiqued because of absence of micro-nutrients sourced from fruits and vegetables. Food from animal sources like eggs, milk & milk products are also prevalent in community based nutrition programmes like Mid-Day Meals and are often lobbied by their respective industries.

Older children aged three to six are given freshly-cooked hot meals at the anganwadi centre as they attend pre-school education (PSE). The PSE is non-formal pre-school education for children between three to six years, intended to be imparted through play-way methods that use aids like pictures or charts, songs and rhymes, stories, art & craft, role play etc. During the PSE session, children are provided with a meal that usually includes cereal-pulse mixes like *khichadi* (rice-pulse porridge), *vatana-rice* (dried pea curry with rice), *moong-rice* (green moong curry with rice), *kheer* (sweetened milk and rice) or *sheera*. The PSE component also includes recording the weight and height of all registered children and plotting these values on growth charts, separately for girls and boys, to ascertain their nutritional status. This has been the official version of programme implementation under ICDS.

The PSE component offered by the AWCs is the backbone of ICDS. It is meant to enhance growth and development of children in areas of physical, motor, language, cognitive, socio-emotional, creative and aesthetic appreciation, and health and nutrition aspects. PSE is known to free older children especially girl child from child-care responsibility and also prepares children for transition to enter the formal schooling system. This aspect of ICDS is implemented by guidelines which are now recognised as a national policy called National Early Childhood Care & Education Policy Draft 2012, in wake of the large private sector and NGOs entering the scene. India has 158.7 million children under ages seven as per the 2011 Census (The Hindu 2012). Of these, about 75.7 million children, i.e. 48 percent, are reported to be covered under the ICDS (Ministry of Women & Child Development, 2012).

To put this statistic in perspective, this population is more than double the population of Canada or higher than the populations of United Kingdom or France. Broad estimations indicate that a sizeable number is also covered by the private sector, in addition to some limited coverage by the NGO sector for which the ministry has no data (Ministry of Women and Child Development, 2012).

Similarly, for the PHCs, service and quality guidelines are laid down by the Indian Public Health Standards (IPHS) for the preventive and curative health services they offer. The services where the two institutions of AWC and PHC converge are the maternal and child health services that include ante-natal check-ups, referrals, post-natal care, new-born care, immunisation, child health and nutrition, family welfare and nutrition, and health education for the mothers.

As per the IPHS guidelines, PHCs are supposed to provide the following 'essential'[3] services in close synergy with the ICDS anganwadi centers (Box 4.1). Therefore, both ICDS and NRHM programmes have policy guidelines and implementation standards in place to ensure universal and standardised maternal and child health and nutrition

3 'Essential' services mean 'Minimum Assured Services' which PHCs are envisaged to provide. There are services which are indicated as 'Desirable', that PHCs should aspire to achieve (Directorate General of Health Services, Ministry of Health & Family Welfare, 2012)

services. In order to understand practices of accountability in service delivery, the first step was to understand the nature of engagement between providers and users.

Box 4.1: Essential package of Health Services required to be delivered by PHCs

- Antenatal check-ups of pregnant women and nutritional counselling.
- Emergency care of sick children including Integrated Management of Neonatal and Childhood Illnesses (IMNCI) strategy. Prompt referral of sick children requiring specialist care.
- Counselling to mothers on exclusive breast-feeding for six months and appropriate and adequate complementary feeding from six months onwards while continuing breastfeeding.
- Assess the growth and development of the infants and under-five children and make timely referral.
- Full immunization of all infants and children against vaccine preventable diseases. Tracking of vaccination dropouts.
- Vitamin A prophylaxis to the children as per national guidelines.
- Prevention and control of routine childhood diseases, infections like diarrhoea, pneumonia and anaemia, etc.
- Diagnosis of and nutrition advice to malnourished children, pregnant women and others. Management of severe acute malnutrition cases and referral of serious cases after initiation of treatment as per facility based guidelines.

Source: Directorate General of Health Services, Ministry of Health & Family Welfare, 2012

4.2.2 Ground Zero Situation

The state of child nutrition outcomes in India however makes even these well-laid entitlements read well, only on paper. There is little local, national, and international reports, as well as papers and studies to show what is not working in ICDS, including the grim situation of child malnutrition in the country. Some well-quoted studies like FOCUS (2006) do report at the national level, and numerous civil society groups and independent authors have continuously pointed enough number of issues of what is not right with ICDS since its inception in 1970s. At the international level, Lancet's writings of child malnutrition have analysed all possible dimensions of this complex issue that is faced not only by India but many developing countries too (The Lancet 2008, 2012). There is a global movement gathering force to end hunger and malnutrition – reflected in the call for a single, standalone food security and nutrition goal in the post-2015 sustainable development agenda and in the United Nations (UN) system's mobilisation behind the Zero Hunger Challenge (Sundaram & Rawal, 2014).

In Maharashtra, there have been numerous challenges and issues associated with the SNP which have been under heavy policy critique and focus since the last decade, owing to growing malnutrition in the state. A study by Support for Advocacy and Training to Health Initiatives (SATHI) found that THR's use and efficacy claims were falsified as the food has barely any nutritional value (Pawar, 2014). As per a newspaper report, even the state government is aware of the problem. The principal secretary of Women and Child Development Department of the Maharashtra government admitted in an interview that there have been several complaints about the quality of THR food (ibid.). Tragically, the government's mid-term correction strategy has been as ineffective as the measure itself. By decentralising the process of making these packets at the local *tehsil* (block) level or asking district collectors to monitor, the production has failed to ensure quality and acceptance of the product with rural households. This is because of a simple reason that the problem is of acceptance and appropriateness first, and then of quality. More qualitative reasons for non-acceptance of THR are mentioned later in the chapter.

The latest report on child malnutrition for Maharashtra was the Comprehensive Nutrition Survey of Maharashtra 2012 by the NRHM Maharashtra and Rajmata Jijau Mission in partnership with UNICEF focusing on children under two years and their mothers. Many studies that have studied governance of the ICDS and NRHM schemes, cite issues of the lack of convergences between nutrition (implemented by Ministry of Women & Child Development) and health (implemented by Ministry of Health & Family Welfare). They also cite inadequate incentives of frontline workers and the lack of public action behind their deficient performance. Sinha (2006) argues that the ICDS needs to become a site for contesting power and demanding rights.

However, a recommendation becomes nothing more than a wish list when juxtaposed against the fact that nutrition and health issues are, politically, the least important or talked about, starting from the village level gram panchayat to even the Parliament. In fact, the quantum of such studies has systematically given the state enough reasons to roll back support. These include reduction in priority and funding, as well as arguments made that there is a decline in access and use of services by the poor, without drastic improvements in health outcomes, especially in a scheme like ICDS.

The Government of India has already decided to implement ICDS into a 'Mission Mode' since the state realizes that the scheme has failed to reduce malnutrition. Therefore ICDS Mission Mode's recommendations are a case in point. Such a scenario is leading to backdoor entry of multinational corporations and the packaged food industry into these schemes (Ray, 2014; Sharma, 2014; Deccan Herald, 2015; Gupta, 2012). For example, three private firms were meant to be excluded from a new Rs 560-crore tender for supplying anganwadi take-home rations. But they won the contracts anyway (Johari, 2020).

4.3 Choice of Providers

Engagement between users and providers can be studied through the concept of 'choice', as per the conceptual framework of the study (Figure 2.7). Owing to the proliferation of the private health sector, users exercise choice in approaching frontline health providers, even in rural areas. Choice in turn can be studied from how households are accessing frontline providers. Common frontline health providers in rural areas are anganwadi center, PHC, rural hospital, private doctors, doctors from alternative systems of medicine like ayurvedic doctors, and finally unqualified village quacks. The rural hospital forms the secondary level of health service delivery, yet it was included here as many respondents accessed RH directly, with or without a referral.

4.3.1 Access to services

Literature points to the fact that throughout the world, the poor experience obstacles – both fiscal constraints and a combination of elite capture and bias – that limit them from fully benefitting capability enhancing services like education and health care that is provided by the state (Goetz & Jenkins, 2005). The capture of service delivery is most common through staff absenteeism where doctors, nurses, and teachers collect their public sector salaries and then moonlight during clinic and school hours (ibid.). In order to understand the nature of these impediments in this study, it is first important to know the extent of access.

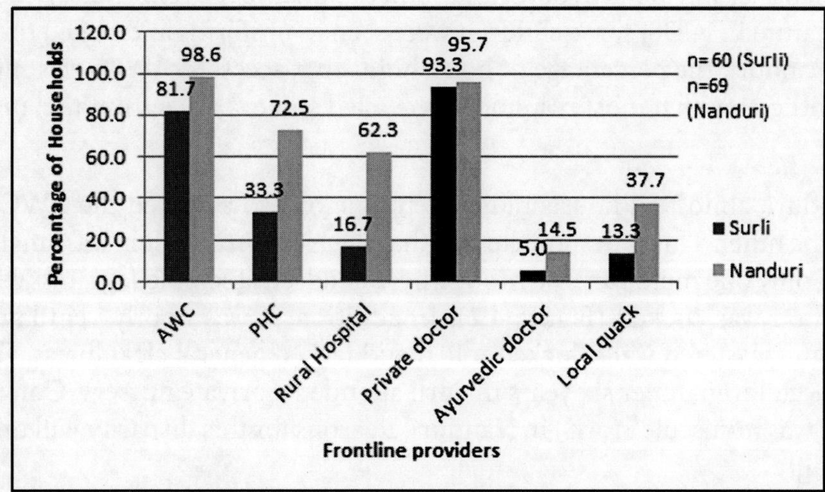

Figure 4.2: Access to Frontline Providers for Maternal and Child Health Services

Note: Access to providers during last episode of illness / pregnancy. One household may have accessed more than one provider for a health issue. Example for ANC check-ups, the pregnant women visit the AWC for check-ups and also visit the private hospital for sonography tests.

Source: Field data, 2012

Users access public health providers for maternal and child health (MCH) services in addition to services for general population. These services include out-patient treatments for snake or dog/snake/scorpion bites, common ailments like cold and fever, as well as communicable diseases like tuberculosis, malaria, and dengue. During household interviews, respondents - the head of the household and mother – were jointly asked if they had accessed common health care providers for women or children in their family during the last episode of illness, in the last six months. (Figure 4.2). The rationale behind the question was to understand how the users engage with various frontline health providers especially when they are located within an accessible distance from government-run PHC. Surli village was 3.5 km away from Wathar Kiroli PHC and Nanduri was 7 km away from Mangrol PHC, but there was a common accessibility factor for both the villages. A busy, well-maintained tar road connected both villages to their respective PHCs, with state buses and private vehicles plying between them. The result of this question was not devoid of surprises (Figure 4.2).

An anganwadi centre is the foremost institution for maternal and child health services at the village level. In the previous chapter, there was already an evidence to show that a higher percentage of children were not accessing AWC in Surli as compared to those in Nanduri. The trend is reaffirmed here too. About 81.7% households in Surli accessed AWC at least once, which meant that a sizeable number of households (19%) did not access any service of the anganwadi, even once. To note, AWC in Surli had a toilet, hand washing area, and a separate area for cooking inside its building (Figure 4.3). The looks of the centres were neat, and they were beautifully decorated with children's crafts, wall art, picture charts, and pictures of regional and national social reformers. Although not a desirable feature in ICDS, some children were seen in uniforms and seated on chairs and tables. In Nanduri, the percentage of households that accessed AWCs was much higher at 98.6%, indicating that most respondents availed some service from the anganwadi at least once.

In Nanduri, almost all households except one or two accessed the AWCs for some service or the other. This is despite the fact that the AWC in Nanduri was smaller in floor space, with only one multipurpose room where children assembled, grains were stacked, and even food was cooked (Figure 4.2). In addition, it was poorly ventilated with no electricity, un-plastered walls, locked toilet, and lacked general cleanliness. On average, almost 15% children under six years in Surli attended a private nursery. Conversely, this percentage was miniscule (1.4%) in Nanduri. Reasons for this disparity will unfold as the chapter progress.

Access to PHC was again low at 33.3% in Surli, while the same was 72.5% in Nanduri. It is interesting to note here that Surli was located merely 3.5 km from its PHC at Wathar which was once a PHC that ran 24 hours a day, seven times a week. At the time of this survey, this PHC did was not open all the time. Nonetheless it had the proven potential of offering all essential and desirable health services. In addition, according to health functionaries, this PHC at Wathar had won an award for the third best PHC in the state, as per the Indian Public Health Standards (IPHS) in 2010. Although both village PHCs had a full time Medical Officer, the one in Wathar, whose MO was staying at staff quarters in the PHC premises, had been working there for more than three years when the survey took place. Despite such favourable conditions, a majority of the households in Surli did not visit the PHC. According to the literature, it is well established that proximity of services to the poorest quintile has a significant impact on their utilisation of services. In Bangladesh, for example, the presence of a health centre in close proximity to a village is associated with the reduction of underweight children in that village, with a disproportionate positive effect on the poorest quintile (Joshi, 2006; The World Bank, 2004). However, this does not seem to have a positive impact on child malnutrition rates in Surli, despite having most of the favourable conditions of a nearby PHC with presence of doctors and staff, a well-functioning AWC, and the presence of toilets.

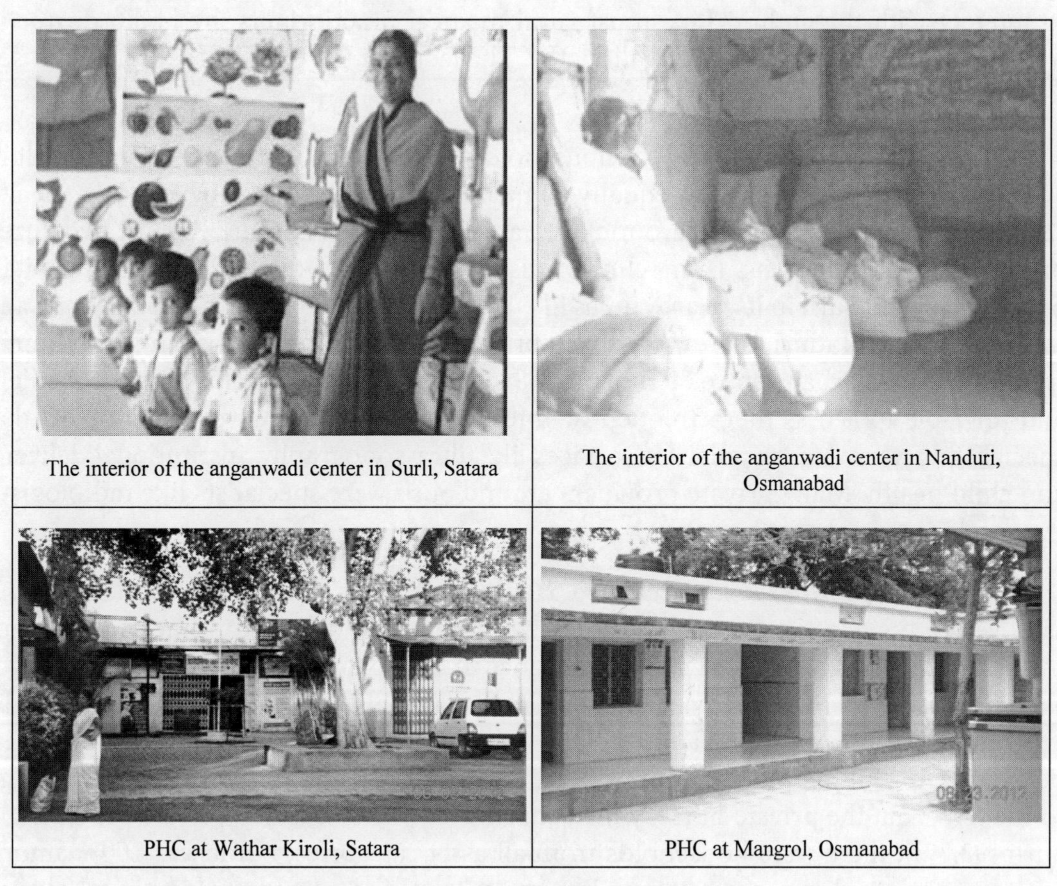

The interior of the anganwadi center in Surli, Satara

The interior of the anganwadi center in Nanduri, Osmanabad

PHC at Wathar Kiroli, Satara

PHC at Mangrol, Osmanabad

Figure 4.3: AWCs and PHCs in Satara and Osmanabad, 2012

Source: From author's fieldwork

In comparison, Mangrol PHC was further away from Nanduri and was not so endowed or acclaimed as the Wathar PHC. Yet, a higher percentage of households in Nanduri accessed the PHC as compared to Surli. The reason for this trend is found in the nature and spread of the private sector development around both the villages. This finding also raises questions on the common argument in health policy circles which attribute persistent poor health outcomes in rural areas to inadequate access, ailing infrastructure, and lack of doctors in government health facilities. The aspect is probed further in the qualitative analysis.

A high percentage of households in Nanduri reportedly visited rural hospital or civil hospital (62.3%), while it was quite low for Surli at 16.7% (Figure 4.3). Both the villages reported low access to ayurvedic doctors (5%) while Nanduri had a higher percentage of those visiting local village quacks[4] (37.7%) as compared to Surli (13.3%). Both Surli and Nanduri had two village quacks each. Of these four, only one from Surli agreed to interact with the author. Like most rural medical practitioners, he had a degree in homeopathy, but he had practiced allopathy. The fact that the other three simply refused to meet the author.

In both villages, the majority of households, 93.3% in Surli and 95.7% in Nanduri, accessed private doctors, as it is equally comparable to the trend in urban areas. Health services were highly privatized around Surli as compared to Nanduri. Almost two dozen private providers ranging from clinics, dispensaries, nursing homes, and hospitals operated around Surli in its nearby areas like Wathar, Rahimatpur, Koregaon, Karad, and Satara city. For Nanduri, there were seven private doctors running their nursing homes from the nearest urban centre of Tuljapur, 18 km from Nanduri, making it inconvenient and unviable to access them frequently. Interviews from HH surveys also reveal that specialist doctors were popular for services like ultra-sonography, institutional delivery, and child health. Many private providers around Surli were specialists like radiologists, gynaecologists, and paediatricians.

Economic Quintiles and Access to Health Providers. For the respondents who said 'yes' to the question on whether they had visited any of the frontline providers for maternal and child health services at least once in last six months, their asset category is shown in Table 4.2. A majority of the households from all asset categories, including the rich, used AWC services in Nanduri. This was not the case in Surli where a substantial percentage of children (20%) from middle, upper middle, and rich categories do not go to the AWC but the private nursery instead. Of those who accessed private providers in Surli (93.3%), there were households from all asset categories, but it was 100% among both the poor and rich asset categories. In contrast, the percentage of households in lower middle and middle asset categories were comparatively less.

Clearly, the private sector is accessed even by the poor asset categories, despite there being an accessible and well-functioning PHC near the village. Of those who accessed PHC (at least once) in Surli (33.3%), the poor and lower middle asset categories were

4 Village Quack is a name coined by mainstream allopathic practitioners to a person who is not a registered medical practitioner (RMP) and yet dispenses allopathic medicines. The term refers to a self-proclaimed doctor who does not have an MBBS degree but practices allopathy illegally, without a licence.

among the majority (85.7% & 50%). Conversely, the middle, upper middle and rich asset quintile households were within 20%. As evident, PHC was preferred only by a miniscule number, and was 'not' the choice for a large majority of the households, including the poor, middle, and rich asset categories.

Table 4.2: Asset Quintile of Households that Accessed Frontline Providers

Study Village	*Asset Category*	*Total HH in village*	*Anganwadi Centre*		*PHC*		*Private Hospital*	
		Count	Count	%	Count	%	Count	%
Surli	Poor	7	7	100.0	6	85.7	7	100.0
	Lower Middle	12	8	66.7	6	50.0	9	75.0
	Middle	21	18	85.7	4	19.0	20	95.2
	Upper Middle	10	8	80.0	2	20.0	10	100.0
	Rich	10	8	80.0	2	20.0	10	100.0
	Total	60	49	81.7	20	33.3	56	93.3
Nanduri	Poor	17	17	100.0	14	82.4	16	94.1
	Lower Middle	15	15	100.0	11	73.3	14	93.3
	Middle	19	19	100.0	15	78.9	19	100.0
	Upper Middle	13	12	92.3	8	61.5	13	100.0
	Rich	5	5	100.0	2	40.0	4	80.0
	Total	69	68	98.6	50	72.5	66	95.7

Note: Access to providers since last episode of illness.
Source: Data from fieldwork

Possible reasons for this trend were revealed in in-depth interviews with frontline providers like medical officers and ANMs. The frontline providers were asked about the high use of private services for maternal and child health despite easy access to the PHC. Childbirth and delivery constitute a major chunk of maternal and child health services offered by the public health system through its PHCs. Despite this, a majority of the poor choose private health providers for child delivery. However, at-risk deliveries, usually involving C-section, are referred to government civil hospitals. This is because both PHCs and its sub-centres have neither a mandate nor are equipped to conduct C-section operations. An ANM mentioned that,

> *'We cannot tell a delivery patient in advance if it will be a normal delivery or a C-section. What we do tell them is that if you come to us, we will ensure a safe and normal delivery. We cannot do anything further. If our sahib (a respectful term like sir, meaning Medical Officer) feels that the patient is at risk, he refers them to the civil hospital. Most of the time, the civil hospital is far from village and is in the city. Also, if there is an operation delivery, the family has to stay there for 10 days. So, people see the distance, time, and travelling costs of coming and going from the hospital. It becomes expensive and tough to*

sustain, especially for a poor family. So, they prefer a nearby private hospital for delivery.' – ANM, Surli

Besides the economic reasons, there were social reasons to explain this trend. A Medical Officer shared his views,

'I have spoken to many people in the village who know that PHC services are free and good. Yet, they have a mindset that they associate PHC with status. They feel it is below their status to use government facilities. The cause behind this mindset is the following. For deliveries, the trend in Maharashtra is that most women go to their mother's house for delivery. The family finds that if they come to the PHC for delivery, the in-laws may ridicule them as being stingy. Although they know that they will get good service here, that doctors are available, and staff is friendly, there is a pressure from the in-laws. The people think that there is uncertainty during child delivery till the last minute and in the medical field no one knows what would happen after one minute. God forbids if something happens. The family fears that in-laws would mud-sling them and say that in order to save money, the girl's parents went to the PHC. That is why even the poor go for the private facility, especially if it is the first delivery of the woman. They do not want to take the chance.' - Medical Officer, Wathar PHC

Clearly the argument that 'supply' is a problem in public health service delivery is questionable, for which there is unmistakable evidence in this study. Despite the well-functional PHC, that is accessible and has availability of doctors, paramedical staff, and medicine, users in Surli still choose private health providers. An ASHA had a different take on this and believed that there is a positive change towards public facilities. She said,

'In the last few years since ASHA has been actively working in the village, there has been a visible change. From this year, almost 28 deliveries happened in government hospitals while only five were in private. Home deliveries have also reduced because of ASHA's work in the village. Now even the ambulance van comes to the doorstep of the house in the village to ferry the pregnant woman. Since the time this ambulance scheme has come, people are opting for public hospital. Patients have started benefitting. So, the number of people going to private facilities has reduced and many people have started accessing government facilities.' – ASHA, Surli

In Nanduri, the trend was similar where majority of households in all asset categories accessed private providers, but all middle and upper middle households also accessed PHC at least once. Also, the trend of who was accessing various health providers was a bit different. Of those who accessed PHC services (72.5%) in Nanduri, a majority of households from all the asset categories accessed its services. However, here too, like

Surli, the utilisation among the poor, lower middle, and middle asset categories were above 70%, while the upper middle and rich were at 61.5% and 40% respectively.

As compared to Surli, Nanduri had a higher percentage of the middle, upper middle, and rich asset categories accessing PHC at least once. This was despite the fact that the PHC was further away in distance from Nanduri. As mentioned earlier, the negligible or miniscule presence of private health providers in the vicinity of Nanduri can also be the reason for why even the affluent visited the PHC, while the same categories in Surli opted for private health providers. Secondly, Nanduri was equidistant from another PHC in the adjoining village of Katgaon. Katgaon PHC was again one that was awarded the best PHC in Maharashtra in 2009.

4.3.2 Access to Maternal and Child Health Services

There was also a need to also understand how households were accessing specific maternal and child health services with the frontline providers. Households were asked which provider they accessed for each of the given maternal and child health services since last childbirth (Table 4.3). Answers were categorised into four categories – Public, Private, Both and None. 'Public' category included all the institutions that are funded by the State like the AWC, PHC, rural hospital, civil or district hospital, and municipal hospital. Category of 'private' included all for-profit providers like nursing homes, dispensaries, doctors, private hospitals, and even quacks. Category of 'both' included access to both public and private health providers for certain services like antenatal care where a pregnant woman visits a private clinic for sonography tests and also visit anganwadi center for immunisation and IFA tablets. The category of none included neither public nor private, in case like childbirth at home.

Results show that most of the preventive public health services like birth registration, immunisation, water quality management, ECCE (Early childhood Care & Education) and family planning operations are dominated by the public providers in both Surli and Nanduri. The ECCE is primarily a service provided by the anganwadis under ICDS that includes supplementary nutrition, growth monitoring, pre-school education, medical check-ups and referrals. In Surli, a majority of the households send their children aged between three to six years to the anganwadis (73.3%). This percentage was much lower at 59.4% in Nanduri. This finding seems to be in contrast with an earlier one which pegged percentage of households accessing AWC services to be higher in Nanduri as compared to that in Surli (Figure 4.2).

On closer analysis, there was no discrepancy since earlier figure was for all beneficiaries like mothers and children combined, and for all services of AWC. This figure is only for children who are either given THR or who come for pre-school education. As compared to Surli, there was a higher percentage of households in Nanduri that use some services of the AWC (mainly by women). Many however, do not send their children under six years to the AWC on a regular basis.

Table 4.3: Households' Choice of Frontline Providers

Village	*Health services used*	*Public*		*Private*		*Both*		*None*		*Total*	
		n	%	n	%	n	%	n	%	n	%
Surli	Ante Natal Check-ups	8	13.3	14	23.3	38	63.3	0	0.0	60	100.0
	Birth registration	60	100.0	0	0.0	0	0.0	0	0.0	60	100.0
	Delivery	14	23.3	44	73.3	0	0.0	2	3.3	60	100.0
	Family planning services	17	28.3	9	15.0	0	0.0	34	56.7	60	100.0
	Immunisation	53	88.3	4	6.7	3	5.0	0	0.0	60	100.0
	Post-natal & breastfeeding	19	31.7	22	36.7	10	16.7	9	15.0	60	100.0
	Post-partum home visit by ANM	22	36.7	0	0.0	1	1.7	37	61.7	60	100.0
	Treatment of childhood diseases	12	20.0	35	58.3	12	20.0	1	1.7	60	100.0
	ECCE (Early childhood care & education) Prevention of malnutrition	44	73.3	8	13.3	0	0.0	8	13.3	60	100.0
	Water quality monitoring promotion of sanitation	47	78.3	0	0.0	0	0.0	13	21.7	60	100.0
Nanduri	Ante Natal Check-ups	14	20.3	9	13.0	45	65.2	1	1.4	69	100.0
	Birth registration	69	100.0	0	0.0	0	0.0	0	0.0	69	100.0
	Delivery	29	42.0	29	42.0	0	0.0	11	15.9	69	100.0
	Family planning services	21	30.4	5	7.2	0	0.0	43	62.3	69	100.0
	Immunisation	64	92.8	0	0.0	5	7.2	0	0.0	69	100.0
	Post-natal & breastfeeding	31	44.9	11	15.9	9	13.0	18	26.1	69	100.0
	Post-partum home visit by ANM	39	56.5	0	0.0	0	0.0	30	43.5	69	100.0
	Treatment of childhood diseases	11	15.9	37	53.6	18	26.1	3	4.3	69	100.0
	ECCE (Early childhood care & education) Prevention of malnutrition	41	59.4	4	16.7	0	0.0	24	34.8	69	100.0
	Water quality monitoring promotion of sanitation	50	72.5	0	0.0	0	0.0	19	27.5	69	100.0

Note: n means count. Access to providers considered last illness and/or childbirth.
Source: Data from fieldwork.

Antenatal check-ups (ANC) form a major service provided under maternal and child health under the public health system. In both the villages, women reported to visit both public and private providers for ANC, constituting 63.3% in Surli and 65.2% in Nanduri (Table 4.3). Private providers were the choice for delivery and childhood diseases which forms the main component of public primary health services. A higher percentage of households (63.3%) in Surli opted for private providers for conducting delivery, as compared to that in Nanduri (42.0%) where an equal percentage of women delivered in public and a high percentage still delivered at home (15.9%). In addition, more than half the households in Surli (58.3%) and Nanduri (53.6%) accessed private providers for treatment of childhood diseases. Reasons given by households were extensive, but the main one was that the PHC does not keep medicine that are child-friendly, in the form of liquid syrups or chewable tables. A Medical Officer of a PHC gave another explanation for this trend,

> *'Our PHC is halfway to Tuljapur which is a taluka headquarters and has its district hospital. Why would a patient come to a medical officer in this PHC when there are specialist doctors like paediatricians, gynaecologists, and anaesthetist available at private hospitals in Tuljapur? There is a direct bus to Tuljapur, so people prefer to go to Tuljapur than come here.' - Medical Officer, Mangrol PHC*

There were two services where the majority of households in both the village did not access either public or private providers. These were home visits and family planning operations. Under the NRHM guidelines, a health worker, usually the ANM, is supposed conduct home visits for the lactating mother a couple of times in the first three months. However, the majority of households in Surli (61.7%) and 43.5% in Nanduri responded that ANMs did not visit the mother and child for counselling. In 2014, the deaths of many neonatal babies in Dharmapuri district of Tamil Nadu brought this weak link of the ICDS to focus and scrutiny.

There is a growing discontent that ICDS continues to focus primarily on pre-school children, ignoring the most critical and vulnerable groups such as pregnant, postpartum mothers and children up to 24 months age (Balaji, 2014). Family planning services was another component that was not accessed by a majority of the households in both the villages. Conclusively, for major maternal and child health services like the delivery and treatment of childhood diseases, private providers are the preferred choice of providers for a majority of households in both the villages. These findings are not new but are in line with the trend towards large-scale privatisation of healthcare, even for reproductive and child health services that have already become a norm in urban India. This is a trend that rural India has also followed suit.

Literature points to the fact that barriers to access can limit and discipline the claims the poor make on public services (Goetz & Jenkins, 2005). This has a disproportionately negative impact on the poor who not only suffer from a declining public service, but also incur higher costs of private provision if they choose to exit. As Goetz and Jenkins also elaborate, 'because of their low social status and relatively low capacity to press complaints or expose corruption, the poor often have to pay bribes than rich users who might object or report corrupt officials. These bribes form a greater proportion of their merger incomes than those made by affluent users (Goetz & Jenkins, 2005:58)'.

4.4 Voices from Below: User' Rating of Services

Accountability is often paired with the term 'voice'. In the World Bank's Voice and Accountability Index, political systems that score highly are deemed to be more democratic than those that score poorly (Goetz & Jenkins, 2005: 27). Using voices of citizens in rating common public services, through instruments like citizen report cards or social audits, have been championed by civil society organisations like the Public Affairs Centre (PAC) and MKSS, respectively. Ratings of anganwadi and PHC services by the respondents was part of this study to find reasons behind households' choice of health providers.

Households were asked to rate providers on four criteria (Figure 4.4 and Figure 4.6). These were location or distance in terms of safety for women and children to travel, the promptness in treatment or referral, behaviour of the provider and its staff, and finally infrastructural facilities like beds, water, toilets, cleanliness and a place for waiting. Households were also asked to give a consolidated rating for the provider on a three-point scale, with 'poor', 'satisfactory', 'good', and 'don't know' as options. Households who mentioned the option 'don't know' were usually those who could not rate the service as they did not access those services.

4.4.1 Rating of Anganwadi Centres

On the aspect of location of the AWC in terms of convenience of distance and safety, a higher percentage of households in Nanduri (65.2%) rated it as 'good' as compared to 48.2% in Surli (Figure 4.4). On the criteria of staff behaviour, a higher percentage of households in Nanduri (68.1%) gave it 'good' rating as compared to 40% in Surli. A majority of households in Surli (45%) rated the behaviour of anganwadi staff to be 'satisfactory' and 40% as 'good'.

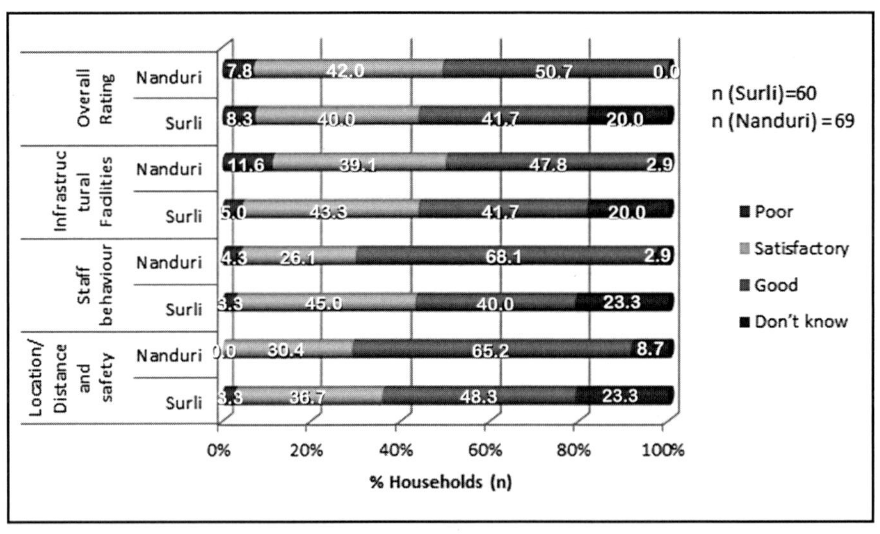

Figure 4.4: Rating of Anganwadi Centers on Select Criteria

Source: Field data, 2012

On infrastructure, surprisingly, a higher percentage of households in Nanduri (47.8%) rated facilities to be good while a majority of households in Surli (43.3%) rated their anganwadi infrastructure to be satisfactory. A higher percentage of households in Surli (more than 20%), as compared to that in Nanduri, opted for 'Don't know' on various rating criteria. This implied that they did not use ICDS services at all. Although the AWCs in Nanduri had poorer infrastructural facilities like toilets, neat rooms, its households still gave better ratings for it on most counts as compared to those in Surli.

On the overall ratings, contrary to the situation on the ground, almost 50% households in Nanduri rated the AWCs to be good, while this was low at 41.7% in Surli. In both the villages an equal percentage of households gave the rating of satisfactory to its AWCs and miniscule rated them as poor. This finding can be explained with the concept of 'perception of quality', which is a subjective issue and can differ even collectively from one context to another. This also happens when users are either not aware of the benchmarks of service delivery, in the case of ICDS, or that their benchmarks are too high, especially if they tend to compare the AWC with a private nursery.

The fact that there are many private pre-schools around Surli, that many households were accessing, could have influenced their responses. It is clear that users were not satisfied with the anganwadi services even in Surli which supposedly was a well-endowed and functioning centre. One speculative reason for this was that households do not know what to expect in terms of quality. In Nanduri, because of the absence of private pre-schools, households were probably not aware of their standards of services and hence gave a high rating to their AWCs. This issue is probed further in a subsequent section on mother's voices.

It is also interesting to note what ratings AWWs gave to their own anganwadi centers. Workers were asked during in-depth interviews on how they would rate their centres on a three point scale of poor, satisfactory and good and the reasons for doing so. Workers in both the villages rated their anganwadi centres as poor, with high scope of overall improvements. Workers shared their reasons for rating,

> *'Our children should be given more care to make them healthier. There should be proper uniform for them, chairs, tables, and better play equipment, as well as toys for playing and new learning aids. There is also a need for palna ghar (crèche) facilities since many mothers work in the fields. We cannot make them stay back. Hence they just roam around here and there.' - AWW, Nanduri*

> *'Currently we do not have our own building but work from a room in the primary school. I feel our anganwadi will improve if we teachers improve. I feel we teachers need to go further and be trained more. I did receive training two months ago on pre-school education. It will be good if these trainings happen regularly to sharpen our skills and keep us motivated.' - AWW, Surli*

While workers in Nanduri emphasised more on infrastructure-related improvements, those from Surli felt that training of workers were more crucial in improving anganwadi services. It is here that the role of 'standards' hold importance. According to the literature on role of standards in accountability, unless users are aware of their entitlements, they cannot demand the same from the provider.

While NRHM has formulated 'citizen charters' which publicly displays minimum basic services, their quality and grievance redressal, there are no such standards laid down for AWCs. To be fair, the Maharashtra ICDS brings out a monthly newsletter '*Amchi Anganwadi*' (meaning our anganwadi) where it reports centres that are given recognition as 'Model Anganwadi centres'. In one of the newsletters, it mentions about an award given to an AWC of number 143 at village Tekadi, Mool block, and Chandrapur district of Maharashtra (Figure 4.5).

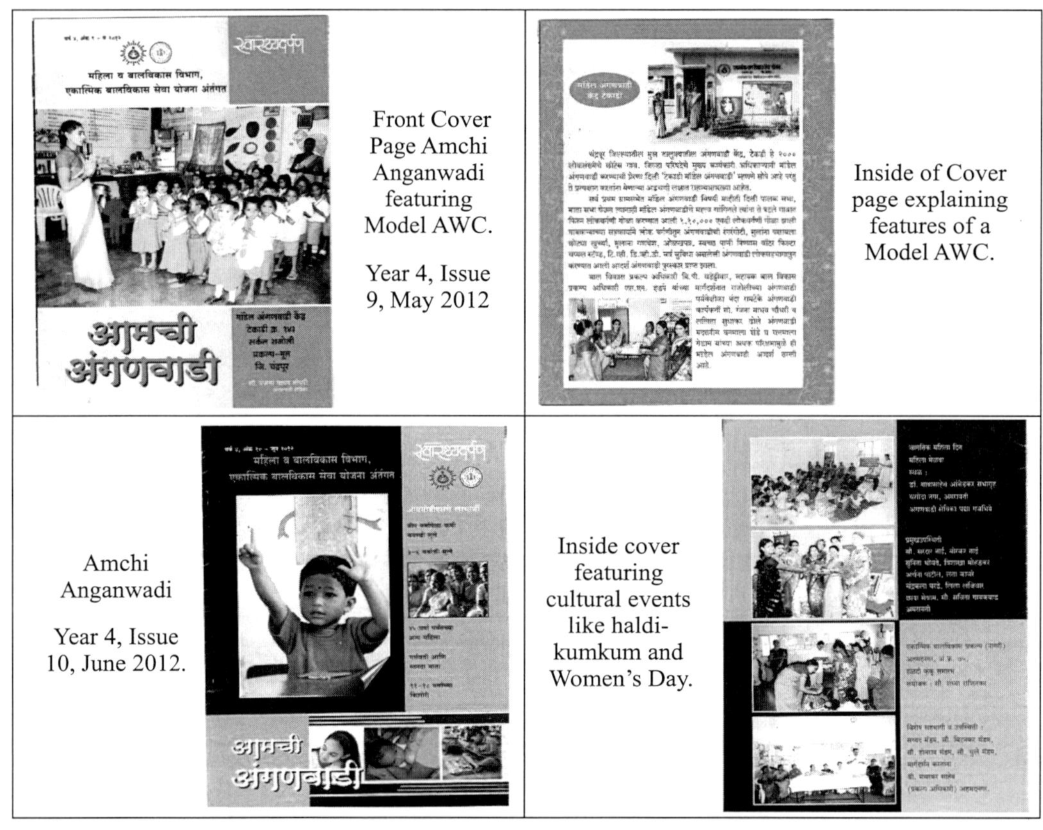

Front Cover Page Amchi Anganwadi featuring Model AWC.

Year 4, Issue 9, May 2012

Inside of Cover page explaining features of a Model AWC.

Amchi Anganwadi

Year 4, Issue 10, June 2012.

Inside cover featuring cultural events like haldi-kumkum and Women's Day.

Figure 4.5: Monthly Newsletter of Maharashtra State ICDS programme '*Amchi Anganwadi*' (our anganwadi)

Source: Documents procured from CDPO Tuljapur Office during fieldwork 2012

As per the description of the Model centre at Tekadi village, it has a population of 2000 as per the 2001 census. This means that the village is similar to the study villages of Nanduri and Surli. Quite surprisingly, the number of beneficiaries accessing its services, a direct success parameter of an anganwadi, (if not a complex local indicator of child malnutrition) was not an indicator to judge it. In fact, indicators like painted walls, chairs & tables, uniform, ID card, water filter, shoe rack, TV, DVD, etc, determined its status of being a model centre. These are infrastructure related indicators that may not directly improve outcomes like reduction in incidence of common childhood diseases or malnutrition.

Nonetheless, experts agree that infrastructure related issues form the pre-requisite to a well-functioning AWC, but these are not a central determinant for improving child malnutrition. Also, users were not involved in this rating exercise, but it seems to be conceived and implemented by the managerial functionaries. This again points towards the techno-managerial nature of governance, which is not only divorced from the users and community but also lacks intrinsic 'outcome' value.

Amchi Anganwadi newsletter is published in Marathi by the Department of Women and Child Development, ICDS under the aegis of *Swasthya-darpan* (Health Mirror) that is based in Ahmednagar. It covers interesting topics like banking advice to women, healthy diets for adolescent girls, yoga during pregnancy, and common problems of caring for new-borns. It also has a special section on seasonal foods available every month, common health problems, and the commemoration of significant health days.

This newsletter mentioned in clear and bold that its readership is not only limited to the ICDS functionaries like AWW, but also for beneficiaries like mothers of children, pregnant women and adolescent girls. However, these booklets do not reach the intended readers in the community. These booklets were not found in any AWCs visited or was referred in any of the narratives shared by interviewees. Therefore, AWCs were rated poorly in Surli and well in Nanduri, as contrary to the conditions visible on the ground.

Mother's voices on Anganwadi Centers. There were other reasons to explain the poor ratings of AWCs. Households revealed these in their replies to an open ended question. Households were asked about the reasons for their dissatisfaction with the anganwadi services and what they would like to improve. Many pressing concerns became known in the qualitative analysis of their responses. The most common reason for dissatisfaction of services in both villages was that quality, variety, and age appropriateness of cooked food that was poor.

To note, children less than two years are given THR, while those between three to five years of age are given hot cooked meals at the AWC. Majority of mothers of young children who were given THR in both villages rejected it. Cooked food also lacked variety according to them. They were either given *khichdi* or cracked wheat sweet porridge (*sheera*) alternatively. Parents in both the villages also complained of bad quality of grains used. They feel that grains remain uncooked and caused either stomach pains or dysentery among children. A woman belonging to the lower middle asset category and OBC family shared,

> *'I am aware about nutritious diet. My daughter does not eat AWC food. She gets diarrhoea. Home food is fine for her.' – A mother during HH interview*

However, there were some issues specific to two villages. In Nanduri, mothers identified infrastructure as one of the most common issues identified by mothers.

Mothers acknowledged absence of basic facilities like water, electricity, open space, sanitation and cleanliness. Mothers also cited lack of toys, books, play equipment and common medicines in the center as a major reason for their dissatisfaction. Another mother from poor asset quintile belonging to general category mentioned,

> *'Upma (Take Home Ration or THR) given by anganwadi has a smell. No one likes to eat that. We feed it to animals. More than quality, we do not cook separately for us or for our children but use everyday foods like mash dal and rice together to make gruel. This is more nutritious than packaged food.' - A mother during HH interview*

Another mother from lower middle asset quintile and OBC category shared,

> *'My daughter is three years old, but she has weight of a six months old child. They (anganwadi staff) do not weigh my child when I take her for immunisation. AWW says it is very crowded now, come later.' - A mother during HH interview*

Also, often frontline providers impose demanding entry point rituals and barriers for users, with an aim to limit their work burden (Goetz & Jenkins, 2005). Examples of barriers include information barriers, calling at odd timing, queuing up, and frequent referrals. Middle asset quintile households get encouraged to exit out in presence of these barriers, with options available in private sector. Responses from the affluent asset quintile were also similar. A pregnant mother from upper middle asset quintile and general category revealed,

> *'I am not aware that packets of food are given to pregnant women. I have never got it. I did not ask the weight of my four year old daughter, so I don't know if she is normal or underweight.' – A mother during HH interview*

In all, mothers in Nanduri pointed out many issues with its AWC services that were either poor needed urgent improvements. Yet, they gave favourable ratings to it as compared to Surli. A possible explanation of this trend is provided later, when more data unfolds. In light of these voices, it is not appropriate to argue that in the absence of standards which households are not aware, that they give higher ratings for public services.

This analysis has three significant conclusions. First mothers in both villages were aware of optimum services that AWCs should provide for their children even though there are no formal standards for these services or wide-spread awareness about it in the community. Second, despite being aware of the prevalent shortcomings in the services, a higher percentage of households in Nanduri not only accessed AWC services (as compared to Surli) but also gave better ratings for it.

Finally, and most importantly these voices show that mothers, despite being aware of the gaps in services, do not demand improvements from the anganwadi workers because of lack of institutional processes for the same (discussed in Chapter V). There is no apparent role of mothers in the VHNSC which in Nanduri was not functional. These observations are significant to the larger argument of the thesis about how and why communities do not demand better services from the service providers. Yet, these conclusions still fall short of explaining the observation in the previous chapter as to why children with any form of malnutrition in Surli improved over a period of time while those in Nanduri deteriorated.

There were some more insights from the interviews of mothers. In Surli, while most mothers, regardless of their asset quintile, rejected the THR. There was a distinct difference in the opinion of mothers from poor asset categories as compared to rich ones with regards to the functioning of the AWC. Mothers from poor asset quintile were somewhat satisfied with the services. For instance, a mother from lower middle asset quintile OBC category shared,

> *'ANM conducts meetings of all the mothers and we are shown demos on cooking. She also counsels us regarding diet.' – A mother during HH interview*

Another mother from middle asset quintile and general category who was aware of her child being under-nourished mentioned,

> *'Anganwadi tai asked me to give boiled potatoes, almonds and dates to my child. He is underweight but she assured me that it can be corrected.' – A mother during HH interview*

Another mother from middle asset category also shared,

> *'We mix all dry grains like wheat, rice and jowar and make them into powder. This is what we feed our children. The THR given by AWC is either thrown away or fed to hens and animals. Home-made foods like moong dal, rice kheer, nachini are more nutritious than ready-made foods.' – A mother during HH interview*

Another mother from lower middle asset quintile and OBC, who had under-nourished child revealed,

> *'We give cerelac or rice-based food to our child. She does not eat what is prepared at AWC. She has bowlegs but doctors told me that it is normal. I go to the AWC when they call me for a meeting where they give information on foods and feeding for infants.' – A mother during HH interview*

A mother from rich asset quintile and OBC category said,

> *'At home we give moong dal, rice kheer, and nachini. We used to eat THR previously but not anymore. We either throw it or feed it to animals.' – A mother during HH interview*

Mothers from poorer backgrounds were either satisfied with services or chose not to comment. Those from rich and middle asset categories exited out of these services by sending their children to private nurseries. It is also interesting to note the responses of the frontline providers on how they respond to rating given by community and the possible reasons for the same. Anganwadi workers in both villages were aware that the THR is being thrown or fed to animals and that many children are going to private nursery. However, one of them defended by saying,

> *'I tell mothers to be more creative with the THR and use it to make innovative dishes like puris and chakli. I work hard to convince them. Still, if they throw or return the packets, I ask them to give a complaint in writing, but they don't want to do that either.' - AWW, Surli*

This practice reveals that there is a pressure above from the AWWs to distribute THR despite resistance. They are held accountable if THR remain undistributed, so they ask for written complaints from mothers. Another worker mentioned the reason behind the preference for private nursery. She said,

> *'Some houses have money and feel they can send their child to English medium school. They feel that what we teach is not of much value as we do not even make children teach ABCD. Secondly, this service is free while they give money at a private nursery so that has more value.' - AWW, Surli*

On the issue of not sharing the child's growth chart with the mother, an AWW explained,

> *'I show growth charts to all mothers in my area. Some women understand it quickly but others, especially those who work in fields, tend not to understand the logic of red, yellow, or green colours. So during the breastfeeding week held every year from September 1 – 7, we try to make the community aware about this issue. Our children and all of us take out a prabhat-pheri (morning march) with red, green, and yellow cloth flags. The campaign helps us to communicate the levels of malnutrition to the community.' - AWW, Surli*

It is evident that most AWWs blame the mothers for either not have time or capacity to understand or follow their instructions. It is a clear excuse to hide their own inability to engage with mothers. They also cited the reason behind households opting for private nursery. It is the importance rich households attach to the English language. In a way, it was clear that they do not place the onus of households exiting AWC services on themselves. Rather, they attribute it to factors that are beyond their control, justifying the poor ratings by shifting responsibility to the households instead.

Academic literature is rife with critiques on the current status of AWWs & helpers. These however seem unjustified given the heavy workload, responsibilities of AWWs who are yet held accountable for child nutrition outcomes. Many experts employ the human rights framework to voice concerns over their position of an honorary worker, who is a woman, is underpaid (with some experts having even argued that AWWs earn lesser than daily wage worker) and have hardly any opportunities for state benefits or promotions (Bhatia, 2014).

Anganwadi worker unions have also raised critiques along similar lines. However, another set of literature views it differently - that both AWW and ASHA are, in-spirit, volunteers from the community who work for community development by selfless choice and are hence regarded as para-professionals to be paid in honorarium. This literature cites history and empirical evidence on the role of community workers, justifying their existing workload and honorariums. It mentions that they are not supposed to be qualified, are locally hired and trained personnel who can work in remote areas, costs less for large scale programmes and are not prone to absenteeism (Joshi, 2006).

Despite these two perspectives, the institutional processes of ICDS and NRHM, in practice, are required to be accountable to the state machinery and also to the community. Evidence shows that strong political commitment is needed for success and sustainability of this community health worker (CHW) initiative because it faces biggest opposition from teacher and health worker unions who have repeatedly protested against heavy workloads against paltry honorariums. Further, issues of ensuring quality of service remain a challenge. This approach thus needs to be coupled with periodic training and monitoring of such staff (ibid). Therefore, while workload assessments must be a regular feature, there are well document impediments like the lack of opportunities for growth, inadequate training, irregular and under-paid honorarium. These conditions continue to exist under which these community health workers like AWWs and ASHAs are not only expected to function efficiently but also be accountable to the community.

4.2.2 Rating of PHC services

In the context of PHC services, a majority of households in Surli (46.7%) gave it 'good' rating on the criteria of location, distance, and safety, while 31.7% felt it was 'satisfactory' (Figure 4.6). In all, almost 78.4% households in Surli were satisfied with PHC services. Yet, as per a previous finding, a majority do not have the same access for any service. In Nanduri, almost 40% households were not completely pleased with the location of its PHC, choosing 'satisfactory', while 31.9% gave it 'good' rating. Also, a substantial percentage of households responded 'don't know' when asked to rate the PHC. This was higher in Nanduri (26.1%) than Surli (18.3%). This was so because the question was context specific to Mangrol PHC and not any PHC in general. There is evidence that more households in Nanduri also accessed Katgaon PHC than Mangrol PHC.

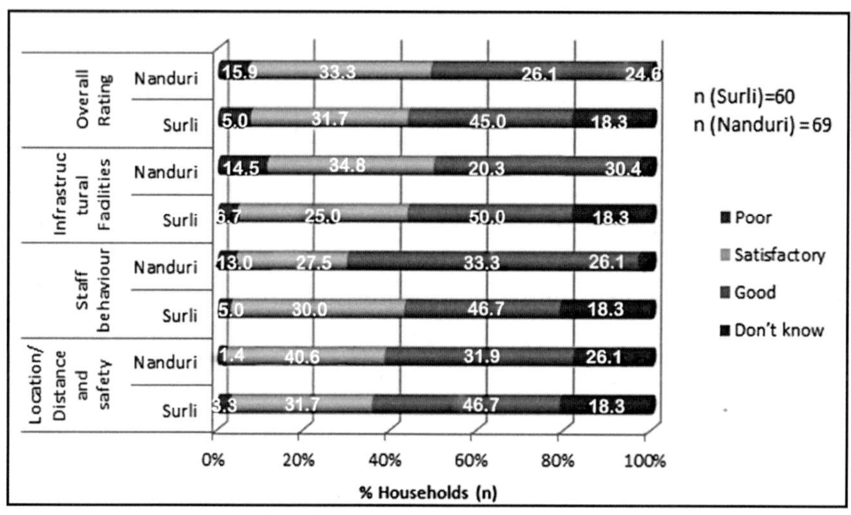

Figure 4.6: Rating of PHC on Select Criteria

Source: Field data 2012

Interaction and behaviour of PHC staff also have a bearing on the choice households make to select providers. A higher percentage of households in Surli gave a 'good' rating for staff behaviour in the PHC (46.7%), as compared to Nanduri (33.3%). A mother in Nanduri explained the reason,

> *'PHC staff need to be caring and sensitive to the needs of the patients, which they lack. They see patients quickly and their care for pregnant women is not proper.' – A woman during HH interview*

Another Nanduri resident, a man from lower middle and SC category shared,

> *'Staff behaviour is bad and they do not pay attention to us. I was once bitten by a dog and was supposed to take 14 injections, but they made me wait for long hours' – a respondent during HH interview.*

Staff behaviour was a most cited reason for dissatisfaction with PHC services, with a higher percentage of households in Nanduri (24.6%) reporting this reason as compared to that in Surli (8.3%). On infrastructural facilities, about 50% HH in Surli gave a rating of 'good' for its PHC while it was only 20.3% in Nanduri. Clearly, as seen on ground too, infrastructural facilities of PHC in Wathar Kiroli was perceived to be above average by a majority of households (75%) while almost 45% households in Nanduri either rated it as 'don't know' or 'poor'.

The difference between the two PHC was visible on ground too. Of all the times the author visited the two PHCs, there were long queues, commotions, and large groups of people seen at Wathar Kiroli PHC while the one at Mangrol was less crowded and often had a deserted look. In terms of overall ratings, a higher percentage of households in Nanduri rated its PHC to be poor (15.9%), while only 5% did so in Surli. Also, a higher percentage of households in Surli gave it 'good' rating (45%) as compared to only 26% in Nanduri. It is obvious that households in Nanduri were not happy with the PHC at Mangrol.

In Surli, the most common reason for households not accessing or being dissatisfied with PHC was that they were made to wait for long hours which was off-putting. In addition, they also complained about the inconvenient timings of the PHC that did not match their occupational routine. Another reason which was cited was lack of facilities like specialist doctors and sonography which are easily available in private sector. Because of this, many choose private providers over the PHC.

In Nanduri, the most cited reason for households not accessing or being dissatisfied with PHC was insensitive behaviour of the PHC staff. Another common reason for dissatisfaction cited was that most of the times PHC referred the patient to civil or rural hospitals and hence they did not want to approach PHC in the first place. Lack of infrastructure and ineffective treatments were other frequently cited reasons for households not prefer going to PHC in Mangrol. However, Figure 4.2 reveals that a huge percentage of households in Nanduri still chose to go to the PHC. This anomaly was explained by an ASHA worker. She said,

> *'Nanduri people usually go to Katgaon PHC since the MO there, stays in its quarter and is always available. If by chance they are unable to manage the case, they have an ambulance through which patient is transferred to a hospital in Solapur city. Therefore, people trust Katgaon PHC more than Mangrol PHC.' – ASHA, Nanduri*

An ANM shared the reason for high rates of referrals in Mangrol PHC. She said,

> *'People in Mangrol are notorious for shunning out medical officers from the PHC. They have been violent in the past with pelting stones and have done similar acts with the current MO madam too. So, she has stopped staying in her quarter in PHC premises. If the delivery patient comes, she is weary to take full responsibility and hence refers the patient. In last month, I am aware that she referred four normal delivery patients to Tuljapur. Trust has gradually waned.' – ANM Nanduri*

To be fair to the MO, the author asked for reasons behind the r miniscule deliveries happening at the PHC. She replied,

> *'Now even the village people have realized that they need specialists for health issues. So, if children are sick, they need paediatricians. For pregnant women they need gynaecologists and others like surgeons, sonologists, etc. Because of this they are resorting to private hospital. At times even we feel that if I am an MBBS, it amounts to nothing. Specialization is required even in rural practice.'*
> *- Medical Officer, Mangrol PHC*

During the interview with the same MO, it was revealed that people who come to Mangrol PHC were either poor, elderly, or women. These form the most vulnerable population and are politically the weakest who are least likely to question or demand better services from this PHC. The rich or productive males were either accessing Katgaon PHC or private health providers. Frontline providers who are related to the PHCs like the ASHAs and ANMs were also asked to rate the services of the PHC on same scale of poor, satisfactory and good and their reasons for the same. While Surli ANM was quite positive about PHC services, the one in Nanduri felt a large scope for improvement. They shared,

> *'I would rate PHC as satisfactory. It needs to be improved. For instance, medicine for children should be available in liquid form. People tell us you do not keep proper medicine for children. That is why we go to private.' - ANM, Nanduri*

> *'I would rate our PHC as good. We have three ANMs in this PHC, so the services will be good. We ensure to take full care of pregnant women with complete ante-natal services and well equipped for delivery patients. We try to give free medicine even though at times we do not have much in stock.' - ANM, Surli*

This revealed that even the frontline providers related to the PHC perceived their service as per the ratings given by the users and reflected the situation on ground. ASHA workers however did not rate the PHC in both villages. They shared,

> *'I have been working as ASHA since 2009. Even we have expectations, yet our salary has not come in. We hope it will begin some day and, in this hope, we keep on working.' - AHSA, Surli*

> *'My work is good and is of great significance to the people. Because of ASHAs like me, people get the right information and they feel free to approach me anytime of the day. That is why people of this village trust me. It is a full*

> *time job and I cannot calculate the number of hours in a day or week I work. Government officials need to understand our importance and pay us some salary.' - ASHA, Nanduri*

ASHA workers are conscious and aware of their importance in the health system. Yet, they are extremely concerned about their status of the state not paying them even basic honorariums. Their comments revealed that they do not feel a part of the health services to be able to rate their PHC. This can have implications for their own notions and practice of accountability to their seniors and to the users, and also the state's expectations of ASHAs to be accountable.

4.5 Nature of Relationship

Households in both study villages were asked about few critical aspects of their relationship with the frontline providers at the village level, mainly the AWW, ANM and ASHA. This concept would provide explanations as to why households access and choose certain frontline providers over others. One of the important aspects of provider-user relationship is availability of the provider when needed, rated on a three point scale – always when required, sometimes, rarely and don't know (Figure 4.7).

4.5.1 Providers' Availability

Staff absenteeism is one of the most common impediments that users face to access public health services. This is especially true of PHCs where ANMs and doctors are unavailable during work timings, a phenomenon often cited as 'capture' as they try to make extra money in private practice while retaining their office. Absenteeism is rare for community workers like AWW and ASHA as they usually reside in the same village. A majority of households in both Surli and Nanduri felt that AWWs were 'always available when required' (Figure 4.7).

This percentage was much higher in Surli (58.3%) as compared to Nanduri (47.8%). A high percentage of households in Nanduri (30.4%) answered 'don't know' to this question which means that they never asked for help from AWWs. Of all the three providers, Nanduri had the highest percentage of households (84%) who responded that ASHA was the one provider who was 'always available when required'. In contrast, only 20% of households in Surli gave the same answer about ASHA while a majority, 38.3% choose don't know. ASHA was the only provider in Nanduri who was seen as the most reliable health worker when compared to others. Interactions with households demonstrated this. She was a pro-active worker, chosen by the village leadership and was trained by the famous 'Bangs of Gadchiroli'. Everyone in the village knew her and had positive feedback about her as compared to the ANM and AWWs. During an interview with Nanduri ASHA, she shared her motivation,

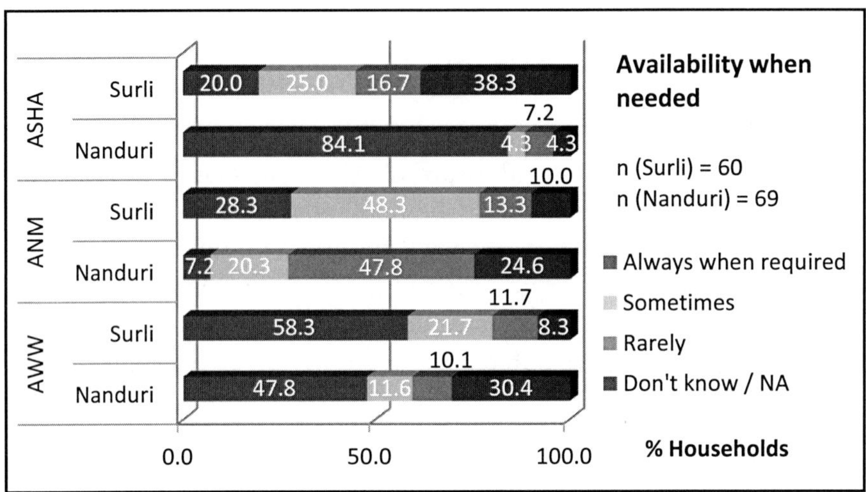

Figure 4.7: Health provider's Availability when Needed by Households

Source: Field data 2012

'I have been working as a community worker for 15 years. The village headmen felt that the whole village will benefit from my experience in maternal and childcare, so they forwarded my name for ASHA, although I am only ninth standard pass. I was not even aware that my name was given. I like doing my work as I feel nice helping people. I do not think about money, much.' – ASHA, Nanduri

Although AWW is also a resident of the village and conducts functions of AWC, it was the ASHA who was more active in Nanduri. In Surli, there were two ASHAs and most households were not aware about them since the ANM was more popular in Surli. About 48.3% households in Surli felt that the ANM was sometimes available and 28.3% households felt that she is always available when need arise.

Surli's ANM has been working as an ANM for 11 years, of which she had spent seven years has been in Surli. She regularly conducts immunisation for pregnant women and children and also awareness sessions with mothers because she is a known name and face of health programme in Surli village. However, her popularity is overpowered by that of Nanduri ASHA, as suggested by the numbers. The main reason for this is that unlike ASHA, ANM do not stay in the village, and visit fortnightly only. ANM's availability is restricted to the days she comes for immunisation or special camps. Also, most households were not aware of their position (ASHA) which was asked in the question but probably knew them by their actual name since they have been residents of the village before being appointed as ASHAs.

4.5.2 Attending community meetings

AWWs in Surli were favoured more than other workers as the voice of the community. Evidence of this explanation were household perceptions of frontline worker attending community meetings like gram sabha. (Figure 4.8). A higher percentage of households in Surli, as compared to Nanduri, felt that AWW (8.3%) 'always' attended while 13.3% felt that ANM 'sometimes' attended community meetings. Although a majority of households in both villages (80% or above) responded with 'don't know' on the same issue, this percentage was over 90% for all frontline workers in Nanduri. Only 7.2% households in Nanduri responded that their ASHA 'always' attended community meetings.

There was a general lack of communication between health frontline workers and the panchayat. This was more pronounced in Nanduri as compared to Surli. As per the GRs (Government Resolutions) of ICDS & NRHM programmes, AWW, ASHA and ANM who are the frontline workers of public health programmes, are supposed to regularly attend gram sabha meetings and share their work. However, despite an institutional mandate for this in the panchayats, in the form of VHSC, there was a disinterest on issues related to AWCs.

Frontline workers from both the villages were unanimous on one issue however, that if the GP did not call them for meeting, they would not attend. AWWs in Surli shared that they are present in the gram sabha meetings and also share their problems. The worker shared,

> *'People of the village are good and if we utter any requirements, they make sure they are met. Recently, in the GS meeting, they gave us the permission to buy chairs and tables from the VHSC funds. We do get the opportunity to talk' - AWW, Surli*

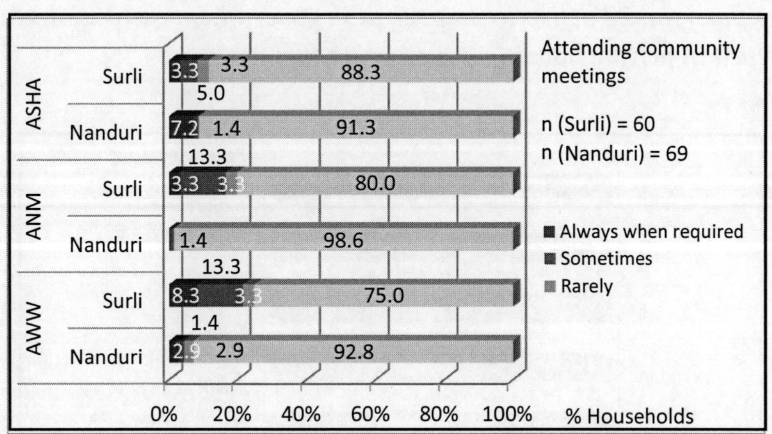

Figure 4.8: Households' Perception about Health Providers Attending Community Meetings

Source: Field data 2012

While another AWW from Surli was of the view that although they did have a voice in the GP, the GP do not in general take interest in the work of the AWC. In Nanduri, health workers did not attend gram sabha meetings. Nanduri AWW mentioned,

'The village people say that you get food stuff from the government, why should we contribute. People never volunteer to give anything here. Gram sabha happens but I have never gone, and they too have never called me. As it is, it is only for men. Women don't go there.' - AWW, Nanduri

While there were opportunities for dialogue between the providers and the community in Surli, community participation link was extremely weak in Nanduri.

4.5.3 On Trust

Finally, households were asked to rate their feelings of trust and confidence in the three frontline providers at the village level (Figure 4.9). Of all the providers, the ASHA from Nanduri elicited maximum trust since 76.8% households felt a 'high' feeling of trust for her. During an interview with Nanduri ASHA, on the question of why people preferred her, she shared,

'Earlier, most deliveries used to happen in private. This was so because the woman's in-laws used to think that staff were absent in public hospitals and that they would be harassed. Now they feel assured that the ASHA is with the patient. Now because of ASHA's work and PHC's ambulance which comes to the door-step of patients, the trend has reversed. Because of the ambulance, transportation costs have reduced, and this has benefited families. From January this year, 28 deliveries happened in government institutions and only 5 happened in private homes.' - ASHA, Nanduri

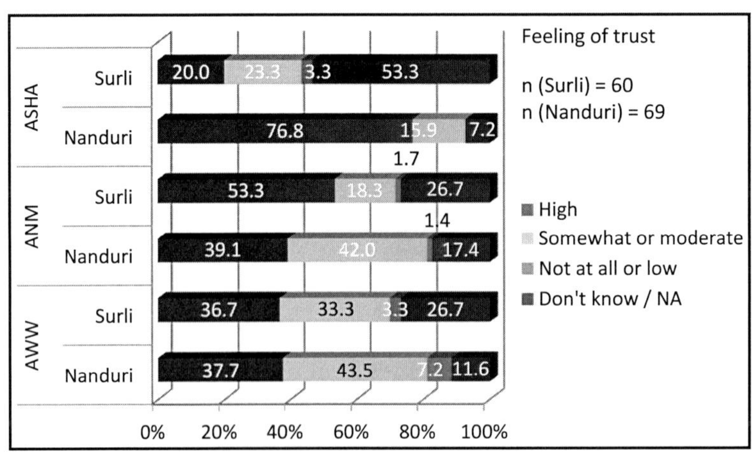

Figure 4.9: Households' Feeling of Trust toward Health Providers

Source: Field data 2012

Incidentally, ASHA worker of Nanduri was not paid any honorarium by the village's VHSC and was held in high respect by the community at large. The reason for her popularity is in the nature of being a voluntary worker and getting non-monetary incentives like respect, trust, and being heard by the community. Also, since there are no payments or honorariums to be paid, there is no tendency to reduce workload by posing barriers for users. In contrast, a majority (53.3%) of households in Surli answered 'don't know' when asked to rate their feeling of trust on the scale for ASHA. When Surli ASHAs were asked during interviews to explain why households were not aware about their work, they expressed denial about this lack of awareness.

The most alarming observation was that only 36.7% and 37.7% of households in Surli and Nanduri, respectively, had 'high' trust and confidence in their AWWs. This meant that a majority of households in both villages had moderate or low trust in AWWs. This percentage also seems to match with the percentage of households that were actually availing AWC services. The reasons for this trust deficit with the AWW, who is one of the central frontline workers for maternal and child health services. This came to light in the answers of mothers when asked in an open ended question on what improvements they would like to see in the AWC. A mother from the rich asset quintile, OBC family in Surli shared,

> *'The anganwadi worker needs to come to our house to give information. I was not aware of health day, for instance. A lot of information is not shared with us and we don't know what to expect from them.' – A mother during HH interview*

Another mother from the general category and rich asset quintile in Nanduri revealed,

> *'I am not sending my child to the AWC. Tai (AWW) keeps calling us to take weight of the child again and again. What is the benefit for me and my child? I don't know what purpose it solves for me?' – A mother during HH interview*

It seems that growth charts are also not shared with mothers, because mothers probably did not see any value in getting their children weighed. Such a gap renders growth charts useless despite it being a crucial tool linking ICDS programme with the community in terms of building communication, trust and confidence. Mothers from upper-middle and rich asset quintiles and general category in Nanduri shared,

> *'Anganwadi sevika does not give medicine to me when I asked it for my child previously. If I am accompanied with Meena tai (ASHA), she gives. Once, sanitary pads had arrived for distribution, but the AWW did not give these to any of the adolescent girls in the village. I have stopped going to her for anything'*

'The AWC staff needs to pay good attention to all children. My child had fallen and hurt himself on his knee. She did not pay any attention or give him first-aid till I complained to her and also to the sarpanch.'

'They (AWW) do not make food tasty for children to like it. My child takes tiffin from home which he eats there. Children do not like the food at the centre and many times, workers force feed them.' – Mothers during HH interview

Only one mother cited this issue about the lack of information on diet, food or growth charts not being shared with them, although most experience it on everyday basis. None of the other mothers mentioned anything about this. Nutrition education is one of the most crucial activities of ICDS yet it is the most neglected. Further, households also cited indifference on part of the AWW as another weak area in the services. A mother explained that, if for some reason the child is absent due to sickness, the AWW does not follow up or conduct home-visits for the child.

Some mothers were also concerned about the educational inputs that their children receive at the AWC. They felt that less importance was given to English. Learning in general was not viewed satisfactorily. If one adds those households who responded 'somewhat or moderate' feeling of trust with those having 'high' trust, AWWs in Nanduri commanded more trust and community's confidence than those of Surli. This observation is particularly interesting given the fact that physical conditions of the centres and service standards of ICDS in Nanduri 'looked' poorer to those in Surli.

Incidentally, most of these women who expressed the above issues about AWWs in both villages were from rich or upper middle asset quintile. It seems that they justify their decision to exit by sharing issues like not given timely information, or that workers did not visit them at home, or follow up if their child was not attending sessions, or if workers did not facilitate them when they visited the centre. Same practices may also be present for the poor but in the absence of alternative choices (private nursery), it is the rich who gradually gets discouraged and finally exit out.

Literature also points to providers imposing information barriers. It is reported that health care workers in rural Maharashtra routinely provide less information on contraceptive choices and side effects to their poorer women patients (Goetz & Jenkins, 2005: 60). Although ICDS is a universal programme, its institutional process seems to be encouraging the exit of rich and upper middle populations. When the Surli AWW was asked the reasons as to why households are opting out of AWC services and sending their children to English medium pre-schools, she responded,

'We visit the homes of parents who opt for English school and try to convince them that at the AWC, we take care of physical, motor, and mental developments

of children, an approach which is not adopted by private schools. Yet, many of them do not understand. Our gram sabha selects us for this job and we have a responsibility of making children responsible citizens.' – AWW, Surli

It shows that although they are aware of households opting out and claim that they do reach out to such households, they do not hold themselves responsible for the trend. In Nanduri too, AWWs were aware of households opting for private school but their reasoning was different. The AWW shared,

'In private schools, children are kept till 3pm while our AWC closes at noon. That is why households who can afford it send their children to English schools.' - AWW, Nanduri

Absence of crèche facilities was also cited as a main reason for households to exit ICDS. Number of households opting for private pre-school was much fewer in Nanduri than in Surli, owing to poor accessibility as well as long distances between the village and nearest city of Tuljapur. It is for this reason that a greater number of households pursued AWWs in Nanduri, as compared to Surli.

In Surli, a high percentage of households (53.3%) felt a 'high' level of trust in ANM while it was 39.1% in Nanduri. At the same time, a substantial percentage of households (53.3%) in Surli answered 'don't know' for ASHA as they probably did not interact with ANM or use her services. This means that, other than AWW, either of the two health workers – ASHA & ANM were approached and trusted by households. While ASHA was active in Nanduri, it was ANM in Surli. AWWs in both villages elicited similar responses, although it was slightly better in Nanduri. Mothers' responses for PHC services also revealed issues which discouraged some to exit out. Issues ranged from frequent referrals, long waiting time, lack of basic sanitation, medicine, and diagnostic infrastructure. A mother from upper middle asset quintile, from a family belonging to SC category in Nanduri, shared,

'We do not go to the PHC as they always refer delivery case to Tuljapur. So, we directly go to Tuljapur or Osmanabad.' – A mother during HH interview

For some services like family planning operation, public provider has a monopoly and as a result the user has no choice but to access a PHC. A woman from upper middle asset quintile and general category in Nanduri revealed,

'There was drinking water available at the PHC but not in its toilets. Its toilets are not clean at all. When I did my family planning operation at Mangrol PHC, I had to go out in the open to do it.'

A mother from rich asset quintile from OBC family in Surli shared,

> *'If any information comes to gram sevak or ANM, it does not reach us. We need better treatment at the PHC. Right now, the PHC staff does not pay good attention to patients. That is why even the poorest have shifted to private facilities.'*

A mother from upper middle asset quintile from general category in Surli shared,

> *'There is a long wait at the PHC, which is a big turn-off. So we have stopped going to PHC. Also, once there were no medicines for rabies and snake bite. They also don't have a separate lady doctor for women patients.'*

– Mothers during HH interview

The rich exited out of the PHCs owing to its institutional processes that shape actions of public service providers. Humphreys (1998) see the exit of the rich from public services, as serving the interests of the public providers as they prevent additional workload within the same remuneration. In addition, any articulation or demand to improve services will also not arise when the rich exit. This practice is by design part of the nature of public service delivery (Humphreys, 1998).

Other studies have also shown that when services are only intended to serve the poor, they tend to rapidly deteriorate. Exit of the middle quintiles from public services can reduce state commitment and lead to a downward spiral. This is especially of danger in contexts where alternatives exist (Kumar, 2007). Evidence in this chapter shows how the institutional processes of public services like ICDS renders them to be continually poor and how this gets operationalised at the frontline of service delivery. It also shows that the choice exercised by the non-poor groups to exit out of a public programme is a result of institutional processes and not because of individual decision making.

Therefore, institutional structures that build common interests between the poor and the better-off are more likely to lead to quality improvements that are sustainable in the long run (ibid.). Also, existing policy on child nutrition needs to prevent the exit of the upper middle and rich asset quintiles as much as it needs to include disadvantaged social groups.

4.6 Discussion and Conclusion

Village is an important context in a web of accountability relationships that exist between users and the state, which at the frontline of service delivery, comprises of multiple health workers. The objective of this chapter was to identify relationships of accountability between various actors at the frontline of service delivery and how these relationships are enacted. This objective was operationalised by understanding the nature of engagement between the users and providers, and by extension the nature of their relationship.

The way in which users exercise their choice in accessing various health providers is the first step in measuring how users are engaging with providers. Data revealed that a higher percentage of households in Nanduri, from a poor HDI rank district, assessed the AWC to be good, in comparison to those in Surli, a high HDI rank district. For PHCs, a higher percentage of households in Surli gave it a good rating, as compared to those in Nanduri, even though a majority do not access it. This observation is counter-intuitive since the literature reveals that rural population will use public health facilities if they are accessible and of high quality. Both villages defied this logic to a great extent.

This observation can be explained since it is in line with the literature on health seeking behaviour and preference of private providers. Studies have shown that consumers make their decisions on which provider to use on the basis of price, available income, their knowledge of different providers and their preference for service with different characteristic, particularly relating to quality (Mills et al., 2002).

The fact that private health providers are preferred despite a well-functioning and accessible public health facility is largely dependent upon two conditions - when a person or household has the resources to access and pay private health and when health needs are not met by the largely preventive public health services. This is especially true for developing countries like India.

Since Surli village had a higher percentage of upper middle and rich asset households, they had the purchasing power to patron private health services and hence they preferred private providers despite having a good PHC nearby. This was not so for Nanduri that had a higher proportion of middle and poor asset category households who accessed and utilised public health services more than those in Surli.

Private pre-school was the choice for a substantial percentage of families in Surli while a majority of households in Nanduri accessed the AWC. A high proportion of households in both the villages also accessed private health providers for maternal and child health services which also included poor and low middle asset quintiles. Another study points out that some private providers are also popular among the poor because they are adjusted to the purchasing power of the client and hence are cheap, such as when partial doses of drug are sold (Patouillard et al., 2007).

In a multi-state study of Indian villages, it was found that village-level literacy is significantly enhanced if households choose private schools over public and Panchayat-run schools (Joshi & Nagarajan, 2013). Growing access towards private services has implications on the capabilities of the communities to demand accountability since there can be none expected from the private sector. This also includes the heterogeneity of not-for-profit NGOs and civil society organisations.

In addition, there is evidence to show that a rapid rise in private providers of healthcare, with a subsequent increase in its utilisation can in turn influence the quality of care in public facilities (Awofeso & Rammohan, 2011; Peters et al., 2002). This means that with the growing presence of private sector, public health faculties are known to deteriorate. However, focusing on the supply of government services still remains a key strategy for improvements in access and quality for many countries. Facilities like schools and primary healthcare centres is still essential, particularly to address issues of exclusion from such services for those groups who cannot afford private providers, or who do not prioritise the treatment or education of women, and for extension of preventative healthcare (Joshi, 2006). The data from the study show that in addition to the supply, public policy must also encourage 'demand' for public health services in combination with regulation of private health sector.

The data from this chapter also supports this fact that people who accessed PHCs largely comprised of the poor, elderly and women. Young men and children even from the poor and lower middle chose private health services, as seen in Surli and to a lesser extend in Nanduri. Another explanation to this trend is that when welfare nets in form of public distribution systems, wage labour, social security benefits etc. are weak, the poor tend to utilise whatever public services are available even if it is of inferior quality. The study did not factor in these welfare nets to claim with confidence, but can speculate that since higher population in Nanduri were agricultural labourers than those in Surli, they had no choice but to access poor services.

This chapter provides evidence that mere supply of public health services in terms of access and perceived quality may not be the only factor that can guarantee their use by rural populations. Experts are now making a similar observation that the provision of high-end equipment in primary health centres will not yield satisfactory results. Effective training of healthcare workers, early diagnosis, and management capabilities will make primary health centres patient-friendly (Hasib, 2014). Strengthening the provision and supply of public health services needs to be accompanied with control and regulation of private health sector in tandem, to make them effective.

To sum up, the nature of relationship between the frontline providers and users was found to be shaped by institutional processes, both monetary and non-monetary incentives, or lack of it, rather than on a one-on-one, need-based relationship, that is dependent on pro-activeness of the worker. Anganwadi workers in both villages had equal ratings that were much lower than ASHA or ANM. This seems to be a bit surprising given a fact that AWW is responsible for early childhood care and education of the children in village. Her position has the potential to command high respect and trust from the local community. However, as data revealed, AWW is least popular and quite equally so in both villages.

The reason for the same has been explained by scholars. On the 'ethnography of state' and 'governmentality', Gupta (2001) provides evidence that ICDS is one of the most appropriate models of governmentality. Its bureaucratic surveillance aimed at regulation by means of surprise checks; enumeration and accountability through maintaining information registers has not achieved what it set out for. This kind of monitoring did not translate into discipline and workers did not conform or police themselves to rules. In fact, such a culture has created tension and friction between higher-ranking officers and AWW workers, as well as between AWWs and 'served' population (Gupta, 2001).

Low popularity of AWWs can also be explained by the fact that the poor, despite having access these services, remain disengaged with low capacity to articulate their demands. In contrast, the middle quintile or rich choose to exit out and hence disengaged altogether. This is one of the central observations on the nature of engagement between the users and providers. According to perceptions about all health workers attending community meetings, households' responses revealed low interactions in Surli, with none in Nanduri. These observations have implications on the way users can formally or informally demand answerability and impose sanctions on the providers to improve their services.

***

References

1. Awofeso, N., & Rammohan, A. (2011). *Three decades of the Integrated Child Development Services Program in India: progress and problems.* INTECH Open Access Publisher.
2. Balaji, P. (2014, November 25). Lesson from Dharmapuri: Strong primary health care. *The Times of India.* Retrieved on November 27, 2014 from http://timesofindia.indiatimes.com.
3. Bhatia, K. (2014). Performance-based incentives of the ASHA scheme. *Economic and Political Weekly, 49*(22), 145–151.
4. Citizens' Initiative for the Rights of Children under Six. (2006). FOCUS or Focus on Children Under Six Abridged report. Right to Food Campaign. New Delhi.
5. *Deccan Herald.* (2015, January 31). Anganwadi workers to stage State-wide protest. Retrieved on February 3, 2015 from http://www.deccanherald.com.
6. Global Development Network. (2009). Varieties of governance: effective public service delivery, concept note ninth global research project. Retrieved on March 28, 2014 from http://gdn.int.
7. Goetz, A. M., Jenkins, R., & Shaw, T. M. (2005). *Reinventing accountability: making human democracy work for human development* (First). London: Palgrave Macmillan.
8. Gupta, A. (2001). Governing population: the integrated child development services program in India. In Hansen, T. B., & Stepputat, F. (Eds.) *States of imagination: ethnographic explorations of the postcolonial state* (pp. 109-136). USA: Duke University Press.
9. Gupta, A. (2012). *Red tape: Bureaucracy, structural violence, and poverty in India.* USA: Duke University Press.
10. Hasib. N. I. (2014, November 21). Quality public health must for UHC: Gita Sen. *B D News,* Retrieved on November 27, 2014 from http://bdnews24.com.

11. Humphreys, P. C. (1998). *Improving public service delivery.* Dublin: Institute of Public Administration.
12. Johari, A. (2020). How three tainted companies retained their grip over Madhya Pradesh's nutrition scheme for children. *Scroll.in*. June 28.
13. Joshi, A. (2006). Institutions and service delivery in Asia. *IDS Bulletin*, *37*(3), 115–129.
14. Joshi, O. & Nagarajan. H.K. (2013). Varieties of governance: varying outcomes. *Global Development Network GDN Working Paper Series.* Retrieved on March 28, 2014 from http://gdn.int.
15. Kumar, A. S. (2007). Why are levels of child malnutrition not improving? *Economic and Political Weekly*, *42*(15), 1337–1345.
16. Kumar, S. (2007). *Parallel bodies & the Panchayati Raj Institutions: A study of village based special committees in three districts of Maharashtra* (Unpublished). Tuljapur: School of Rural Development, Tata Institute of Social Sciences.
17. Mills, A., Brugha, R., Hanson, K., & McPake, B. (2002). What can be done about the private health sector in low-income countries? *Bulletin of the World Health Organization*, *80*(4), 325–330.
18. Ministry of Women and Child Development, Government of India. (2012). Draft National Early Childhood Care and Education (ECCE) Policy. Retrieved on September 24, 2014 from http://wcd.nic.in.
19. Patouillard, E., Goodman, C. A., Hanson, K. G., & Mills, A. J. (2007). Can working with the private for-profit sector improve utilization of quality health services by the poor? A systematic review of the literature. *International Journal for Equity in Health*, *6*(1), 1-17.
20. Pawar, Y. (2014, March 16). Governments Rs 300-crore plan to tackle malnutrition in Maharashtra a waste of money: study. *Daily News & Analysis*. Retrieved on March 17, 2014 from http://www.dnaindia.com.
21. Peters, D. H. (2002). *Better health systems for India's poor: findings, analysis, and options*. Washington DC: World Bank Publications.
22. Ray, K. (2014). Govt planning backdoor entry of MNCs into kid's scheme. *Deccan Herald*. July 29, Retrieved on August 1, 2014 from http://www.deccanherald.com.
23. Sharma, D. C. (2014, August 31). Fit for the malnourished? *Daily News & Analysis*. Retrieved on September 11, 2014 from http://www.dnaindia.com.
24. Sinha, S. (2006). Infant survival: A political challenge. *Economic and Political Weekly*, *41*(34), 3657–3660.
25. Sundaram, J. K., & Rawal, V. (2014). Nutrition: what needs to be done? *Economic and Political Weekly*, *49*(42), 46–53.
26. *The Hindu*. Early childhood care and education policy proposed. (2012, March 26). New Delhi. Retrieved on March 26, 2012 from http://www.thehindu.com.

27. The Lancet. (2008). Maternal and child under nutrition series. *371*(9608), p177–274.

28. The Lancet. (2012). The Global Burden of Disease Study 2010. *380*(9859), p2053–2260.

29. The World Bank. (2004). *World Development Report 2004 Making Services Work for the Poor*. Washington DC: The World Bank and Oxford University Press.

CHAPTER 5

Answerability and Sanctions: Getting Services Delivered

5.1 Introduction

Answerability and sanctions are concepts in addition to engagement that are central to study accountability relationships. These are central in the conceptual framework of the study in Chapter 2, Figure 2.7. Conceptually, answerability means to not only to answer for one's action or inaction through providing information but also to give justifications or explanations for those actions (Figure 2.3). The most fundamental tool in ushering in the culture of accountability through information from state agencies and functionaries was the Right to Information enacted through RTI Act, 2005. In a democracy like India, even this took more than fifty years to come in effect. Conceptually, this instrument caters to only a part of answerability that is giving information and hence can achieve 'partial' accountability. The other part of answerability that allows information to be used to demand accountability is 'justification'.

Ideally, a gram sabha is a site for confrontation and providing justifications in a rural setting where frontline functionaries like ANM, an Anganwadi worker, a gram sevak, a talathi and a medical officer needs to be present, report their work and respond to questions from the community. However such a practice, although mandated in the Panchayati Raj Institution Act, is far from reality. Justification also includes a minister providing answers to questions in a parliament. This, however, is regarded as a long-route of accountability or vertical accountability according to the literature by the World Bank.

Long route of accountability has been regarded as ineffective for improving service delivery and reducing corruption for the common man. Literature points at many newer forms of engagement to demand accountability from public institutions that are emerging other than the traditional ones like elections, ombudsmen, public interest litigations and CAG (Comptroller & Auditor General of India) Audits. Involving citizens in monitoring of services has been successful with citizen report cards and Mazdoor Kisan Shakti Sangathana (MKSS) led campaigns in NREGA using public hearings and social audits. Other instruments like User Satisfaction Surveys and Community-Based Monitoring (CBM) have also been experimented with some degree of success in India, while Participatory Budgeting are success stories from Latin America.

Finally, even if information and justification is achieved through answerability, practically, accountability cannot be delivered to the people unless these processes are followed up by sanctions. Sanctions give teeth to the notion of accountability. Existing institutions of ombudsmen, active in few Indian states like Kerala and the much controversial Jan Lokpal Bill are attempts to create such sanctioning institutions, mainly with financial-legal authority that can formally punish government servants who have been proven guilty of corrupt malpractices.

This chapter deal with concepts of answerability and sanctions at the frontline of service delivery. This is also aligned to the study's second objective. The second objective of the study is to analyse how users, especially the poor, demand or negotiate better services and entitlements through informal mechanisms when the formal mechanisms of accountability fail or exclude them. What are the formal mechanisms of accountability available to users at the frontline of service delivery? To what extent are these effective and if not, then what are the reasons? Are there informal ways in which users demand accountability and impose sanctions? How are these exercised and with what implications? On the other side, what do providers perceive about whom are they accountable to? Is such a perception an issue of the individual actors or the institutional norms and rules that shape actions and perceptions of frontline actors?

These are some of the questions that link the concept in the conceptual framework with the objectives of this chapter. This second objective has two sub-objectives. The first part aims to identify and compare various institutionalised and formal accountability mechanisms like elections or debate in parliament with informal forms of accountability, like authority or patronage. And the second, to examine whether informal forms of accountability have a comparative advantage over formal ones or vice versa.

In order to understand how users demand their entitlements for nutrition and health services, it is imperative to understand existing institutional processes for accountability as part of the ICDS and NRHM programmes at the village level. This is attempted in the following section.

5.2 Tools to Question: A Peep into the Anganwadi

The ICDS has an extensive framework of monitoring (MIS) for its functionaries to be answerable and accountable to its bureaucratic and political leadership. Its institutional framework does allow, to some extent, the user-community to also engage with the providers. These tools are the Growth Charts and the Village Health & Sanitation Committee (VHSC). Officially, growth charts are not considered upfront as tools for users' engagement with providers. However, they were introduced and provided by agencies like UNICEF for the very purpose of mothers tracking the growth of their children on prescribed standards.

Growth charts have a high potential to be a key tool in linking beneficiaries with the ICDS programme. Doctors from the PHC are also meant to use the growth charts for explaining mothers their children's nutritional status during health check-ups and referrals mandated under ICDS. However, as revealed in the following section, it has largely been interpreted as, yet another record-filling, bureaucratic activity of the frontline workers with minimum interface with the users. Some civil society organisations claimed to have conducted social audits and community based monitoring surveys in ICDS in select districts in Maharashtra, but these were isolated incidents and hence their validity and partisanship is questionable.

5.2.1 Growth Charts: A Bottoms-Up Tool, Reduced to a Farce?

In the case of child nutrition, one of the ways in which the mothers of the children can keep a track of their nutritional status is by the growth chart. The growth chart is a visual record prepared for each child by the anganwadi worker under the ICDS programme. Plotting the child's weight, taken every month or quarter, on this chart and joining these points forms the growth curve, makes the growth of the child visible as against the standard norms (NIPCCD, 2010). At the anganwadi centre, a growth charts book is separate for boys and girls with each page exclusive for a growth chart of one child. Anganwadi workers are required to fill these regularly to ascertain grades of malnutrition. Also, this resource is exclusive to a public programme like the ICDS and most private nurseries, both in urban and rural areas are not equipped to do so.

The idea of the growth chart is that it enables anganwadi workers to communicate, educate and counsel mothers if their child is underweight and needs exceptional care and feeding at home, in addition to supplementary nutrition received at the anganwadi centre (ibid.). Ideally, a growth chart can be a crucial link between the institution of ICDS, its frontline provider anganwadi worker and the parents of children. A growth chart is a standard against which parents get to know information about their child's physical growth progress, data which is aggressively collected by the ICDS. The question is whether mothers or parents consider the growth chart as a tool in their hands to monitor and question the frontline providers on the nutritional status of their children and also whether it is considered in the same intent by the institution of the ICDS. In either case, it is not so.

The irony of the institution of the ICDS is that the weight and the height of children are meticulously recorded and extensively shared for bureaucratic monitoring, but the same is not demanded by the mothers or shown to them, defeating its very purpose. It is a common observation that growth charts are the most under-emphasised, under-utilised and ignored aspect of the ICDS from the context of both users and providers. Though children are weighed more or less regularly by anganwadi workers, their growth charts are not maintained properly, nor is their classification into different grades done accurately. This undermines the basic purpose of maintaining growth charts (Khullar, 1998).

In Surli, growth charts were found to be filled with information. Strict top-down monitoring from supervisors and CDPOs ensured that anganwadi workers in Surli updated these records in a timely manner. However, that does not guarantee that they are also shared with mothers, as revealed during household interviews. In Nanduri, growth charts were grossly incomplete and hence it is fair to assume that they are never shared with the mothers.

Mothers in both villages were largely unaware about the growth charts when asked during the household interviews since none had seen their child's growth-chart. This is no surprise and is a common trend with anganwadi centres across India. It resembles a situation where mothers do not ask, providers do not share, and everything continues without a glitch. To note, anganwadi centres in Nanduri & Surli had started functioning in 1983 and 2001 respectively, and therefore this issue should not be labelled as 'lack of awareness'. It is to do with the way existing institutional processes work within the ICDS.

The reason for this trend lies within the NPM framework of managerial accountability where for few activities like sharing growth chart with mothers there are no indicators to measure and monitor if this actually happens or not. So, it is blatantly skipped. This also does not mean that activities that are monitored by the MIS, happen regularly. It only means that the existing processes in the ICDS do not provide space for users to use these instruments and ensure their implementation.

> *'When mothers come, I show them the book and point at red, green and yellow to show if their child is normal, mild, moderate or in severe malnutrition. I show this to all mothers of children in my area. Women who are smart, they understand what I say. But women who work in fields, if I tell them about red, yellow, green, they don't tend to understand. So during Sept 1 to Sept 7 when we have breastfeeding week every year, we organise prabhat pheri (morning procession) by our children where they hold red, yellow or green colour flags with our (ICDS) logo. Then on the way women ask about these colours and then we share the meaning.' - Anganwadi worker, Nanduri*

> *'This time when the Supervisor madam had come then she had told both of us to fill that book. She came again and asked, so I told her that book is lying in house of the worker who is on delivery leave and that is why it could not be completed. Madam asked us to jointly complete it as soon possible. She kept following us and told us and told we should get the completed book in our forthcoming meeting on the 28th of this month.' - Anganwadi worker, Nanduri*

It was clear that although workers claim to share the growth charts with mothers, but the fact that these were incomplete in Nanduri, the claim falls flat and in Surli too, mothers had not seen any.

Workers seem to use the premise of lack of awareness and poor educational status of some mothers, as a pretext for not sharing. Such a prejudice is merely an excuse and is not backed by evidence. Many workers claimed that they show growth charts to mothers who come to the centre on immunisation days. In practice, on those days, anganwadi workers usually take a back seat since the meeting is conducted by the ANM of the PHC whose agenda is conducting immunisation and counselling mothers on specific health issues. The ANM is neither responsible not mandated to share growth charts. Therefore, this claim too is falsified.

For mothers who are present, anganwadi worker takes their signatures as a proxy for 'mothers' meeting', which is one of the indicators monitored by ICDS MIS for nutritional counselling. These observations are not novel to this study. However, what is significant about this finding is that this study locates this disconnect within the institutional process and accountability relationships in the ICDS, which has not been discussed in the mainstream literature on child nutrition programmes in India.

Usually, the dominant NPM discourse attributes this to an overburdened anganwadi worker who is under-paid and therefore not filling the growth charts or not sharing with mothers, which to an extent, is justified. One is again barking on the wrong tree. Anganwadi workers diligently and regularly record every child's weight in the numerous formats and registers required as per top-down supervision by their supervisors and CDPOs. The present institutional framework of the ICDS fails to recognise mothers or parents of children as stakeholders in the process. And this is worse than exclusion.

5.2.2 Village Health, Nutrition, Water & Sanitation Committee: A Site for Contestation?

At the household level, the growth chart was one tool to elicit the confidence and value of the ICDS among the parents. At the village level, in order to create bottoms-up accountability and community ownership on nutrition, health and sanitation, the NRHM in 2005 envisaged and institutionalised Village Health, Sanitation Committee (VHSC). In Maharashtra, way back in 2006 and within an year of launch of the NRHM at the centre, this committee was renamed with 'nutrition' added and hence re-organised as Village Health, Nutrition, Water & Sanitation Committee (VHNWSC) at least on paper (Dhumaal, 2006). The Ministry of Health & Family Welfare, Government of India acknowledged nutrition in VHSC only in 2011 (Pradhan, 2011). The idea behind this committee was to synergise three key features.

First, there is a multi-departmental convergence of centrally sponsored health and nutrition programmes implemented at the village level which includes government departments like Rural Development, Water & Sanitation, Public Health, Women & Child Development and at times Social Welfare. These convergences needed to be reflected at a village-level public institution within the Panchayati Raj system.

Second, social determinants of health and nutrition such as education of mothers, food security, access to health services, availability of drinking water, and sanitation jointly influence health and nutrition outcomes. All these concerns are required to be addressed jointly and not individually. Earlier there were separate committees in the panchayat for water and sanitation and for health which did not serve the purpose, hence, a need for an overarching mechanism.

And lastly, a community process would bring in transparency, accountability and hence a demand for health services. A Village Health Sanitation & Nutrition Committee (VHSNC) fitted the bill on these three counts.

The Maharashtra government's amendment to its Panchayat Raj Act of 1958 sub-section 49 clearly articulated merging existing Water and Sanitation Committee of the panchayat with Village Health Committee to constitute this new committee which included nutrition in its mandate (Dhumaal, 2006). A Government of India notification to all states and UTs in 2011 and again in 2013 stipulated that VHSNC should be made as a sub-committee under the panchayat, to function under its supervision and be accountable to both gram panchayat and gram sabha (Pradhan, 2011; Jhalani, 2013; Yaden, 2013).

Therefore, the state did institutionalise a bottoms-up accountability and community monitoring mechanism of child nutrition at the village level through VHSNC within the NRHM implementation framework. The NRHM 2005 guidelines stated that the VHSC should comprise of Anganwadi worker, ANM, ASHA, representatives of the village panchayat including a female member, women non-governmental organisations, backward social classes like SC/ST/OBC/BPL representatives and self-help groups. The objective of this committee is not only to plan, and fund programmes related to curb child malnutrition in the village but also to act as a grievance redressal mechanism. Since child nutrition, as a subject, is not directly delegated to the Panchayati Raj Institutions, panchayat is not mandated to demand accountability from the anganwadi. It is only through the VHSC that the anganwadi centre will be accountable to the gram panchayat (Husain, 2011).

In Maharashtra, within an year of launching the NRHM nationally in 2005, VHSC was renamed and re-organised as Village Health, Nutrition, Water & Sanitation Committee (VHNWSC) in 2006 (Dhumaal, 2006). Policy progression happened in Maharashtra much before the central Ministry of Health & Family Welfare acknowledged it in 2011 (Pradhan, 2011). However, the practice despite the presence of a state policy was grossly under-implemented, at least in the study villages. The VHSC was formed and functioned in Surli as an independent committee, but not within the panchayat, as stipulated by the state and central governments. And in Nanduri, its panchayat water and sanitation committee never included nutrition as its mandate and also did not form any separate VHSC. Therefore, in both study villages, 'nutrition' was not part of the Panchayati Raj Institution despite a Maharashtra government policy stipulating that it be so since 2006.

In practice, the VHSC was formed and functioned in Surli as a duplicate committee (since a water and sanitation committee already existed at the panchayat) and not as a part of the panchayat. In Nanduri its water and sanitation committee in the panchayat never included nutrition as its mandate and also did not form any separate VHSC. However, Surli stood out as there was a consensus between the gram panchayat and anganwadi workers on the spending priorities of VHSC funds. The VHSC seems to function in Surli, as I could access minutes of the meeting recorded along with statement of expenditure as per consensus of its members (Table 5.1). Annually, Surli's VHSC received a Rs. 15,000 grant which was used in buying chairs/tables for children, paying honorarium to Accredited Social Health Activist (ASHA), conducting health survey, and sanitation.

It was for this reason that the anganwadi centre probably 'functioned' better in Surli than in Nanduri. But the fact that it was a stand-alone committee, not under a panchayat's purview defeated its very purpose. In addition, a worker shared her challenges of calling VHSC meetings. She said,

> *'I have to go and call each one of them for a meeting. It causes me a lot of problem as some of them don't come despite repeated requests. We have divided this money into four parts – arogya (health), bachat (savings), anganwadi and pani-purowtha (water & sanitation). We do not use this money arbitrarily but as per jointly decided norms. That is why work in our village is good.'*
>
> *– Anganwadi worker, Surli*

The situation in Nanduri was opposite where the VHSC was not formed and funds not utilised for anganwadi because of in-fighting between the sarpanch and anganwadi workers. One common observation in both villages was that actors, both providers and users were confused as to if the VHSC was a separate, stand-alone committee or the same as the water and sanitation committee of the gram panchayat. Therefore, while policy created a bottoms-up formal mechanism of accountability for child nutrition services at village level, institutional processes allowed local actors to misinterpret it and with no sanctions levied against them for not including nutrition at par with water and sanitation.

Table 5.1: Accounts of the VHSC, Surli from 16/09/2011 to 11/03/2012

Sr. No.	*Particulars*	*Amount in Rs.*			
		Opening Balance	Funds received	Expenditure Incurred	Balance
1	Village health survey	548	15,000	100	554
2	Organisation of health and nutrition day				
3	Meeting of gram sabha related to health issues				
4	Nutritious food for children at Anganwadi				
5	Pregnancy related services				
6	Allied services				
7	Destruction of mosquito breeding sites (Banner for Tobacco Control)			900	
8	Health awareness programmes				
9	Buying of TCL (bleaching powder)				
10	Maintenance of water supply system				
11	Improvement of Anganwadi centre				
12	Buying of furniture for Anganwadi (table/chairs)			9,800	
13	Play equipment for Anganwadi centre				
14	Honorarium for ASHAs			2,250	
15	Sanitation of common/public toilets			950	
16	Stationery and others			1,000	
	TOTAL	548	15,000	15,000	554

Source: Anganwadi centre, Surli during fieldwork, 2012

Whatever little VHSC functioned in Surli, it too was reduced to a farce owing to local politics and power of caste and gender. During the in-depth interviews with the anganwadi staff, a worker shared her opinion when asked about monitoring of their work by the gram panchayat. She said,

> *'The gram panchayat does not take interest in this work (anganwadi). They are more political in nature. Also, this is to do with health and child nutrition which does not come under their jurisdiction.' – Anganwadi worker, Surli*

The functionaries too had a flawed notion and expectations from the gram panchayat and seemed to be ignorant and misinformed about the VHSC. During the in-depth interviews with the anganwadi workers on their role and functioning of the VHSC, there was a distinct contrast between the two villages. In Surli, an anganwadi worker shared,

> *'The gram sevak gives us money as if he is doing a favour. It is our money and the gram panchayat cannot use it to clean gutters as they already collect money for that from each house. This year we did not give any money to the gram panchayat but used it to get chairs-tables for children. We had bought 10 kg*

peanuts and jaggery to make nutritious sweet. We also gave some money to the ASHA workers.' – Anganwadi worker, Surli

The ASHA worker in Surli was also supportive of VHSC functioning. She said,

'ASHA workers and Anganwadi staff have to do the household survey together; listen to the problems of the people and regularly check for leakages in water and sewerage pipelines. We are given water testing kits and if we find the water contaminated, we report it to the gram panchayat to take immediate corrective steps.' – Anganwadi worker, Surli

The Anganwadi worker in Nanduri shared,

'The VHSC money has been lying in the bank unused because of a dispute between the other Anganwadi worker and the Sarpanch of gram panchayat.' – Anganwadi worker, Nanduri

When the other Anganwadi worker was asked about this matter, she explained,

'I am the secretary of the VHSC, and we get money from the PHC to be spent on nutrition, health of the children and water & sanitation issues of the village. I and sarpanch hold a joint account in the bank. Last year, the sarpanch took out the full money and spent it on installing a slide and a swing in the school premises and in constructing a water tank. However, there is no water in that tank, so money went waste. We got a paltry sum for buying nutritious food for children. This year he is neither using it nor allowing us to use.' – Anganwadi worker, Nanduri

In Nanduri the friction involved other actors too. ASHA worker echoed similar fears when she said,

'The VHSC is supposed to pay me an honorarium of Rs. 1000 annually for all the mobilisation work, but till now they haven't paid anything. Whenever I have asked the sarpanch, he says that they have utilised all the funds. But he would not share the accounts on how the money was spent. When I ask Anganwadi worker, she says that this money is only meant for the Anganwadi centre. I came to know that higher official had sent a letter to the Medical officer (medical officer) instructing them that ASHA needs to be paid. medical officer sent that letter to the sarpanch. But he did nothing. Now he says there is no money in the bank. What can I do now?' – Anganwadi worker, Nanduri

It was evident that functioning of the VHSC in Nanduri was mired into conflicts and was not functional at all. A reason for ghost names on anganwadi centre lists is also related to this fact that the attendance registers at the anganwadi centre are checked only by the ICDS supervisors and never by the local village authorities like the sarpanch, gram panchayat member, gram sevak or any member of the VHSC. It was found that the sarpanch had little say in the matters since he was only the rubber stamp for the deputy sarpanch who had a strong influence on all matters of the village. Although the ANM did not mention this but it was not difficult to find that Nanduri sarpanch was from Scheduled Caste (SC) community while the deputy sarpanch was from the upper caste.

The elite capture of such local institutional bodies that were meant to be accountable was a grave issue in Nanduri which was not seen in Surli. In Surli, there was a female sarpanch from Other Backward Class (OBC) community. Studies have shown that female sarpanchs are mere rubber stamps in the hands of males and upper caste political leadership. This cannot be totally ruled out in Surli, however functioning of the VHSC indicated a positive impact from local political leadership, despite there being a female sarpanch. During an interaction with the Surli sarpanch, she shared that she often went to the anganwadi centre to taste the food and show her solidarity with the workers. This was also confirmed by the anganwadi worker. Political capability of the community in both the cases could explain underlying causes of political consensus or lack of it that affect institutional processes like VHSC.

5.3 Users' Political Spaces

Accountability is intricately linked to political capability of actors, especially the users. In order to access political capabilities of the people in both the villages, the heads of the households were asked questions on their awareness and nature of participation in community organisations during the household survey. There are many community organisations (CO) in a village like gram sabha, gram panchayat, political party, bank society, and self-help groups (*bachat gath*). Households were asked if they are aware of these community organisations and if they participated in these in the last one year (Figure 5.1). In addition, households were also asked the nature of their participation like holdings posts, attending meetings, volunteering or taking any benefit (Figure 5.2).

5.3.1 Panchayati Raj Institutions (PRIs)

Almost 100% households were aware about the gram sabha and gram panchayat in both the villages (Figure 5.1). However, only 66.7% households in Surli and a bit lower percentage (65.7%) in Nanduri attended gram sabha meetings. Informal discussions had revealed that the gram sabha is called thrice in a year at most and is scheduled on important dates like January 26 (Republic Day), August 15 (Independence Day) and October 2 (Gandhi Jayanti).

It is attended largely by men, while women's participation is culturally seen as non-conformist. If at all women participate, it is an exception rather than a norm. Reasons shared by households on why they do not participate in gram sabha were largely confined to statements like –

'don't get time; don't feel the need to go there or not interested and don't know.'

Households that attend and participate in gram sabha meetings go for select issues mainly involving development of local infrastructure either for agriculture related activities or related to water and sanitation. Some also go there for educational improvements, government scheme implementation or just for gaining information.

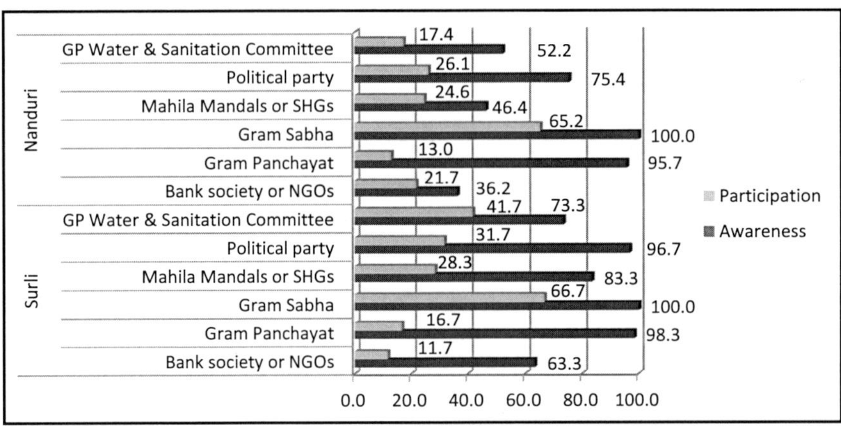

Figure 5.1: Awareness and Participation in Community Organisations

Source: Field level data 2012

Of all the respondents, on an average, 5-10% heads of the households or any of its members currently are or have occupied position of either members or office bearers in some committee of the gram panchayat of both villages (Figure 5.2). The office of the gram panchayat in Surli had displayed names and office bearers of the current committees like tax collection committee, village education committee, forest committee, bandh-kaam (brickwork) committee, dakshata (security) committee and even *pani-puravtha* (water and sanitation) committee. It was not so in Nanduri.

It is common to see that health and nutrition, is not a community issue unlike education, water and sanitation despite it being brought together under one roof in VHSNC. There is similar evidence in other researches that show that health and child nutrition is not an issue at all that draws people to attend gram sabha meetings. According to Joshi (2006),

> *'local governments put education on the agenda of gram sabha meetings in close to 10 percent of the meetings, with water and sanitation following at 8.8 percent. Between 4.8 to 9.3 percent of individuals attend gram sabha meetings because one of these services is on the agenda. In some cases panchayats allocated a lower proportion of resources to health than that allocated by the state government prior to decentralisation. Active panchayat support for primary healthcare centres existed only in a few cases; however, when it did, the result was positive.'*

To probe further, an open-ended question was asked from the households to directly ask them on how they perceive the gram panchayat's role in the functioning of the anganwadi centres (Figure 5.2). Answers to this question were analysed qualitatively to identify households' perceptions of the gram panchayat 's role in anganwadi centres. The convergences or divergences of the responses could explain the difference in the nature of political participation in Nanduri and Surli. Clearly, a majority of households in both Surli and Nanduri either didn't know that their gram panchayat played a role in functioning of the anganwadi centre or they were of the opinion that it played no role (Figure 5.2).

There was however a distinct difference seen in Surli where its gram panchayat played an engaged role in its anganwadi centres as compared to that in Nanduri. One of the most noteworthy features which households in Surli mentioned was that their gram panchayat contributed funds to the anganwadi centre.

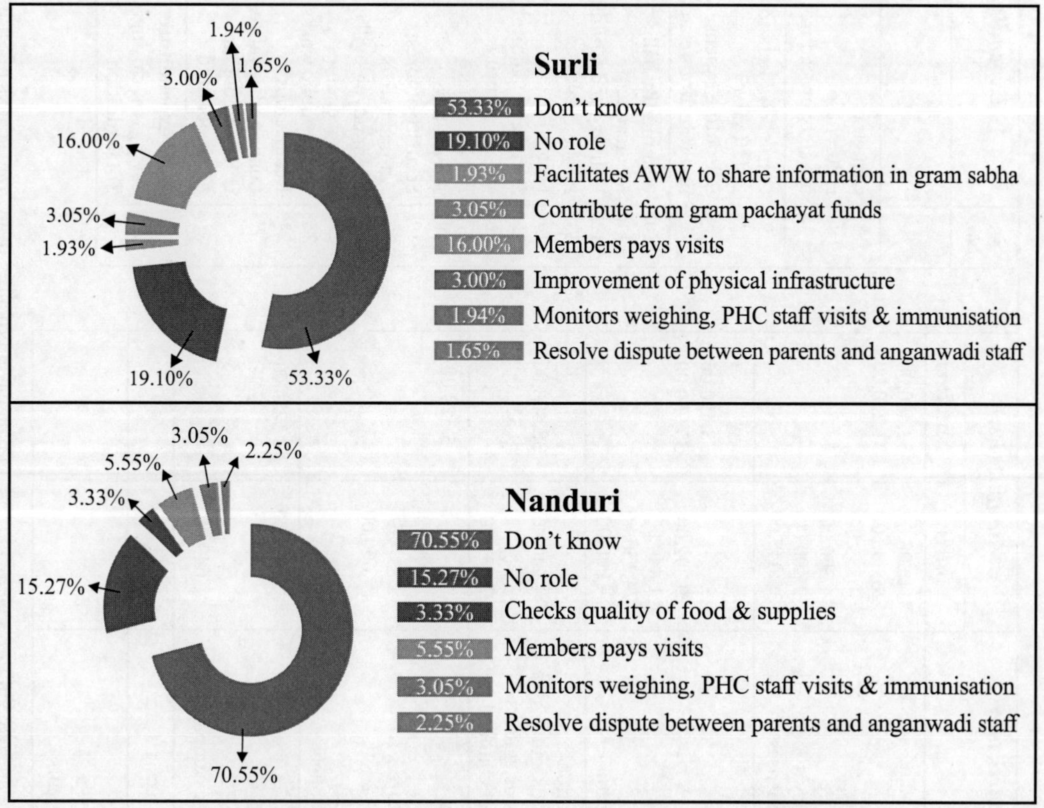

Figure 5.2: Households' Perception of Gram Panchayat's Role in Anganwadi

Source: Household survey, fieldwork 2012

Table 5.2: Comparison of annual expenditure of gram panchayats of Surli and Nanduri, 2011-2012

Expenditure particulars	*Amount (Rs.)*	
	Surli	*Nanduri*
General Works	24,508.00	30,460.00
i. Workers salary	26,806.00	31,200.00
ii. Travelling allowance	4,735.00	
a. For office staff	4,300.00	
b. For gram panchayat members	2,400.00	
iii. Office monthly expenses	36,045.00	
Water Supply		
i. New connections		58,490.00
ii. Repairs	9,392.00	35,950.00
a. Ponds	1,440.00	
b. Wells	74,150.00	
c. Culvet construction	4,000.00	
Means of communication		
i. Construction of roads, gutters	4,940.00	38,408.00
ii. Maintenance of roads, gutters		9,530.00
iii. Telephones and net connection	2,532.00	
Health and Sanitation		5,370.00
i. a. Staff salary	8,600.00	
b. Montly expenditure		
ii. a. Gutter cleaning	19,600.00	
b. Filling of pot holes		
c. Construction of toilets		
Electricity	36,563.00	27,250.00
i. Staff salary		
ii. Disel/oil		
iii. Any others (Village campaigns)	1,640.00	
Site for pilgrimarge, bazaars etc.		
Abbator		
i. Construction		
ii. Maintenance & repairs		

Sr. No.	*Expenditure particulars*	*Amount (Rs.)*	
		Surli	*Nanduri*
8.	Cemetry	550.00	
	i. Purchase		
	ii. Safety procedures		
9.	Cattle Pen / Rent for Anganwadi room	800.00	
	i. Staff salary		
	ii. Routine expenses248.00		
	iii. Protection related		
10.	Community hall	3,66,630.00	
11.	Medical help	6,080.00	
12.	Delivery and Child Development	6,400.00	
13.	Public Health		
14.	Education	5,000.00	
15.	Social and Cultural activities	1,527.00	
16.	Village security	500.00	
17.	Public welfare	35,000.00	
18.	Agriculture		
19.	Security of forests		
20.	Animal care & protection		
21.	Gram udyog - village cottage industry		
22.	Tools n engines	21,410.00	
23.	Other public works		
24.	Retail shops	1,241.00	3,230.00
25	Loans and advances	1,845.00	
	i. Return of loans	33,250.00	
	ii. School fund	20,000.00	
	Total expenditure	**7,69,582.00**	**2,39,858.00**
	Savings on closing	4,26,818.00	17,290.00
	Total addition	11,96,400.00	2,57,148.00

Source: Annual income and expenditure statement of gram panchayat procured from gram sevaks of Surli and Nanduri gram panchayat s during fieldwork in 2012. Data was in form of photocopied papers and was in Marathi. It was translated and typed for this comparison. Income comparison is not included here.

To note, funding to anganwadi centres by a gram panchayat is neither stipulated by the ICDS or NRHM scheme, or even by the panchayati raj institution's list of subjects & spending priorities since it is a vertical programme funded directly by the state through the ICDS. Surli households also mentioned that their gram panchayat contributed in improving physical infrastructure of the centres. I checked the quantum and frequency of the gram panchayat 's contribution to verify these claims (see Table 5.2).

According to the income and expenditure statements of Surli's gram panchayat, the panchayat did contribute some amount (although little) towards rent and miscellaneous expenditures of the anganwadi centre. In addition, it also spent exclusively on heads like 'medical help' and 'delivery and child development'. There was no such category of expenditure in Nanduri where even spending under the head 'health and sanitation' was much lower as compared to that in Surli.

Therefore, the fact that the Surli gram panchayat spent funds on Anganwadi centre, meant that it did occupy a political space in the village. Another distinguishing feature of the gram panchayat mentioned by households in Surli was that it facilitates anganwadi workers to attend and share their work at the gram sabha meetings. Such a practice shows that there were opportunities for information dissemination and answerability between providers and users in the institutional spaces of panchayati raj institution in Surli. Since such a feedback was coming from households, it had high credibility and weight. All these features were not present in Nanduri and were neither shared by its households. In Nanduri, when VHSC funds itself remained unutilised owing to ` clash between the sarpanch and anganwadi workers, the gram panchayat contributing funds for anganwadi centre looked far-fetched.

In Nanduri, there was one distinct practice seen which did not exist in Surli. Households in Nanduri mentioned that its Village Education Committee (VEC) members (and not gram panchayat members) who were active not only in paying visits to the anganwadi centres but at times tasted the cooked food and checked supplies. To note, the VEC has an institutional mandate to check mid-day meals in schools but not at the anganwadi centre. In practice, the VEC was also checking food at anganwadi centre in Nanduri.

This shows that the absence of VHSC was, to an extent, filled by the VEC. Household interviews revealed few common features about the gram panchayat 's role in anganwadi centres, which were equally so in both the villages. For instance, the gram panchayat ensured health services like immunisation and weighing happened regularly. Another significant feature commonly cited by households in both villages was that gram panchayat members pitched in to resolve any disputes arising between parents and anganwadi centre staff. It means that there were confrontations happening between users and providers in both villages, the nature and extent of which is discussed in the last section on 'User's Claims to Answerability'.

Another institution at the village level which is also linked to political participation in general and participation in panchayati raj institutions in particular are political parties (Figure 5.1). Awareness of local political parties was higher in Surli (96.7%) than Nanduri (85.3%), also, a higher percentage of households in Surli (31.7%) than in Nanduri (26.1%) were involved with local political parties. Participation in political parties included activities like taking part in its cultural events like haldi-kum kum for ladies, local protest campaigns for instance on farmers issues, organising a rally or a mass meeting for a contesting, candidate and volunteering in election campaigning.

Households were also asked if they had participated in a political rally nearing the time of elections. A higher percentage of households in Surli said they did not participate (78.3%) in any political rally or a function as compared to those in Nanduri (71%). Reasons for keeping away from local politics ranged from not being interested, not wanting to be seen as partisan, not having time, and not knowing. Households in Nanduri were politically less active than those in Surli in everyday local politics but more active during time of elections. At the national level, there are studies to suggest that child health as an issue is considered insignificant in electoral calculations (Sinha 2006). Rural electoral culture at the frontline does not look any different.

When asked about awareness and participation in the VHSC, a majority of households mistook it for Water & Sanitation committee of Gram Panchayat which is an active arm of the gram panchayat and has a high interface with households. It is obvious that they do not know about the VHSC since by design it does not have a mass reach. Therefore, I allowed them to respond even if they mistook it for the gram panchayat 's Water & Sanitation committee (gram panchayat -WSC).

The survey results showed that a higher percentage of households in Surli were aware about gram panchayat -WSC (73.3%) as compared to Nanduri (62%). There was a striking difference in the participation between the two villages. While a high percentage of households (41.7%) in Surli participated in this committee, this percentage was low at 17.4% in Nanduri. Participation was sought mainly for providing suggestions or being informed about government schemes related to water. Households who did not participate in this committee especially those from Nanduri cited that since the committee was already doing decent work, there is no need for them to participate while others even mentioned lack of confidence in participating in such forums.

5.3.2 Community Organisations

On an average, 'awareness' of all community organisations was found to be higher in Surli (85.8%) as compared to Nanduri (68%) (Figure 5.1). However, when it comes to 'participation' of households in community organisations, it was higher in Nanduri (43%) as compared to Surli (37.6%) on an average. This was because a higher percentage of households in Nanduri used the bank's society for agriculture loans (21.7%) as compared to Surli (11.7%), on an average. In Surli a higher percentage of households participated in SHGs (28.3%) as compared to Nanduri (24.6%). SHGs are known as *bachat gaths* (small saving groups) where members save and take small loans, largely for consumption expenditure like hospitalisation, marriage, buying consumer durables etc.

Clearly households in Nanduri availed loans for livelihood while those in Surli for consumption. In Nanduri, few SHGs were dissolved as there were complaints of corruption and many had lost their savings. The finding matches with the patterns of asset ownership which show higher percentage of households in Surli falling in rich and upper middle asset quintile than those in Nanduri. In rural areas, bank society includes credit-based community-based organisations (CBOs) which give agricultural loans to farmers, for instance in Nanduri these were called *Osmanabad Sahakari Bank, Nanduri Vikas Society, Padamsingh Mazdoor Sahakari Society Ltd. Tuljapur* and the one in Surli was called *Surli Cooperative Bank.*

In addition, there were non-credit CBOs based on culture or sports like the one called *Shraddha Bahuudeshiya Sanskritik Kreeda Mandal* for *Ganesh* festival and a reading club called *Mahatma Phule Vachanalaya.* Nature of participation in community organisations in Surli was low and largely on the fringes by either attending meetings for the sake for being informed while that in Nanduri was of active engagement. It is equally important to understand who participates in various community organisations, especially from asset categories (Figure 5.3).

Clearly, elite capture is seen in most community organisations, particularly the rich asset quintile participating in Gram Panchayat and local political parties which was similarly high in both villages. What sets the two villages apart is that the poorest in Nanduri were more active in participating in majority of community organisations like gram panchayat, political party, *mahila mandal* and in bank society as compared to the poor of Surli. Also, there was a higher participation of lower middle asset quintile in Nanduri as compared to those in Surli.

In addition, the middle asset quintile in Nanduri had the highest participation in the gram sabha as compared to all other categories. Participation of the poor-most asset quintiles in local political institutions can impact the way answerability is demanded and sanctions imposed on the providers. An implication of this will be revealed as more data unfolds. Such level of participation in community organisations by the poor and middle asset categories in Nanduri has implications on people's ability to sanction providers. Another indicator to access political capability of users is their access to multiple power holders at the frontline of service delivery. This is discussed in the following section.

5.3.3 Local Power Holders

Political capabilities can also be understood in terms of people's capacity to approach and interact with those in positions of power for common community or personal issues (Table 5.3). Households were asked if they have ever approached few listed power holders for personal or community work in last three months. These power holders can be persons holding positions, both at village level and higher levels like members of gram panchayat, political party representative, politicians like zila parishad (ZP) member of MLA, bureaucrats and even local NGOs.

A staggering 90% of households in Surli had approached politicians for some personal or community work while this percentage was the lowest at 8.7% for Nanduri. In Nanduri, a majority of households (88.4%) approached gram panchayat members to some work as opposed to 70% in Surli. Also a higher percentage of households in Nanduri approached bureaucrats (37.7%) than those in Surli (2.7%).

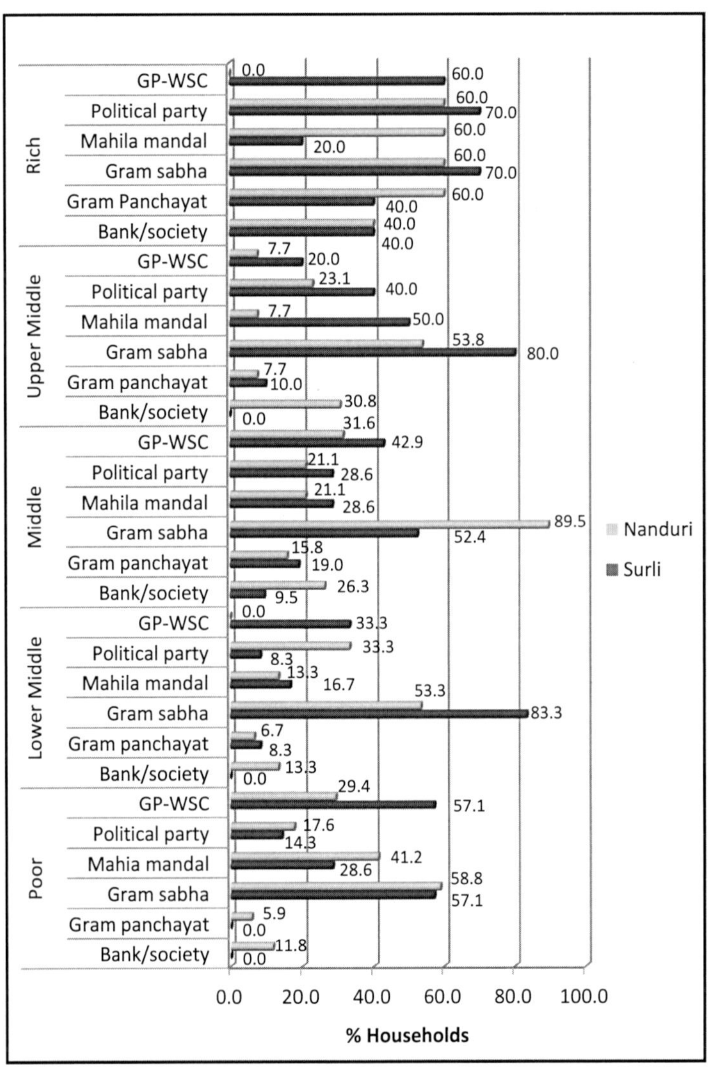

Figure 5.3: Participation in Community Organisations by Asset Categories

Note: Participation in last one year. Source: Household survey during fieldwork, 2012

This implies that households in Nanduri opted for state-related power holders in gram panchayat and bureaucrats, while those in Surli were more inclined towards non-state actors in political parties and politicians.

This observation can be explained by the social composition of the two villages. In Surli, high percentage of rich and upper middle asset households warrant asking and giving favours to local politicians. In Nanduri, higher middle and poor asset households could access state functionaries.

Table 5.3: Households' Capacity to Approach Power Holders

Power holders	***Households that ever approached 'Yes'***			
	Surli (n=60)		Nanduri (n=69)	
	Count	%	Count	%
Activist or NGO member	3	5.0	5	7.2
Bureaucrat at taluka or zila level	16	26.7	26	37.7
Gram panchayat member	42	70.0	61	88.4
Mahila mandal member	12	20.0	14	20.3
Political party member	18	30.0	19	27.5
Politician at village/zila/district/state	54	90.0	6	8.7
VHSC member	26	43.3	17	24.6

Note: Approached in last one year. Source: Field level data (2012)

The question is which of these strategies yield results for the poor? Recent studies on participation by and representation of the urban poor vis-à-vis service provisioning suggest a kind of reluctance on the part of the government to improve the access of the poor to basic services (Pande, 2008). A study revealed that it was unclear whether the needs being highlighted genuinely reflect the priorities of slum residents, or get inadvertently replaced or otherwise by the priorities of Government or NGOs, in a hurry to show results' (ibid.).

Therefore a contradictory trend seem to be emerging in India as a whole - that the needs and interests of the poor are now being met more effectively through the 'new politics' of social movements, rather than through trade unions, burgeoning non-governmental organisations (NGOs), associations of civil society, or indeed political parties (ibid.).

5.4 To Question and To Claim Answers

Hirschman classifies 'voice' as one of the three strategies through which people seek to exert influence (Goetz & Jenkins, 2005). Over the past two decades, increased participation to bring the 'voices of the poor' to the ears of the policy makers have been undertaken in the developing countries. Initially welcomed, these initiatives have been increasingly dismissed as tokenism unless there is a shift in focus from merely capturing the voices of the marginalised to actually using them to hold the powerful accountable (ibid.).

It is equally true that voice and accountability are conceptually distinguishable, but inseparable in practice. In fact in Sen's 'Development as Freedom', Sen identifies three benefits that arise from political freedoms of which voice's constructive role is integral to human development (ibid). Voice can be expressed individually or collectively. In the context of this study, evidence on how communities in Nanduri used voice to hold providers to account are documented (See Box 5.2 and Box 5.3).

5.4.1 Formal Instruments

According to scholars,

> *'Conventional forms of political voice and accountability – two of the defining features of liberal democracy, have not been able to safeguard the interests of the poor. Voting in elections, joining political parties, expressing preferences in community forums – none of these channels of voice has been adequate to the enormous task of sanctioning governments for failing to promote human development' (Goetz & Jenkins, 2005: 28).*

However, formal instruments are still the mainstay of accountability mechanisms in India. Therefore, there is a need to access them in the context of this study. The formal institutional mechanisms for eliciting answerability and hence accountability at the frontline of service delivery in a village are elections at various levels of governance including panchayat elections, Right to Information Act, Citizen charters and VHSC. Other mechanisms like Rogi Kalyan Samitis (RKS) although existing at the bottommost level of health service delivery at a PHC, was out of the authority of a village or a panchayat.

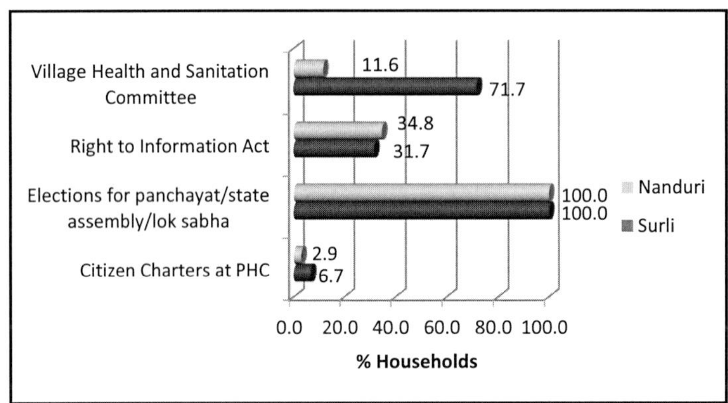

Figure 5.4: Formal Institutional Instruments of Accountability

Source: Household survey during fieldwork, 2012

Respondents were asked if they were aware of these instruments (Figure 5.4). If they responded with a 'yes', then I asked how they participated or used these instruments and their perceptions on impact these instruments have had on their lives and on their village.

Elections – Almost 100% respondents in both villages were aware about various elections and majority of the respondents (heads of households) participate through voting in elections (Figure 5.4). Informal conversations with the head of the households revealed that many women do not have their voter identity cards made and are also not encouraged to vote. When asked about any impact of elections in an open-ended question, households in Nanduri mentioned that elections had resulted in creation of village infrastructure like roads, light and water availability. Such a feedback was also present in Surli but not significant, probably because such a development had already happened there. In Surli, households did attribute better implementation of housing schemes like Indira Awas Yojana (IAY) to elections.

Literature also confirms this finding that information deficiencies lead voters to giving more credit to politicians for initiating public works projects (construction) as these public resources are easily and directly targeted to supporters (Goetz & Jenkins, 2005). Also, there is a growing understanding that long established relationships between elite patrons and poor in clientelist system may prevent voters from punishing errant politicians at election time, for fear of losing whatever benefits they receive as loyal clients (ibid.).

In fact, it is interesting to note that households in Surli felt that elections had no impact on their lives and on their village as compared to those in Nanduri. Issues related to improvements in agriculture, healthcare, school education were hardly identified in relation to elections. These findings are in line with the literature, as mentioned by scholars - "It is difficult for voters to coordinate in assigning rewards or penalties to politicians for their performance on public services, particularly primary health and education, because these are complex services and outcomes are hard to attribute to any representative's (or government's) term in office (ibid.).'

Right to Information (RTI) – As a counter-intuitive trend, a higher percentage of households (34.8%) in Nanduri were aware about RTI as compared to Surli (31.7%). Also a higher percentage of households in Nanduri filed an RTI query (six households) than those in Surli (two households). Key issues on which RTI queries were filed were related to records pertaining to land or certificates, schools, anganwadi centre and corruption at panchayat.

One man from Nanduri had filed an RTI query to CDPO's office related to exclusion of his three-year-old niece from anganwadi services in the village. He wanted to know the reasons why the anganwadi centre did not provide any service to his niece who could not walk to the centre as one of her foot was handicap. He demanded information on height and weight of all children registered with the anganwadi centre for year 2010-

2011. He revealed that although he did not get a reply, but he did not regret it since the anganwadi centre started providing all services to his niece.

Few other interesting instances of RTI queries related to nutrition and health services were narrated by frontline workers in Nanduri (Box 5.1). Frontline workers were a reliable source of information on RTIs since they are the ones who compile information on the queries received from the CDPO's office and are also aware of queries pertaining to the village's gram panchayat. The above query was made by a man from SC community belonging to middle asset category since he was working as a clerk in local government and hence aware of RTI provisions.

People too made other queries, belonging to largely from middle, upper-middle or rich asset classes of general category. In Surli, the two RTI queries pertained to issues like personal salary appraisal from a government office, the other one to the village talathi related to farming. Clearly, households in Nanduri were not only more aware about RTI as a tool but were also filing RTIs especially related to ICDS.

Village Health & Sanitation Committee – A higher percentage of households in Surli (71.7%) were aware about VHSC, which was merely 11.6% in Nanduri. This was so because as discussed earlier, most actors were confused owing to duplicity of this committee as the one from the gram panchayat or VHSC (See 5.2.2). Consequently, only six households reported of giving complaints related to water and sanitation in Surli as compared to only four in Nanduri.

When asked about the possible benefits of the VHSC to those who were aware, most did not know how it helped them or their village but some cited benefits like improved water and sanitation, and better water management in the village. In Surli, households mentioned the *Nirmal Gram Puruskar*[1] (Open Defecation Free Village Award) which their village got in 2011. It meant that households associated the award with the work of the water and sanitation committee of their village (Figure 5.5). There was a perceived positive impact of the workings of such committee in Surli, which in Nanduri was only limited to acknowledgement of availability of water. There was no mention of health, nutrition or sanitation issues.

Citizen Charters – The Government of India (GoI) had launched Citizen Charters in 1997 as an important reform to tackle the problem of information asymmetry and the perennial disconnect between the allocation and effectiveness of public expenditure. All central and state ministries and departments are supposed to prepare citizen's charters in order to inform the public about their rights and entitlements in public services, the standards of the services, and the remedies available in case of failure (Paul, 2008). Citizen charters are the benchmarks or standards against which entitled services are to be delivered.

1 *This is an award conceived by the Maharashtra government to a village gram panchayat to recognise its efforts in making the village open defecation free. The award had a cash prize of Rs. 1,00,000 to promote and sustain the status of the village.*

Conceptually, standards have a significant role to play in the process of accountability (See Figure 2.3). Providers are held responsible for their decisions and actions against some 'standards' like rules, norms, outcomes and procedures (Rubenstein, 2007). Under the NRHM, charters meant for the citizens are usually displayed at a public facility like a PHC. Yet, a majority of households in both villages were not aware about citizen's charters even after 18 years of its introduction (Figure 5.5). Awareness among respondents in Surli about citizen charters was higher than that of Nanduri, although their access to a nearby PHC was much lower than those in Nanduri.

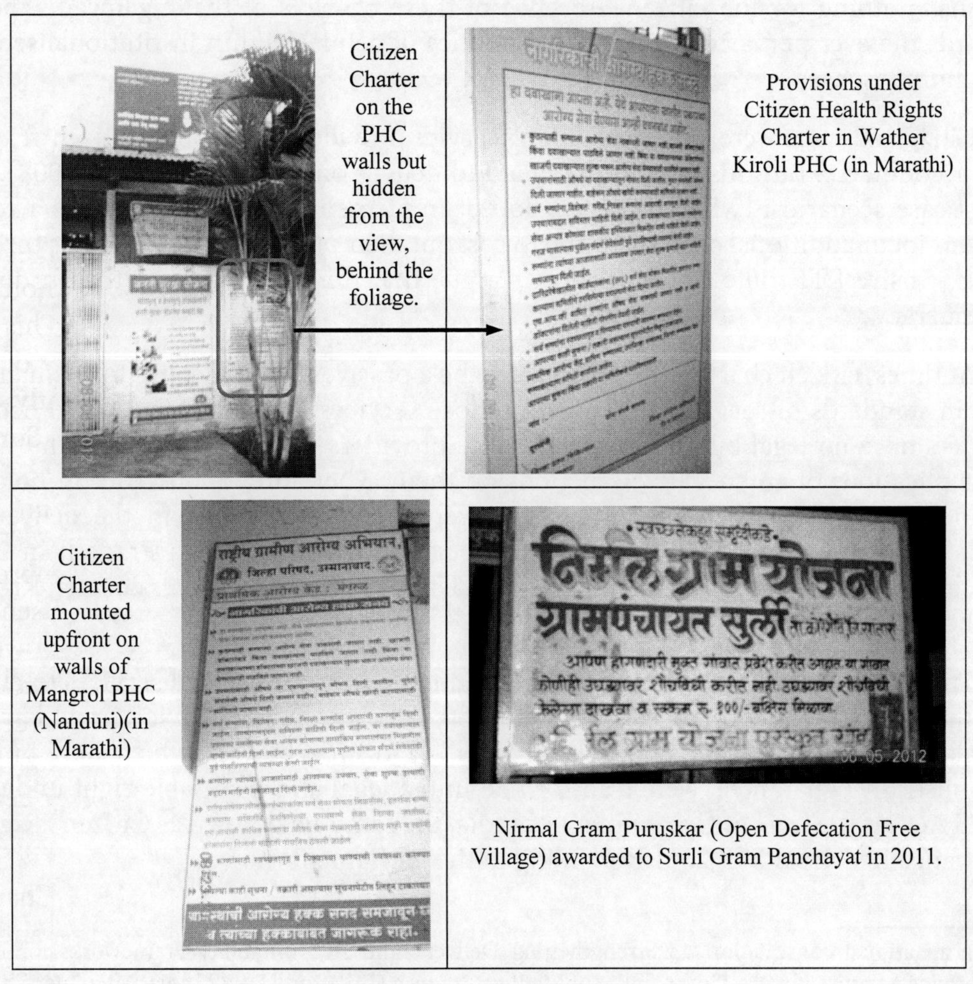

Figure 5.5: Citizen Charters

Source: Pictures from author's fieldwork, 2012

Citizen charter was printed on walls of Wathar PHC, but the irony was that it was barely visible (Figure 5.5). Upon enquiring the reasons about charter looking deliberately camouflaged behind foliage, medical officer said, '*Yes sometimes we have to take decisions which are illegal but karna padta hai* (we have to do it)'. He justified his views by adding that when people come here, they are under physical and mental distress, needing quick treatment. They would hardly read anything of this sort. He added that this charter anyways has no implication even if evaded on any count.

In Mangrol PHC, the citizen charter was seen upfront as soon as one entered the PHC premises. Under the ICDS, there are no citizen charters pasted on the walls of the anganwadi centres, anywhere in the country. The Union Ministry of Women and Child Development that fund the ICDS has drafted its citizen or client charters for the ministry as a whole with no separate charter for the ICDS (Ministry of Women and Child Development 2015). Even this 50 page document is actually meant for the bureaucracy and has nothing for the citizen. Absence of these charters at the anganwadis, points towards the ever pervasive, yet invisible politics of gender within institutionalised and community spaces.

Citizen charters were aimed at making service providers more open, citizen-friendly and accountable. But this reform has failed to deliver on its promise (Paul, 2008). The worst case scenario is where agencies do not implement citizen's charters; as a result, citizens incur additional costs by trying to sort out their public service problems through the expensive RTI route (ibid). Scholars argue that this also increases the burden on bureaucracy.

At times, citizen charters are critiqued to be a passive and ineffective for demanding certain standards of service and ensuring those services are delivered. It is so because charters have no legal binding on the service providers unlike the RTI Act and hence no implications of any negative sanctions on them. Therefore, in order to up-hold the democratic ethos of accountability, transparency and equitability in the delivery of public services, several State governments, beginning with Madhya Pradesh in 2010[2] and followed by Bihar, J&K, Delhi, Rajasthan, Uttar Pradesh and others enacted Right to Public Services Act (RTPS Act).

The Act is intended to guarantee time-bound delivery of selected services to citizen (Mathur, 2012). The Act places the onus of delivery on the service provider with penalties for delays in service provision (ibid.). Citizen's charters, which were only an administrative guarantee, were transformed into a legal and justiciable right under the RTPS Act. At the level of Government of India, the same act, known as Citizen's Right to Grievance Redressal Bill, 2011 is pending in the Parliament.

2 In a national consultation on Strengthening Delivery and Accountability Frameworks for Public Service organised by the Government of Madhya Pradesh (MP) and UNDP India, MP Chief Minister explained why and how they decided to go in for legislation on public services: 'At the time of elections people are the most important. After that the government ignores them. The CM, Ministers, and bureaucrats, all think that they are perfect, and wisdom cannot reside outside this group. In case of MP, we had introduced one-day governance, samadhan ek din mein (solutions in a day) and we had Citizen's Charters. But when we listened to the people, we found that no body looked at the Citizens Charters and nobody bothered about the details. We wanted, then, to introduce a Citizens Charter Act. There were a number of doubting themes. But the question we asked was if we are giving rights through charters why are we scared of fixing responsibility? Thus was born the MP Lok Sewaon Ke Pravdhan Ki Guarantee Adhiniyam (Public Service Guarantee Act).' (Mathur, 2012)

Implementation of the RTPS Act is in fairly initial stages of implementation in various states and there is not enough evidence on its impact for improving public services. Maharashtra government has recently asked for citizen comments on the draft of its Maharashtra Guarantee of Public Services Bill (Marapakwar, 2015). However, activists have critiqued this draft as missing on three crucial components - services covered, time duration and penalties for erring officials. Other state governments like Kerala, Karnataka and Orissa have also proposed the bill.

Box 5.1: Nature of RTI Queries in Nanduri
On Village Health & Sanitation Committee (VHSC)

'A man from Dhanegoan, an adjacent village from Nanduri had filed an RTI query asking the expenditure details of Nanduri's VHSC. Both these villages fall under my jurisdiction. As per my information, the VHSC had got Rs. 10,000. As per the mutual understanding both anganwadi worker and sarpanch divides the amount equally. However, I came to know that the sarpanch took the entire amount and did not give anything to the anganwadi worker. I also told him to give half the amount, but he did not pay heed. Then we told him to give receipts of the expenditure incurred. He didn't give that too. Consequently this man filed an RTI query. In response, sarpanch asked for some time to give all the receipts. In the meantime, the term of this sarpanch ended a new sarpanch took charge. Then he started saying, that he is no longer the sarpanch and do whatever you want to. It was too late to come to the notice of higher officials that money meant for anganwadi centre was spent unaccountably.' – ANM, Nanduri

Candidate's eligibility on two-child norm in Panchayat elections

'Once local elections were about to happen, including that of the sarpanch. There is a rule that candidates with three children cannot become a sarpanch. RTI was the tool in the hands of all rival candidates to find out number of children of those contesting elections. For full one month our head office had many queries and so my seniors asked me to get all birth and death records since 1993 onwards. Such old records were all over the place and it took me three days just to organise them. Our senior put his entire staff on the job to Xerox all the pages. Our office incurred an expenditure of Rs. 4000 on this account but once this figure was told to that person who had filed the query, he never turned up to get it. Later I came to know that the query was made against village's current deputy-sarpanch since he has three kids. He argued that his third child was born before 2001, when this ruling came into effect and hence, he was qualified to hold the post.' – Anganwadi worker, Nanduri

Miscellaneous

'Once a domicile related query had come from Mangrol village. As a rule, if the domicile of the anganwadi helper is not of that village, she cannot be selected as a helper. This was a case of a woman in Mangrol who had worked as anganwadi helper for four years. In the same anganwadi, there was a vacancy of anganwadi worker. She applied for it. Another village resident, a man wanted his MA/Bed wife to get this post and had made her apply too. But that helper bagged the job and this man's wife didn't. So he filed an RTI query to know how a helper can become a worker. He got the reply from our office showing the court order that if a helper fills a form for vacancy of worker, she will be given preference to fill the position. There was a lot of inspection on her background since she was only 12th pass. But her track record was good, and all her documents were valid. We also get RTI queries related to self-help groups or information in the diary of the supervisor as to where she goes for inspection etc.' – ICDS Supervisor

Source: In-depth interviews with frontline providers, fieldwork 2012.

5.4.2 Informal Instruments: An Outlet of Assertion

In the relationship of the user and provider, the balance of power usually favours the provider. In such a case it is unlikely a user in individual capacities or even as a community will raise a voice or sanction the provider. It is all the more true for health services in Indian context where social status and professional power distances doctors from poor patients (Hossain, 2010). Even health providers like ANM and nurses enjoy a higher respect and status than anganwadi worker.

In recent times this balance of power is seen to be tiling in favour of users or patients with increasing incidents of attacks on doctors being reported. However, these are confined to urban areas while rural India continues to conform to the traditional power structure. Mortality and illness, being sensitive issues, related to power and hierarchy, there is a risk that study respondents may not share incidents of direct and informal confrontations or of demanding accountability with health providers. Literature points to the concept of 'rude accountability' which is unorganised and informal pressures that poor citizens exert on officials, ranging from faintly impolite to downright abusive and plainly violent incidences (ibid).

With help of indirect questions aimed at third person, it was possible for me to know about respondents' first-hand experiences of such informal pressures on providers. However, prior to this question, it was important to understand the extent to which households were facing these situations in their routine interactions with health providers.

For this, households were given six situations which are commonly reported as impediments in accessing a public health facility and were asked if their acquaintances have faced them (Figure 5.6). Situations were those that are commonly experienced and complained by people like long waiting time due to queues, unavailability of doctor, poor water and sanitation that often discourages people to access public health services.

Respondents, mainly the head of the household and the woman (mother of child under six), were jointly asked with a yes or no if they have experienced six listed situations in context of accessing public health and nutrition services in last six months. About 10% households in Surli and an equal percentage in Nanduri shared that they have faced long waiting time owing to lack of staff. A majority did not experience these situations because they probably never visited the PHC and had opted for a private health provider. About 21.7% households in Nanduri had experienced a situation where the doctor was unavailable at the time of emergency. This percentage was much lower (10%) in Surli.

Only 14.4% in Nanduri felt that PHC staff made regular home visits for lactating and pregnant women. This percentage was almost nil in Surli which means PHC staff like ANM or ASHA did not home visit any pregnant and lactating mother. About 11.6% households in Nanduri reported the situation of food at the anganwadi centre not being appropriate and children falling sick after eating it. Only one household responded to this situation in Surli. One situation where households in both villages reported a yes response was for a faulty prescription by the doctor causing abnormal reaction and suffering, 11.6% in Nanduri and 6.7% in Surli.

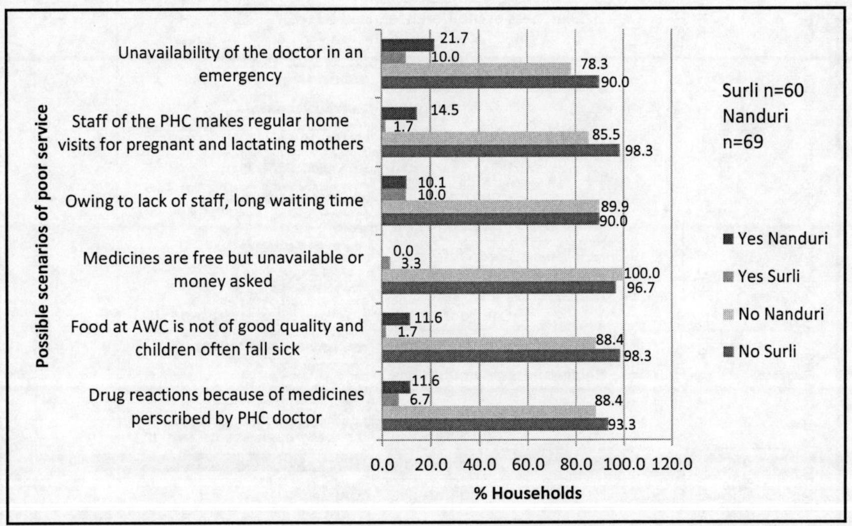

Figure 5.6: Households' Response to Possible Scenarios of Poor Health Services

Source: Household survey during fieldwork, 2012

Finally, most households in both the villages said 'No' to the situation about medicines being free at the PHC but available with bribe of money. In all, the percentage of households facing any of these six situations is certainly not high, nonetheless, it was significant in knowing if respondents faced these situations at all.

There seem to be a low rate of incidence or prevalence of such incidence. So the same situations were presented before the respondents as hypothetical situations to elicit their responses and access their capacities to demand answerability. Respondents were asked six hypothetical open ended questions following from the previous section on instances of poor health and nutrition services (Figure 5.7). They were asked in an open ended question, that if they were to face these situations, what they would do. Responses were later categorised in four main categories – confrontational, exit, helplessness or indifference and finally don't know. Actual responses within each category are explained with the analysis.

The first situation presented to the respondents was unavailability of the doctor in a PHC at the time of emergency and what would they do in such a scenario. A much higher percentage of respondents in Surli (76.7%) than in Nanduri (58%) said that they would opt to go to a private doctor, a response that was considered as 'exit'. Pervious evidence in Chapter 4 too supports this observation. Interestingly, a higher percentage of respondents in Nanduri (15.9%) than in Surli (10%) would confront this situation.

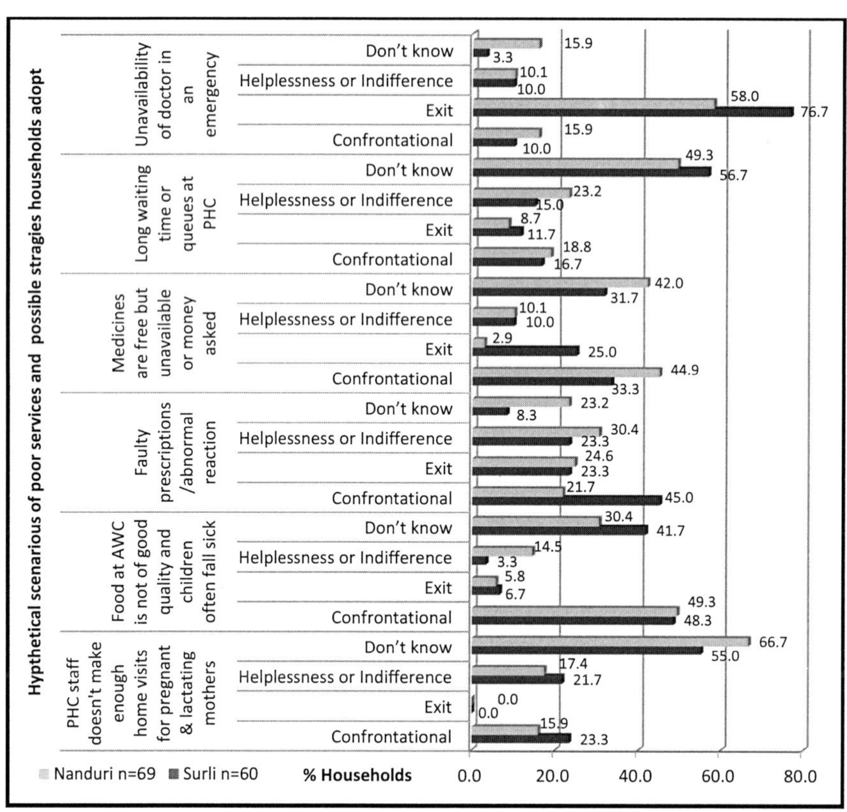

Figure 5.7: Households' Strategies in Case of Poor Health and Nutrition Services

Strategies of confrontation, although hypothetical would provide insights into the nature and the users' potential to confront the providers. Respondents mentioned informal strategies like getting rude with the PHC staff to call the doctor and demanding explanations on why doctor cannot attend to patients during emergency (Box 5.2). Many also cited formal forms of protests like registering a police complaint, or complaining to gram panchayat members or to a higher authority like health officials (Box 5.3). Both formal and informal strategies of confrontation were clubbed ogether because of small numbers

The second scenario given to respondents was long waiting time and queues at the PHC. A majority of respondents in both the villages responded with a 'don't know' response – 56.7% in Surli and 49.3% in Nanduri. It means that an earlier observation is reinforced that a majority of households in both villages do not visit PHC despite it being within its accessible distance and with availability of doctors and staff.

This observation was followed by response of helplessness with respondents mentioning statements like 'we will wait, cannot do anything', which was higher for Nanduri (15%) than Surli (11.7%). Respondents resorting to confrontational strategy were few in this scenario, but higher in Nanduri (18.8%) than Surli (16.7%). Informal confrontation included rude suggestions to staff and medical officer to recruit more people or complaining to the local politician. In Nanduri, there have been instances of local politicians getting involved in protests against doctors of the PHC (see Box 5.2).

Box 5.2: Case of Informal or Rude Accountability

'*People here (Mangrol) are like this – they think that when we come to PHC, what we want, we should get it like give injection and saline. If we tell them that you do not require saline, they insist strongly in getting it. Jo nuke maan mein hai woh hona chahiye (what they expect, they need to get it). They go back to the village and then bitch about us that we don't give saline. We can sense this roughness.*' – ANM, Nanduri

'*People of Mangrol are notorious in scaring and shunning away PHC doctors. They have shown their colours to me too. This incident took place when I used to stay with my husband at PHC staff quarters. It so happened that people came to wake me up at midnight for a patient. But we were sleeping with a noisy table fan; my phone was on low ringer and we also didn't hear knocks on our door. Soon, people got berserk. They started shouting loudly and throwing stones at our house. Next day morning I came to know from our staff that village people had created a big scene and how much they tried to wake me up. Local politicians called me. I regretted and explained that my phone had gone bad. On the same day I got a new SIM card. That patient was a child. He was referred to Tuljapur in my absence as he had fever, but there was nothing serious. That incident had left me feel vulnerable and I decided not to reside in staff quarters. I am at the PHC till 5 pm or 6 pm and then go home in Tuljapur.*' – Medical officer, Mangrol PHC

'*When Ganpati festival comes villagers come to collect donations from PHC staff. Once, our medical officer told them that he would contribute on behalf of all the staff and not allow individual donations. But they argued that all staff must independently donate a minimum amount of 501. The medical officer asserted and asked them to accept whatever he gives as a joint contribution. The result was that same night people marched towards his house and started pelting stones. When he came out, he was even injured by a stone. Later, medical officer asked for transfer and got it too. People had done a similar thing with an earlier doctor too. Most medical officers are weary to stay here for long. People say things to us like tum kyoon nahi de sakte, tum yahan baithe free mein paise khate ho. (Why can't you give, you are paid such salaries, but do you work accordingly?)' – ANM, Nanduri*

Source: In-depth Interviews during fieldwork in Nanduri 2012.

Some even mentioned posting a written complaint in the complaint box kept in the PHC3[3]. It was a revelation of sorts that there was a complaint box kept in the PHC and one respondent was also aware of it. Upon enquiring about this box from medical officers in both the PHCs it was found that the facility was only there in Wathar PHC and not in Mangrol PHC. However, when the I checked the box during a visit to the PHC, it was kept in one corner, surely to be missed from public eye. The medical officer when asked about it, said in a mocking tone that the box is in its ideal position – hidden from

3 Complaints in complaint box at the PHC are formal modes of confrontation (See Box 5.3).

public view. He also added that they would end up spending more time in attending to complaints than seeing the patients, if it was not so. It was not a surprise that there were no complaints posted in the box. A miniscule percentage of respondents said that they will opt to exit, meaning to choose private health providers, percentage of respondents who said so was higher at 11.7% for Surli than Nanduri (8.7%).

Box 5.3: Case of Formal Sanction

'Once, a tubectomy camp was organised in the Mangrol PHC. At that time RK madam was our MO. When RK madam came for operation, she saw that a staff meeting was going on. She was upset as she expected everyone to be inside the operation theatre and things to be ready before she came. She probably didn't see two ANMs who were preparing patients by administering anaesthesia. This made her angry, so she shouted at the supervisor and left the PHC in her car. Two patients had already been given injections for sedations. There were 9 patients in all. We shifted sedation patients to the cots and gave food to all the other patients. We told them that the operation has been cancelled. Patients had fasted a night before and that day also they did not eat till evening. How would their families tolerate this? Children of women in sedation started crying that their mothers are not waking up. In the meantime someone went in the village and told people what was happening in the PHC. Soon relatives of patients came to know about this and they gathered a crowd. An influential local politician, who was a former ZP member, was informed. Soon officials came, cameras were here, pictures were clicked, and it came in papers and news. There was an FIR lodged. Police van came. They recorded statements from us and patients. They asked RK madam also. Everyone felt that it was her mistake and she should not have done like this. She was merely transferred from here. Her private practice is on but now she has been given a bigger posting at a bigger village.' – ANM, Nanduri

'There was a problem with the service regarding a family planning operation. Issue was not so big, but it was projected as a big issue. In such an operation, we usually give sedation to the patient (local anaesthesia). After 5-6 hours the patient becomes normal and conscious. RK madam had agreed to come although she was on leave. As per the routine protocol, madam had instructed nurses to give sedation to patients while she was on her way. The staff gave the sedation and she came in the meantime. Our meeting was going on and my sister just went for a wash. Madam came here and felt that staff was unnecessarily delaying things when they should have been promptly ready. So she yelled at the staff and left in anger. She didn't say anything to the patient. In fact, nothing happened to the patient. Yet, the villagers complained to the District Health Officer in Osmanabad. They did not know that it was not general anaesthesia which can put the patient at risk. I was also here at that time. We explained to the patient and their relatives that the operation will happen tomorrow morning. Madam wanted to punish the staff so that they would not repeat it again. But the whole thing got flared up. Actually people had it against her, prior to the incident as they felt that she is never present in the PHC. She was transferred from here.' – Medical Officer, Mangrol PHC.

As a third situation, respondents were asked what they would do if medicines that are supposed to be free at the PHC are unavailable or money demanded. A high majority of respondents from Nanduri (44.9%) said that they would confront the situation as compared to those in Surli (33.3%). Confrontations included complaint to the *grahak takraar niwaran kendra* (consumer dispute redressal forum) and complaints at Helpline numbers painted at the walls of the PHC. Mangrol PHC had helpline numbers painted on its walls while this was not present at Wathar PHC. Also, the fact that one Nanduri respondent was aware about it implies stronger processes for grievance redressal. When I dialled those numbers, they were non-functional.

Few also mentioned formal confrontations like complaining to the medical officer or gram panchayat members. The advantage of asking the open-ended question was to get insights like these which could not be possible with structured questions. About 42% respondents in Nanduri and 31.7% in Surli were not aware about what to do in such a scenario and an equal percentage (10%) in both villages cited helplessness.

Responses for helplessness included statements like 'will give money'. Interestingly, a high percentage of respondents in Surli (25%) said that they would buy medicine from any other chemist else visit another doctor. It means a higher percentage of respondents from Surli would simply exit. As discussed earlier, reasons were a combination of higher income status and easy access to private health sector. It meant that with increasing financial prosperity, households tend either to give-in to corrupt practices by bribing or paying rents or to get their way by exiting the situation and buying the services from the private sector.

On faulty prescriptions by PHC doctor causing abnormal reactions, 45% respondents from Surli said that they would confront this situation as compared to 21.7% from Nanduri. However, most of their confrontational measures included formal modes of complaints like that to the police, higher officials of health department or gram panchayat members. In Nanduri, a majority of its respondents (30.4%) cited their helplessness in this scenario with statements like 'I will ask the same doctor to rectify, I will not complain'. This observation shows that since higher percentage of households in Surli accessed private providers than those in Nanduri, they probably have faced medicine-induced reactions. An equal percentage of respondents in both villages (24%) cited option of changing the doctor that is, exiting from the situation.

Finally, respondents were presented with two hypothetical situations related to nutrition services. First, they were asked to respond to the case of food at the anganwadi centre not being appropriate because of which children often fall sick. Almost equal percentage of respondents in Nanduri and Surli (48%) said that they would confront the situation. These confrontations included informal ones like asking the anganwadi worker to take care or do a verbal complaint to the ICDS Supervisor. Formal methods like complaint to the gram panchayat and also to the police were also included, especially in light of recent newspaper reports of cases of food poisoning in Mid-Day Meals and even ICDS. In contrast, 41.7% respondents from Surli answered 'don't know' for this situation, which was much lower in Nanduri (30.4%).

This observation matches with a fact that a large number of households in Surli had exited out of the ICDS while this was not so in Nanduri. For the same scenario, about 14.4% respondents cited helplessness by stating phrases like 'cannot do anything, feed that food to animals or will give child home-made tiffin.' A miniscule percentage in both villages, equally so, mentioned to take the child to the doctor, a measure categorised as 'exit'.

The second situation respondents were asked what they would do if PHC staff like ANMs did not make enough home visits to pregnant or lactating mothers. A majority of respondents in both villages, higher in Nanduri (66.7%) than Surli (55%) were not aware on what can be done. Clearly, most households did not know service entitlements they are supposed to receive from NRHM programme. Only about 23.3% in Surli and 15.9% in Nanduri said that they would confront the situation with formal measures like complaining to the anganwadi worker, medical officer or a gram panchayat member.

A high percentage of respondents felt indifference to this scenario in Surli (21.7%) as compared to Nanduri (17.4%). They explained that it is the mothers, be it pregnant or lactating who are supposed to go and visit the anganwadi centre when the ANM is visiting and not vice-versa. Additionally, they felt that since the time ASHA worker comes home to visit, they do not feel the need for any health professional to visit them. The observation shows that presence of ASHA in the village has drastically reduced people's felt need for medical workers to home visit pregnant or lactating mothers. This is one of the significant contributions of ASHA workers towards reproductive and child health.

Of all the six hypothetical scenarios, in four such situations, a higher percentage of respondents in Nanduri reported to confront the providers. Also the strategies they used to demand answerability involved both formal and informal means as seen in Box 5.1, Box 5.2 and Box 5.3. A senior worker in Nanduri also confirmed this trend. She shared,

> *'Nanduri people are quite aware. They would call me or complain to me when I visit the village. They would say things like, 'they (anganwadi centre staff) don't open centre on time; they fight among themselves in front of children; grains provided by the bachat ghat (Self Help Group) is not proper; today food was not prepared properly' etc. Once DP bhaiya (local politician, name changed) also called to say that 'come and taste this food, our children will not eat this food.' I have even prepared a panchnama (mediator's report) for complaints regarding food. It is handed over to the gram-sevak who gives it in gram panchayat office. Once a woman came complaining, that her goat died because of eating (Take Home Rations) THR. I told her that it is meant for children and not animals.' –ICDS Supervisor, Nanduri*

There was a case of THR reported in Surli out of very few cases of confrontation. A worker and medical officer from Surli shared,

> *'Mothers in their village do not prefer THR and instead demand hot cooked snacks all the time. They refused to take THR. So I told them to do signatures of non-acceptance and I called my supervisor. But supervisor said that this will not help, and we needed to write to our sangathana (union of Anganwadi workers). I am a representative from this zila in our sangathana. In our meeting, there was a demand from workers all over Maharashtra that they don't want THR. For us, if we don't distribute it, where will we stack it? We may invite trouble and if we give, mothers don't want to take it. There are incidences of people feeding this THR to animals who die after consuming it.'* – *Anganwadi worker, Surli*

> *'We get many cases of rude patients' behaviour. Once I have had a hectic day at the PHC with three back-to-back deliveries. At 10 pm in night, I had sat down for dinner with my family. I had just taken a bite that a man came and told me that he has a patient who is feeling dizzy and wanted me to see. I assured them that I will come in 5 minutes as there is nothing to worry, it can be tackled and is not an emergency. He went back but no later than a minute he came back and asked me in a rude tone if I was coming or not. He went back and after a while came and threatened me with dire consequences. I also replied to do whatever he wants to and threatened him back on what he will do if I don't see the patient at all. Then he became calm. I also examined the patient, who was his father suffering from hypertension. If I had not replied, he wouldn't have allowed me to live in peace.'* – *Medical officer, Surli*

The informal forms of confrontations in Surli were not rough, rude or violent as in case of Nanduri. Neither frontline workers nor respondents reported any formal form of confrontation in Surli. In addition to user's capacity to demand services, providers' perception and practices of account giving would also add to the understanding of these processes at the frontline of service delivery which is discussed as follows.

5.5 Providers' Account Giving

Michael Lipsky (1980) suggests that, in order to understand public policy in action, we must attend to the everyday work of street level or frontline workers, because policy is enacted through their discretionary practices. Scholars have argued that that one needs to move beyond corruption as a reason why accountability institutions fail to deliver justice to the poor (Goetz & Jenkins, 2005).

Accountability failures seem to derive from two sources – elite capture and elite biases embedded in formal remits, operating procedures and informal practices which can be casteist, sexist and anti-poor (ibid.). The following section illustrates the nature of accountability failures within the state hierarchies and between providers and users.

Frontline providers providing services for early childhood care and education including maternal and child health include anganwadi workers from the ICDS, the ANM and ASHA from the NRHM programme. While the anganwadi worker and the ASHA are key functionaries of the ICDS and the NRHM respectively, they are honorary and are not paid a fixed salary. The ANM on the other hand are government employees and have a fixed salary as well as performance incentives.

However, both the ICDS and the NRHM programmes are predominantly and heavily conceived and dependent upon services of the Anganwadi worker and the ASHA at village level. Hence from a policy perspective, these two functionaries shoulder a high responsibility for service delivery at the frontline level. They are also expected to be accountable both upwards (towards seniors like supervisors and CDPOs) and also downwards (towards the panchayat and community).

5.5.1 Monitoring Excess

The institutional framework of the schemes is such that existing supervision, monitoring and checks are purely managerial in nature, instead of offering mid-term corrections to the programmes at the village level or being supportive to the workers. With the assumption of the existing New Public Management (NPM) framework of monitoring with strict surveillance and control over the functionaries, anganwadi centres can function better.

Literature however, points to the backlash against the proliferation of information and reporting requirements like output targets, performance indicators and service charters which are 'overly bureaucratic, excessively costly and infinitely manipulable' (Goetz & Jenkins, 2005:190).

Both the ICDS and the NRHM have elaborate computerised monitoring mechanisms with information flowing from bottom to top levels of administration. During in-depth interviews with these providers, one common feature that emerged across frontline providers was that they are accountable to their seniors for reporting data by way of filling registers, formats, forms as per the requirements by the department. Some workers do it under coercion while others do it for monetary incentive. The workers shared,

> *'There are 22 registers to be filled. I do not get time here at the anganwadi, so I carry them home. I have to fill these records during my family time. I can't even complain about this to anyone. By hook or crook, whether day or night, I only have to do it.' - Anganwadi worker, Surli*

> *'We have daily, weekly and monthly reporting. Usually we don't get time at work to fill registers since mostly we are in the field and return only by evening. We go home finish our household work and then finish filling the registers. Where is the time?' - ANM, Surli*

> *'If there is a childbirth, we have to report its day, date and time to the PHC on the same day. So, nearing the delivery date, we keep following up with woman's family or her neighbours if she delivered. Even if the woman is at her mother's place, we still have to report as she would eventually return back. We get Rs. 10 to report one such case. But for these 10 bucks we make numerous visits, phone calls, give a written note and get it signed by the ANM and then we get Rs. 10. It is not worth the hassle.' - ASHA, Nanduri*

Broadly they are aware that this data is used for policy tweaking but are alienated about where the data goes what use it is put to and what impact it has on their work. A worker said, '*Data that I collect and collate is fed into the computer and it then goes to Delhi*.' However, workers felt that owing to extensive record filling, attention given to children at the anganwadi has reduced. In addition, there seems to be friction within their families because of spill-over of record keeping work into their homes.

Local manoeuvres – Consequently, these frontline workers have devised their own interpretation of implementing programme activities taking advantage of the very system of bureaucratic monitoring. An anganwadi worker responded to the question on filling the home-visit register,

> *'We are supposed to home visit mothers of 5 children every week. On my way to the anganwadi centre, I meet mothers on the way.' I clarified, 'You mean on the road?' She replied, 'Yes there itself she asks what food is being made at school and I also suggest her few things. That is counted as a home-visit.' - Anganwadi worker, Nanduri*

The worker, on her part, concluded the home visit activity and recorded this information, yet it was grossly ineffective from the perspective of the users or programme objectives. As put by scholars, 'what gets measured gets done' (Goetz & Jenkins, 2005:190). Also for activities like sharing growth chart with mothers and nutrition counselling, the existing monitoring framework was again used to circumvent the activity all together. Anganwadi workers devised their own version of sharing growth charts with mothers. Yet, fieldwork revealed that most mothers in both villages had not seen growth charts of their children.

A worker defended herself by saying that when mothers come to the centre once a month for immunisation, growth charts are shared with them. In practice, as observed during the fieldwork, it is the ANM from the PHC who leads in conducting the immunisation programme. There is no scope for anganwadi workers to share these charts with mothers. The ASHA supports through outreach of calling mothers while the anganwadi worker takes a back seat. The ANM vaccinates the children and pregnant women and also counsel mothers on specific health issues but she is not mandated to share growth charts. For mothers who are present, the Anganwadi worker takes their signatures as a proxy for mother's meeting (and sharing of growth charts), which is one of the indicators monitored by the ICDS MIS. Therefore, as per the monitoring requirements, activity took place only on paper.

Bureaucratic whip - Frontline provider's actions show that they feel accountable to their immediate seniors, the supervisors, who keep vigilance on their work by making surprise visits and checking registers. Higher officials like the CDPOs, Block Development Officer (BDO), Taluka Medical Officer (TMO), and District Health Officer (DHO) rarely came unless there was a problem to be resolved or invited by the Panchayat for social functions. Workers shared,

> *'Supervisor checks all the registers. It takes her an hour to do so. Senior officials like JT sir and TP sir (only initials used to mask identity) come on surprise visit to see how we are providing nutritious food to the children and how the centre is functioning. They not only inspect our work but also of our supervisor.' - Anganwadi worker, Surli*

> *'Whenever senior officials visit the anganwadi, they give positive remarks in the guest book. We ask our children to recite poems, songs and prayers in front of them. But when we offer them anganwadi-cooked food, they resist. Zabardasti karni padti hai...We have to force them to eat. So we tell them that sir, checking the quality of this food is your right. If we make a mistake, you can correct us.' - Anganwadi worker, Nanduri*

> *'Our supervisor, as well as medical officer both comes to anganwadi centre, once in two months or so. Whenever they come, they call me to the centre. They do not inspect any record but physically inspect the centre and ask questions like if the water samples collected and tested regularly.' - ASHA, Nanduri*

> *'Senior officials come on surprise visits. When they come, work becomes stand still and nothing happens because we all have to give attention to 'him'. They are supposed to receive izzat (respect) every time they come and need to be welcomed by garlands. Who has so much time to do this regularly? Why can't they come for our motivation and guidance?'- Anganwadi worker, Surli*

This suggests a strong top-down vertical bureaucratic accountability practice. Also, importance of this nature of accountability circumvents actual services that are mandated in the programme. The most under-played issue is also of gender-related power-hierarchy.

While all anganwadi workers, Helpers and Supervisors are women in ICDS programme, most of its senior officials like CDPOs or community organisations are usually men.[4] Such unchallenged hierarchy and power imbalance favouring men creates varying discontentment among these workers.

---

4 Number of Anganwadi workers in India (all women) were 12,83,672 and number of ASHAs were 8,34,922 in 2014. Source: www.ashavani.org.

Scholars have argued that such practice has origins in the state's perspective on community health workers, where the assumption is that frontline workers are local women, with low educational qualifications and hired locally. Another assumption is that these women are natural care givers and the ICDS work is an extension of those duties, so they can be paid in honorarium.

The result of such assumptions is that anganwadi workers often remain in their position for years together and continue to extend their altruistic and caring services from households to the community (Bhatia 2014). The institutional, social policy and bureaucratic framework of these schemes dismisses a system of self-development, promotion and growth for frontline workers within the ICDS or the NRHM. This has serious implications on the engagement of these workers both with the bureaucratic machinery as well with the community.

On the other hand, there are services like Family Planning that have continued to be incentivised to such an extent that it has become a source of friction among frontline providers. Although the Health department will deny any kind of targeted approach, interviews with frontline providers revealed the contrary. An ASHA worker shared,

> *'We do a lot of work madam but those above us (ANM) take away all the credit. Our work does not get seen as it is seen as part of their work since it is the data from ANM that goes into the system. We have devised an informal understanding. Sometimes they take the credit, other time we take it. For instance, in one year we are supposed to facilitate three cases of family planning operations. Last month there were two cases- one went under her name and one went under me.' – ASHA, Surli*

The centrality of bureaucratic nature of accountability may achieve certain level of monitoring and discipline in workers, but is largely unsuccessful in prevent localised, micro-level pilferage.

A study on ANMs in Vishakhapatnam district of Andhra Pradesh, examined the impact of a reform, introduced in 1990s requiring ANMs to keep records of local illnesses and demonstrate public health improvements. A punch-card system through fingerprint scans at remote medical sub centres recorded ANMs' visits and measured the time they spent in the field. This system was based entirely on controlling and punishing errant frontline worker rather than sympathetically examining the practical constraints they face. Since attendance became a crude proxy measure of accountable behaviour, this so-called reform did little to improve nature of ANMs' engagements with clients or improvements in human development outcomes (Goetz & Jenkins, 2005:193).

Evidence in this study show that false data, especially bogus or ghost names of children are present on the beneficiary list (see Chapter 3 pg. 20). It allows for practices like siphoning off food supplies and black marketing since food supplies are allocated on the basis of listing of beneficiaries in anganwadi registers. A mother whose house was adjacent to the house of the anganwadi worker revealed,

> *'I know that she (anganwadi worker) gets food supplies home, like matki (pulses), oil etc. She makes small packets and sells it. When I confronted her, she said, I will do it, do whatever you want to. She says that we do so much for the anganwadi, it is our legitimate right to take some part of it.' – Mother during household interview*

Issues of local level pilferage by frontline providers need not be seen in isolation but within the context of institutional framework, their incentives and disincentives as discussed in the following section. Institutions of accountability are often known to suffer from elite and gender biases.

According to Goetz and Jenkins (2005), 'demoralised, underpaid, and poorly resourced workers will seek to control the variety of demands that clients place upon them by limiting the information about services they offer, curtailing their contact with socially marginalised clients and exaggerating rituals of deference in order to augment their own status and power in relation to clients' (Goetz & Jenkins, 2005: 62). Scholars argue that emphasis on surveillance – whether through citizen over-sight, new monitoring technologies, public-private partnerships can minimise scope for corruption, but downplays the importance of building cultures of probity and trusteeship in public services (ibid.).

Discontented engagement – Lack of justified honorariums, social security (retirement pension) and opportunities for growth becomes ingredients in hands of workers to exploit the system. The discontentment of frontline workers, mainly ASHA, Anganwadi workers and helpers was quite evident in the study because their financial expectations, whatever minimal, were not being met. ASHAs did not have a regular and fixed honorarium, at the time the data collection happened.

In Maharashtra, the situation has not changed, although in 2012 few states had announced fixed payments for ASHAs apart from incentives. Anganwadi workers too are generally discontented with their status and honorariums. Workers shared,

> *'We do a lot of work, but no one appreciates. Officials and people say good things about us, but we don't get any monetary incentives or certificates. To tell you frankly, officials have a lot of influence at the village level and there is also village-level politics. Since I am a single woman, staying alone with no family support, I feel I am more vulnerable and I do suffer on that account.' - Anganwadi worker, Surli*

'The ANMs at the PHC do not have much work-load, yet their pay is incredibly good. If we are given even a small proportion of such salary, we can do a better job than them. People today work for money. When I go around roaming the village, my family members taunt me that I loiter around for nothing.' - ASHA, Nanduri

'I am supposed to attend to a pregnant woman, be it day or night. Last year I had facilitated 78 deliveries of which only 30 were BPL women under Janani Suraksha Yojana. I am required to stay two days at a stretch with the delivery patient if it is a seizure (C-section) case. Officials also ask me to wait for two days and do not sign the papers. If I don't wait, I lose 200 rupees. Now you only tell madam, if I stay back for two days for every patient, how am I supposed to run my house?' - ASHA, Nanduri

There is a contrary evidence to show that not paying honorariums for community health workers like ASHAs actually resulted in improved development outcomes[5]. The study by Tendler (1994) studied reforms designed to improve responsiveness of public health service providers to poor clients in Brazilian state of Ceara (Goetz & Jenkins, 2005).

In a striking similarity to the ASHA programme of the NRHM, the Brazilian programme recruited thousands of new basic community health workers (mainly women) to carry out immunisation and child prevention health campaigns. They were non-tenured, low skilled field workers from same communities in which they were to work. This bypassed the patronage system of local institutions like health department or local mayor.

Use of highly visible uniforms, blue packs filled with supplies and their spirit of social mission contributed to their own job satisfaction and create a sense of 'calling'. This instilled a sense of public ownership of the programme. Ordinary people themselves acted as informal agents of accountability by exposing deficient performance in public – a worst form of social sanction and also felicitated sincere workers at community functions. Over time, these health workers were held accountable for higher standards of care – demonstrate empathy, responsiveness and integrity. The biggest advantage was that these workers did not use their extended discretion to limit their workload, which is often a pattern with paid service providers who are over-worked and under-motivated (Goetz & Jenkins, 2005:194).

5 Reformist state governors in Brazil turned around mediocre public agencies in the areas of health, agriculture, public works and small enterprise development. The result was most impressive in rural preventive health service, where within a space of five years, there was an increased preventive health coverage from 30 to 65 percent of state's population and contributed to a 36 percent drop in infant mortality (Goetz & Jenkins, 2005: 193).

In the Brazilian study, non-material incentives helped to develop job commitment and responsible use of discretion (ibid.). Frontline providers reported non-monetary incentives when they shared -

'Last year at a panchayat samiti meeting in Osmanabad, I was felicitated with a shawl (stole) and a coconut. At that time 11 anganwadi workers were recognised for their work. I was chosen because of factors like cleanliness in my anganwadi especially for shiny utensils as if shimmery silver; food given to children was consistently good and weights were also taken regularly. I was also noted for being extremely punctual and not being late in opening the centre.'- Anganwadi worker, Nanduri

'How will we ever get rewarded? We are never able to achieve targets. For instance, we need to report 16 institutional deliveries from our sub-centre in a month. But we had only 11 deliveries. It happened because our sub-centre should cater to a population of 4000-5000 but the current population is only 3000. But targets are targets. My salary is Rs. 27,000 per month. An increment of Rs. 500 happens every year owing to inflation.' - ANM, Nanduri

However, scholars using the rights framework (of workers) and not considering the political-institutional paradigm of service delivery, have pointed that non-monetary incentives are performance-based and these cannot be a substitute for justified and fixed monetary payments to frontline providers especially ASHAs (Bhatia, 2014).

Literature especially from civil society and academic evaluation reports have often taken sympathetic stand for these two workers, citing their overburdened work-load and range of responsibilities against their honorary nature of employment and extremely low honorarium. Sinha (2006) mentioned,

'The ICDS programme relies on the frontline functionary, the anganwadi worker to realise policy maker's dream of a society that respects women, takes care of adolescent girls, gives them dignity and space, rectifies gender imbalance, ensures safe delivery of infants and maintains nutritional status of children until she reaches six years of age. She is also expected to maintain the data that feeds into the statistics of the government and maintain lists of women who could access innumerable schemes of issuance of doles, stipends etc. She is also accountable to layers of official supervising and monitoring at block, district and state level. She is neither qualified nor paid minimum wages. National level consultations continue on what more could be added as activities to anganwadi workers already overflowing timetable.'

In view of such understanding, there have been long standing demands from left-supported unions of ASHAs and Anganwadi workers to realise some of their entitlements which they consider as a right (Box 5.4).

Box 5.4: Anganwadi workers' Union Memorandum of Demands

Key Demands of Anganwadi workers Union

- Stop all forms of privatisation in ICDS. (Privatisation is one of the key recommendations of ICDS Mission Mode, 2014)
- Make adequate financial allocations to ICDS. (need to change the scheme from Plan to Non-plan component of Central Government Budget)
- Improve infrastructure in Anganwadi centres.
- Regularise all Anganwadi workers and helpers; provide them minimum wages and social security benefits.

Source: www.aifawh.org (All India Federation of Anganwadi workers and Helpers).

To be fair, the NRHM created institutional process within VHSNC and mandated it to pay the ASHAs honorarium from its annual budget. The idea behind was to make this a community and joint process. But elite capture and biases together with complexity of the process with a potential of conflict in working of VHNSC defeats its purpose.

The study provides evidence that VHSNC itself was mired in politics of caste, gender and hierarchy, creating enough bottlenecks for ASHAs to claim their entitlements. Functioning of VHSC in Surli showed that two ASHA workers were paid a one-time honorarium of Rs. 1000. In Nanduri, ASHA did not receive any payment from VHSC funds.

Literature too points that the structure of authority at the anganwadi centre level has little scope for the anganwadi worker to have a dialogue with the supervisors (Sinha, 2006). The only interaction they have with the supervisors is for the purpose of data monitoring during their monthly meetings or during 'inspection' visits by the supervisors.

Therefore, there is little such a system of monitoring with existing incentives can do to ensure improvement in outcomes and prevention of corruption. Finally, there was hardly any significant difference in monitoring practices between Surli and Nanduri that could set them apart and issues of frontline workers remained same in both cases.

5.5.2 Perception versus Practice on Answering

Frontline providers were asked in an open-ended question on actors they were accountable to. Most anganwadi workers in both villages shared that they are answerable and accountable to all people of the village, their supervisors and towards senior officials. However, it was found that their being accountable to people was more in theory than in practice.

When asked about the methods they give account of their work to the community, most anganwadi workers replied that they are already doing it through one-on-one interaction with the mothers. Workers shared,

> *'My accountability is towards all – pregnant women, lactating women, women in age group of 15-45 years and citizens of the village. We are strongly accountable to our supervisor. If my register is incomplete, then she questions me, and I am supposed to complete it. We also have to answer the gram sevak, ANM and gram panchayat if they call me. But they don't call me to the gram sabha as only men go there. So I discuss my work with men staying near my house who usually attend the gram sabha. They come back and tell me what happened in the meeting.' – Anganwadi worker, Nanduri*

> *'I do give answer to people when asked. If they happen to ask me why we prepared that food on that day, then I explain them. This is how I sort the issue with people.' - Anganwadi worker, Nanduri*

> *'Yes, we are answerable to the users, but such a situation has not arisen. We do not give any opportunity to anyone to complaint or question us. We work fine, so why should anyone question us.' - Anganwadi worker, Surli*

These were anganwadi workers own interpretation of being accountable. However, it is well known that this is not institutionalised account-giving. Also, workers in Surli perceived accountability as a negative feedback on their work and argued that if their work is good, they are already fulfilling their responsibility and hence cannot be questioned. Probably, there seem to be a semantic confusion between the Marathi translation of words accountability and responsibility. Accountability is translated as 'jababdari' in Marathi and 'jawabdari' in Hindi, which can often mean 'responsibility' or 'uttardaitwa' in Marathi as well. The anganwadi worker in Surli shared that they are present in the gram sabha meetings and also share their problems. The worker shared,

> *'People of the village are good and if we utter any requirement, they make sure we are given. Recently, in the gram sabha meeting, they gave us the permission to buy chairs and tables from the VHSC funds. We do get opportunity to talk.' - Anganwadi worker, Surli*

Anganwadi workers from Surli were of the view that although they have a voice in the gram panchayat, it does not take interest in the anganwadi's work. Other frontline providers like the ANM & ASHA shared that they are aware that they work for the people but actually feel accountable only to their seniors and not the gram panchayat. Most of them were unanimous on one issue, that if the gram panchayat does not call them for meeting, they do not go. Workers shared,

'Gram sabha rarely happens and whenever it happens, I am not called. If they will call me, I will surely go and answer them. I am bold and would not shy away. But let them call me first.' - ASHA, Nanduri

'Yes whenever gram sabha happens, they call me, and I go. Usually it is twice a year, on 15th August and 26th January. There are a lot of people there and many things are discussed like issues related to water and sanitation. But we have no role there. We go, sit through and come back.' - ANM, Nanduri

As per the GRs (Government Resolutions) of ICDS & NRHM programmes, the Anganwadi worker, ASHA and ANM are required to regularly attend the gram sabha and share their work. However, without an institutional mandate for this in the panchayat coupled with politics of gender, it remains in the realm of idea only. The visible disinterest of both villages' gram panchayat s on nutrition shows its poor political outreach. One worker shared,

'Once in the gram sabha, we were supposed to read out the names of children who were in grade II and grade III. It was a big gathering at that time. I had read out the names. Soon parents of these children got extremely angry at this. They said publicly, this is our family matter, we will keep our kids the way we want to, in thick and thin, what is your (anganwadi worker) interest, let our kids remain the way they are. Since then we are rarely invited for meetings.' – Anganwadi worker, Surli.

'When the gram sabha happens, we don't even come to know. When it gets over then we come to know because they come to take our signatures. Many big people gather, but only two to three women are present including our sarpanch who are part of the gram panchayat committee. We women do not go there.' – ASHA, Surli

Naming of children with malnutrition caused embarrassment and shame to their parents. Such a practice is not mandated neither in the ICDS or panchayati raj institution act. Hence, it was yet another form of misinterpretation of processes. The worker clarified that they were prompted by the gram panchayat members to do the same. Possibility of this cannot be ruled out since such a move would favour the gram panchayat members' unchallenged male domination and power hierarchy. However, this action had high political costs for the programme in Surli where parents of the children lost trust on the workers. Another worker shared,

'Village sarpanch, members of gram panchayat and all other people need to pay attention to the anganwadi. Is it only our job to see, madam? After the school gets over, animals roam around this place, elder children come and sleep

> *here; they drink and create a ruckus. Are we exclusively accountable for this? So there is no point talking to them (gram panchayat members). Why should then we listen to them? Sometimes the gram panchayat members come just to check the food prepared. That's it.' - Anganwadi worker, Surli*

While there were opportunities for dialogue between the providers and the community in Surli, the community participation link was extremely weak in Nanduri. Workers mentioned,

> *'The village people say that you get food stuff from the government, why should we contribute. People never volunteer to give anything here. Gram sabha happens but I have never gone, and they too have never called me. As it is, it is only for men, women don't go there.' - Anganwadi worker, Nanduri*

> *'Village gram panchayat does not pay much attention to our work. When we go to meet them, they are never available to meet us, not even the gram-sevak. They are supposed to sprinkle powder on garbage to prevent spread of epidemics. But during my recent visit, I asked sipahi reasons for no sprinkling done, but he said he was not aware and has not been paid salary in the last 14 months. Many households fill water for six months at a stretch and do not empty vessels once a week as per our advice. Our Medical Officer has sent many letters to the gram panchayat listing down activities for prevention of epidemics. When we follow with the gram-sevak, he assures us that he will inform the members. But we know our letters are merely filed with no action taken.' - ANM, Nanduri*

> *'In this village, the gram panchayat has never called me for any meeting. I have never shared my work publicly, but the village people know of my work. People of this village think that we are government employees and get a salary from top. But we have to keep convincing them that we don't get any money. Yes, I am accountable to all, but government needs to give us something to demand accountability from us.' – ASHA worker, Nanduri*

People's representatives from the gram panchayat were reported to visit anganwadi centres in Surli but Zila parishad members rarely visited the centres in both the villages.

5.5.3 Facing Sanctions?

Accountability cannot exist without sanctioning power (Pande, 2008). Frontline providers were asked indirectly if their colleagues or someone they knew faced sanctions from authorities like demotion, transfer, suspension etc owing to user's complaints.

Sanctions can be formal (See Box 5.3) or informal (see Box 5.2) depending upon the nature of forum.

According to theoretical understanding of accountability, sanctions are the defining feature in the web of accountability relationships. The question was asked indirectly and impersonally to frontline providers, it being a sensitive issue. Most anganwadi workers were of the view that they have known workers and helpers who have worked for more than 20 years but such sanctions rarely happen.

However, some frontline workers from Nanduri revealed few incidents of sanctions.

> *'A sister (ANM) in a nearby village had faced suspension. A parent complained against her. When our staff went for inspection there, they found two boxes of expired vaccines meant for immunisation. They click pictures on mobile. Our medical officer madam also went there; she called three more witnesses, did a panchnama (mediators' report) and put up her file. They calculated a fine of Rs. 37,000 because of her negligence. It has been about six months since she was suspended, and her case is still going on.' - ANM, Nanduri*

> *'Recently, in a nearby village, an anganwadi worker claimed that the sarpanch took out the entire money from VHSC funds from the bank and spent on his own. When she asked him to give bills of the expenditure, he never gave. Our office harassed her since according to them it is the anganwadi worker who is accountable for that money. She was so upset over the issue that she applied for a 15 day leave to go to Mumbai. Probably, she may not return on duty as she had mentioned that she doesn't want to be in such a job.' – ANM, Nanduri*

> *'This case had happened five years ago. There was an anganwadi worker in one of my villages. There were complaints from parents that she did not make proper food at the anganwadi centre. I too observed that her behaviour was also not proper. She also remained absent many times. I made sure that she was suspended from the duty.' – ICDS Supervisor, Nanduri*

At times, workers become victims of politics of gender hierarchy and face the brunt of sanctions in form of harassment and scrutiny from officials. In cases of food poisoning reported in the media for schemes like mid-day meal or the anganwadi, it is the anganwadi worker and cook that are blamed and sanctioned and rarely the immediate senior. According to a media report, two employees (helpers) at an anganwadi near Sanand, Gujarat were suspended by the district development office after 20 children were affected by food poisoning. Two others – matron (anganwadi worker) and cook were given show-cause notice (Shastri, 2013).

Frontline workers from Surli denied knowing their colleagues facing sanctions but those from Nanduri had few incidents to narrate. The above examples revealed that most workers have faced formal sanctions while cases of informal reprimanding may not be uncommon. Nonetheless these are challenging to document.

A senior worker added that at times they are unable to act on few anganwadi workers because they are chosen by the panchayat. She mentioned an example of an anganwadi worker from a village near Nanduri who had a physical handicap.

> *'This anganwadi worker is unable to lift and hold any child to weigh; her record is usually incomplete and doesn't take proper care of the children. Yet, she continues despite her inferior performance. Helper has to compensate for all her lags. There were better candidates for the post in the village, but panchayat has criteria in addition to educational qualifications. They have a marking system with points for criteria like education, caste etc. They tend to give points to women who are widowed, divorced, mildly handicapped and from SC/OBC caste.' - ICDS Supervisor, Nanduri*

With a panchayat not sanctioning an inefficient worker despite evidence, again points to the politics of gender and hierarchy. Reasons are evident that it is in the interest of the local power holders to appoint those who do not shake apple carts. Mediocrity in workers becomes a desirable asset in maintaining local power hierarchies.

At times, the sanction is against the entire institution and has financial implication. During the fieldwork, I observed a mother who came to complain to the anganwadi worker in Nanduri. Her one year old infant was suffering from high fever and severe inflammation on his thigh. She shared that two days ago, the ANM had given him a vaccination shot. This mother was anxious since according to her, her child has not slept for two nights, is constantly crying, refusing food and fever medication was also ineffective. The anganwadi worker asked the ANM to visit the village urgently and examine the child. The ANM instead asked the anganwadi worker to get the child to the PHC. The child was diagnosed with severe infection at the injection site. The mother was referred to Civil Hospital, Tuljapur. However, she protested in front of the medical officer and PHC staff. She refused to visit civil hospital and instead demanded them to sponsor her child's treatment with a private child specialist at Tuljapur.

The Medical Officer had to pay for the consultation, medicines and even travel for the mother, her child and the anganwadi worker to visit a private specialist. In addition, it was a blow on PHC's credibility for not being able to treat an infant despite being responsible for his condition. It was a serious sanction with collateral damage both to the institution of NRHM and also to its users. Yet, the process of NRHM largely remains passive to such incidents and treats them as routine and errors of judgement.

PHCs as part of the NRHM framework are also infamous for being lax regarding health check-ups and referrals of anganwadi children, which is an important activity under ICDS programme. A frontline worker in Nanduri cited an incident about AD PHC (name changed). She shared,

> *'AD PHC was surrounded by high incidence of child malnutrition as reported by a local newspaper. During investigation, its anganwadi workers were asked reasons for the same. It was revealed that since last two years, the children didn't have any health check-ups. It became an issue and onus came on the medical officer of AD PHC. However, no action was taken against that Medical Officer.' - ANM, Nanduri*

ICDS services converge with several schemes and government departments like water, sanitation, education and PDS but more particularly with NRHM for health. In such a case, pinning accountability on health staff for deficiency in service within the ICDS is a tricky issue that have been discussed frequently in policy circles, without a solution in sight. The worker also shared,

> *'When our medical officer visits any anganwadi centre for these check-ups, she records data of children but would not touch them. Technically, the anganwadi worker cannot complain that a medical check-up has not happened. Medical officer call parents of malnourished children, show them the chart and tell them how many times they needed to be fed etc. We do not show card of children who are normal. I remember a mother of a malnourished child asking the medical officer,' how is it possible to feed the child 7-8 times in a day when I am working in fields from 10 am to 6 pm? I feed my child twice a day. medical officer stuck to her guns and could not offer any answer.' – ANM, Nanduri*

It shows that although medical officers are responsible for ensuring timely health check-ups of all anganwadi children, they are rarely or never held accountable if the service is not delivered. This shows elite biases even within the bureaucratic hierarchies of the state. It confirms a long-held view that in addition to high politics of the state, there is profound injustice or irresponsibility in the deep politics of society, that is, the relationship between rich and poor, powerful and weak (Goetz & Jenkins, 2005). During the fieldwork, there were only nine children in Nanduri who were officially identified under SAM and MAM, needing admission in Village Child Development Centres (VCDC) for supplementary feeding in 2012.

There were no cases of SAM/MAM or VCDC reported in Surli although the study data did reveal moderate levels of malnutrition in children, about 14% malnutrition in all (see Chapter III, pg. 19). Since the VCDC is funded under the NRHM, it has excluded many under nourished children (like the example above) by supporting a new format of measurement. On the other extreme there was also a reported case of coercion in VCDC programme with negative implications for the programme. A health worker from Nanduri shared an incident,

> *'There was a woman who was not ready to get her malnourished child come for VCDC at the anganwadi centre. An arrangement was devised by which anganwadi helper used to go every time at her house to feed the kid. At times, on my insistence child was brought to the centre and fed eggs. That woman yelled at the worker that she cannot forcefully take away her child and feed him as per their wishes. Helper used to explain that she does not have any personal agenda, and this was required. Then the mother used to question the workers and say that if they took so much tension because of her child, she would rather take her child out of the anganwadi. She actually took the child out. Her argument was that there was plenty of food at home, but her child refused to eat.' – ANM, Nanduri*

Health workers on their part feel that they are responsible and held accountable to increase the weight of children admitted in the VCDC. Most of them blame the parents for not taking care of their children. As a result, the children get better in the VCDC but again slips back to malnutrition soon.

From the perspective of workers, parents needed to take responsibility of their children's nutrition, and it should be imposed on them. To complicate matters, medical officers from Nanduri and Surli shared their perspectives,

> *'Funding of this VCDC should be through ICDS and not NRHM, because the anganwadi worker who is implementing this will not listen to me and my ANMs will not listen to ICDS Supervisor.' – Medical Officer, Nanduri*

> *'I do not understand why this VHSC money comes to us? It should go to the ICDS and they should release it. The problem is that I cannot hold the anganwadi worker to account regarding the spending of VHSC money, as I am not her senior.' – Medical Officer, Surli*

It seems that health providers from the NRHM are questioning the convergent nature of these processes and flow of accountability which probably was intended to formalise these convergences but in reality, is causing conflict in their lines of authority or scope of work. In addition, to clash on the notions of responsibility and accountability between the users and providers, one can also witness it among various providers. Institutional processes encouraging coercion (like the case above) and justifying activities without acknowledging the context of users and their informed consent have resulted in exit of children from ICDS and also diminishing the credibility of the programme.

However, exit of users is neither monitored nor acknowledged within the ICDS policy and processes. Power hierarchy of the profession of medicine has largely insulated them to be answerable and accountable for public health goals like child nutrition. This is a serious gap in the formal accountability processes within the ICDS and NRHM institutional framework at the local level.

Providers were asked about the malpractices like ghost names on the anganwadi lists which was revealed at the time of household survey. Upon confronting a senior worker about ghost names in beneficiary lists of the anganwadi centre, she explained,

> *'If such a thing becomes known officially, then whatever the extra ration comes, it gets compensated from the salary of the anganwadi worker responsible for the same. Yes, it has happened many times and I have fined workers. In SD village, one anganwadi worker used to put 4-5 bogus names on the lists. We used to take that list and go around in the village asking people where these children stay. It was easy to find out. I have deducted salary of five such anganwadi workers. They surely need to be punished.' – ICDS Supervisor, Nanduri*

It is clear that despite threat of real sanctions and monitoring, such malpractice continued unabated as witnessed in both Surli and Nanduri. The ease of such a malpractice gives incentives to workers since they know that official efforts to unearth it are much rarer and more difficult. It demonstrates that a contrast exists - workers at times are victims of hierarchies and at times agency of corruption. All along, institutional processes play a role in these practices not individual workers alone.

Implications of rude sanctions need not always be positive or long-term. As mentioned in Box 5.2, the medical officer of Mangrol PHC stopped staying at the PHC due to an incident of aggressive behaviour of the locals. She also had past evidence of similar instances with previous medical officers to argue her case. This is like a vicious cycle of mistrust where the user loses trust since the provider is not available during need and the provider too treats it like a mechanical duty. A health worker shared how medical officer justified her decision,

> *'If a patient comes at 7 pm for delivery, medical officer madam feels that if something happens then what will she do. She felt why should she take the whole responsibility alone especially when the villagers are so violent? Therefore, she has started referring them elsewhere. So people also now prefer Katgaon PHC over Mangrol PHC since there, the medical officer is always available, as he stays in the staff quarter and his service is nice. Katgoan's Medical officer also manages emergency well as they have a vehicle and driver to ferry patient to Solapur if they are unable to manage. Here it is not like that. Therefore people trust Katgaon PHC more than this place. Even Nanduri people go to Katgaon.' – ANM, Nanduri*

It shows that a well-functioning PHC with a resident doctor instilled trust and confidence in people of Nanduri and this was the reason they continued to access public health services.

However, the PHC near Surli seems to defy the same logic since it also had a resident medical officer and good infrastructure, yet most of its residents preferred private health sector. As explained earlier, a household's higher economic capacity and easy access to a growing private health sector were the factors that can explain this anomaly. These factors were either weak (like fewer households in upper middle or rich asset quintile then Surli) or not present (growth of private health providers) in case of Nanduri. Surprisingly, there the functionaries did not share a single case of negative sanctions reported by frontline workers in Surli.

5.6 Discussion and Conclusion

By design, the ICDS as an institution, has failed to create opportunity for a mother to know the value or purpose in weighing, and monitoring growth and development of their children. The process within the ICDS needs to make users realise the importance of tools like growth charts. Growth charts cannot be used as report cards to hold anganwadi workers accountable for child malnutrition. But one surely needs to question if their purpose is towards the mothers or the bureaucracy. Owing to this, ICDS has been reduced to a 'dole' as many experts have also voiced earlier, which now is also getting increasingly ineffective and even counter-productive when even the poor are opting out of the ICDS.

This is one of the central reasons for disinterest and lack of community ownership in the ICDS programme. Seeing the fall in the beneficiary will give the state enough reasons to justify its recent cuts in allocations for ICDS. The allocation for the ICDS Scheme has been reduced from Rs 18,195 crore in 2014-15 budget estimates to Rs 8,335.8 crore in 2015-16 budget estimates (Zee News, 2015). In 2021-22, budget allocated for Saksham Anganwadi and POSHAN 2.0 (Umbrella ICDS - Anganwadi Services, Poshan Abhiyan, Scheme for Adolescent Girls) was clubbed to Rs 20,263 crore, and cited as a small increase from Rs 20,105 crore from 2020-21. (Economic Times 2022). It is clear that correcting the structures that obfuscate the flow of information is also a political issue and unless local bodies and community see the importance of accurate and reliable data, it would be difficult to circumvent it (Sinha, 2006).

VHSC functioned somewhat in Surli, if not as per the policy norms, which in turn had a role in ensuring better functioning of the anganwadi centres in Surli as compared to Nanduri. To note, child malnutrition was found to be lower, with better improvements towards normalcy in Surli as compared to Nanduri. However, on the flip side, there were higher percentages of households that have already exited out of ICDS in Surli, including the poor, as compared to Nanduri where exit was not so significant. This indicator of exit is a worrisome trend for a well-functioning anganwadi centres of Surli with supposedly low incidence of child malnutrition. Exit, which is a crucial check of programme effectiveness is neither monitored nor analysed and acknowledged in the ICDS policy framework.

Also, despite Maharashtra government's policy and notifications in creating VHSNCs under NRHM in 2006, nutrition is yet to be included as a part of the panchayat's functions and is not a mandate even in one of the most developed districts of Maharashtra. Finally, if I had not used a case-study design and instead drawn a representative sample of fixed households from a block, observation of this exit would never have been revealed. It is so, because I would have focused only on those households that were availing ICDS services.

Low community participation and high personal contacts with state power holders like panchayat office bearers or bureaucracy at village level in Nanduri, points to the practice of paying rents to get one's work done. In Surli, households reported to have higher contacts with local politicians as compared to state functionaries suggesting a culture of 'benevolent feudalism' (Sekher, 2004). Such relationship of patronage does not allow confrontations and hence no cases were reported in Surli. The distinct difference in political participation in both villages has a direct impact in the way users confronted service providers.

Using the present evidence, it is clear that a supposedly well-functioning anganwadi centre or a PHC like those for Surli can be explained with local level processes. It was also a result of large exit of the middle and rich asset quintile. Small numbers of beneficiaries remaining are managed by a system of strict top-down bureaucratic monitoring and to some extent by participation of panchayati raj institution institutions or VHSC. These situations were absent in Nanduri.

In Nanduri, personal interests tend to supersede community interest as most approach state power holders for getting work done. Nanduri instead had higher instances of confrontations with the providers, both formal and informal, yet a higher utilisation of public services amid their 'perceived' poor standards, especially when compared with Surli. While informal methods of confrontation like rude or violent behaviour lead to immediate results, their long-term impact could actually be negative as seen in Nanduri.

However, Peruzzoti & Smulovitz in 2006 claimed that the intensity and visibility of voice through 'symbolic sanctions' can have 'material consequences', therefore it is unfair to dismiss societal accountability mechanisms altogether (Pande, 2007). For instance, if a voice protest incident, even if it is at individual level, gets reported in the media, it becomes a political issue and formal action follows.

In addition, experts speak of need-based negotiations, where the poor rely heavily on political representatives as the initial form for redressal or service provisioning (ibid.). Formal mechanisms of sanctions like transfer of officials, fines, suspension do act as a strong deterrent for unjustified or corrupt practices. A possibility of a theory emerging out of these observations is explored in the following chapter.

***

References

1. Bhatia, K. (2014). Performance-based incentives of the ASHA scheme. *Economic and Political Weekly, 49*(22), 145–151.
2. Dhumaal, V. S. (2006, December 6). Maharashtra VHSNC: Notification. Retrieved on December 19, 2014 from http://nrhm.gov.in.
3. Goetz, A. M., Jenkins, R., & Shaw, T. M. (2005). *Reinventing accountability: making human democracy work for human development* (First). London: Palgrave Macmillan.
4. Hossain, N. (2010). Rude accountability: Informal pressures on frontline bureaucrats in Bangladesh. *Development and Change, 41*(5), 907–928.
5. Husain, Z. (2011). Health of the National Rural Health Mission. *Economic & Political Weekly, 46*(4), 53.
6. Jhalani, M. (2013, September 13). Letter to mission directors of NRMH (States/UTs) on enhancing role of panchayat in centrally sponsored schemes from Ministry of Health & Family Welfare, Government of India. Retrieved on December 19, 2014 from http://nrhm.gov.in.
7. Joshi, A. (2006). Institutions and service delivery in Asia. *IDS Bulletin, 37*(3), 115–129.
8. Khullar, V. (1998). Integrated Child Development Services: A Critique of Evaluation Techniques. *Economic and Political Weekly, 33*(10), 537–545.
9. Lipsky, M. (1980). *Street-Level Bureaucracy: Dilemmas of the Individual in Public Services*. Russell Sage Foundation: New York.
10. Marapakwar, P. (2015, January 28). Draft right to services bill lacks clarity. Retrieved on January 28, 2015 from http://timesofindia.indiatimes.com.
11. Mathur, T. (2012). *Right to Public Services: A Comparative Perspective of Implementation of Guarantee of Public Services in Select States of India* (p. 19). Centre for Organisation Development.
12. NIPCCD National Institute of Public Cooperation & Child Development. (2010). *Growth Monitoring Manual.* Retrieved on August 26, 2014 from http://nipccd.nic.in.
13. Pande, S. (2007). The right to information and societal accountability: the case of the Delhi PDS campaign. *IDS Bulletin, 38*(6), 47–55.
14. Pande, S. (2007). The right to information and societal accountability: the case of the Delhi PDS campaign. *IDS Bulletin, 38*(6), 47–55.

15. Paul, S. (2008). India's citizens' charters: in search of a champion. *Economic and Political Weekly*, 43(7), 67-73.

16. Pradhan, P. K. (2011, July 25). Order from Ministry of Health and Family Welfare, National Rural Health Mission for Village Health Sanitation Nutrition Committee. Retrieved on December 19, 2014 from http://nrhm.gov.in.

17. Rubenstein, J. (2007). Accountability in an unequal world. *Journal of Politics*, *69*(3), 616–632.

18. Sekher, M. (2004). Indigenous institutions and forest conservation: user-group self-initiatives in India. Working Paper No. 140, Bangalore: Institute for Social and Economic Change.

19. Shastri, P. (2013, January 14). Anganwadi food poisoning: two suspended, two given show-cause notice. *Times of India*. Ahmedabad. Retrieved June 17, 2013, from http://articles.timesofindia.indiatimes.com.

20. Sinha, S. (2006). Infant survival: A political challenge. *Economic and Political Weekly*, *41*(34), 3657–3660.

21. Tendler, J. (1997). *Good government in the tropics*. USA: Johns Hopkins University Press.

22. Yaden, L. (2013, September 13). Letter to all NRHM mission directors on guidelines for village health sanitation nutrition committees. Retrieved on December 19, 2014 from http://nrhm.gov.in.

23. Zee News. (2015, March 10). Budget cut will expose children to greater vulnerability, say activists. Retrieved on March 18, 2015 from http://zeenews.india.com.

CHAPTER 6

Rethinking Accountability

6.1 Introduction

The dominant Neo-liberal framework of governance and new public management practices has made accountability a rhetorical and paradoxical idea for improved public service delivery. A recent development provides testimony to this trend, when the Bill & Melinda Gates Foundation offered to partner with the Ministry of Women & Child Development to develop a software for ICDS monitoring (Press Trust of India, 2015).

The move included equipping anganwadi workers with tablet-like devices and weighing machines so that the nutrition status of children can be monitored through geo-positioning system (GPS) in real time. The assumption here is that the lack of bureaucratic monitoring is one of main reasons for continued poor nutrition outcomes. Such an assumption, however, belittles the extensive, regular, and ritualistic MIS which programmes like ICDS and NRHM is infamous for, especially in the context of the workloads this activity bears on frontline workers.

Lack of accountability is increasingly cited as a reason for poor service delivery outcomes in a democracy like India. Such a notion has also been exploited for political gains during elections, especially in the discourse on corruption. A review of perspectives from public administration, democratic participation and the World Bank's governance framework, from which accountability has been studied, misses three major elements:

- Local institutions[1] and processes that determine how, why and which strategies citizens use to question and confront providers of public services from below?
- When users do not confront providers, what are the reasons for the same?

1 Institutions are social structures comprised of rules, codes of conduct, and norms which play a significant role in our daily lives by influencing social, political and economic behaviour (Ostrom, 1990). Some of the institutional processes like position, boundary, authority, information, collectives, payoffs like incentives and sanctions, and information are embedded within social institutions like family, PRIs, and the Anganwadi. Political science scholars have argued that, until recently, policy analysis has often ignored the role of institutions.

- How institutional processes exist in a contrasted context of development where these process work in one place but not in another, despite both places sharing similar governance structures?

The process and practice of accountability assume significance when services appear to be poor or satisfactory, as the two villages of the study demonstrate. The study attempted to fill this gap by enriching existing theory with empirical evidence.

The core objective of this study was to understand how accountability is enacted through various processes and institutions between users and providers in a public service delivery setting. Institutional and Development (IAD) framework from the discipline of political sociology was used to link main concepts of the study – accountability processes (visible through engagement, answerability, and sanctions) between users and providers; households and their capabilities; and finally public service delivery (in terms of outcomes like child malnutrition, access and user satisfaction) (See Figure 2.6 & 2.7). This framework aided in understanding how accountability processes get influenced and also shapes contrasting developmental contexts.

The conceptual framework led me to choose two study sites. This first was Nanduri village in the poorly ranked district of Osmanabad, in terms of human development outcomes. The second was Surli village in a better ranked district of Satara in the Indian state of Maharashtra. Maharashtra was chosen as it is infamous for child malnutrition outcomes amid large income disparities. Child nutrition is an important developmental issue for which the Indian state has often been scrutinised for accountability by local judiciaries, multilateral financial institutions, sections of academia and media. This is so because the state funds large-scale universal child health and nutrition programmes like ICDS and NRHM. Therefore, it is imperative to explore its service delivery linkages with local institutions and processes of accountability at the frontline level. Since the ICDS and NRHM converge on child health outcomes in a rural setting, they formed the context of this study.

The study was located in an exploratory research design and hence used a comparative case study approach, within a deductive framework. The study used the triangulation of both qualitative and quantitative data and data collection tools. Methods of primary data collection included household survey interviews and semi-structured interviews from providers. Secondary data was collected in the form of children's records of age, weight, height and malnutrition grades from anganwadi centers. Secondary data also included panchayat income and expenditure statements, Village Health and Sanitation Committee (VHSC) income and expenditure, as well as minutes of meetings and district and block level ICDS MIS data from CDPOs and ICDS supervisors.

Key respondents were the heads of the households. These were mothers of children below age six, various frontline providers, and panchayat representatives. The sample from both the villages include 129 households, 157 children, and 16 frontline providers.

6.2 Main Findings

This concluding chapter recapitulates broad findings of this study. It attempts to do so by linking its findings to the conceptual framework, thereby providing answers to the questions it had set out to ask and also asking further questions on the nature of reality of governance and accountability at the frontline of public services in India. These insights offer several implications on policy for public service delivery in general, and for child health and nutrition services in particular.

On Local Institutions: The issue of malnutrition is often linked to factors like water and sanitation, mother's literacy and education, as well as economic and social development. Yet these factors were rarely connected with local institutional processes like information barriers, reasons for choices, hierarchy, elite capture, elite bias, gender bias etc. Local institutions can only be understood within their local context, as this book attempted in Chapter III through the profiling of the two villages – Surli and Nanduri. This came in terms of socio-economic and demographic profile using indicators like household composition, gender, sex ratio, caste, occupation, literacy, education, economic class, and also nutrition outcomes.

Change in the grades of malnutrition between two time periods in a child's life in the two study villages revealed that a majority of children in Surli had some form of malnutrition at birth and also at six months, but most were in mild or moderate forms. In Nanduri on the other hand, many children, despite being born normal, had deteriorated to severe malnutrition by six months. In terms of the rate of change in nutrition, children in Surli were nutritionally better-off than those in Nanduri with progressing age - from birth to one year, to 18 months of age.

I had assumed that the factor of breastfeeding was a standard practice common to children of both the villages. This is known to play a role in child nutrition especially till six months to one year of child's age. Hence, this analysis sought to understand nutrition status and its change among children in both study villages. This evidence supports the fact that children in higher HDI ranked district (Satara) have a better start. They also do not drastically slip to severe forms of malnutrition within first six months as compared to the children in a poor HDI ranked district (Osmanabad).

Secondary data from other studies revealed that the status of malnutrition does not vary significantly with asset quintiles or even among caste 'within' the villages, while there is evidence that malnutrition varied 'between' the two villages. This meant that children who were malnourished in Surli and Nanduri belonged to all asset quintiles and caste categories. The finding matches with a study based in rural Maharashtra that also provides evidence to this trend in which overall malnutrition amongst children, adolescents, and married women in the study area is substantial and does not differ significantly between different socio-economic groups (Parasuraman & Rajaretnam, 2011).

At the macro level too, there have been studies to support the disassociation between economic growth and child malnutrition (Vollmer et al., 2014; Subramanyam et al., 2011; Baragona, 2014). Scholars argue that there is a break-down of causal chain determinants of child malnutrition and that a disjunction exists between prosperity and malnutrition (Walton, 2009). Walton (2009) cites reasons like the behaviour of mothers (even those better off or educated) that may be inconsistent with recommended practices; rising wealth may have modest effect on food spending. While 80% may have access to anganwadi centre, most do not use it. In addition, despite access to safe drinking water, only one third treat water to make it potable etc.

Therefore, just making the anganwadi centre work better will not work alone to tackle local child malnutrition. In fact such a strategy has failed (ibid.).

This is so because malnutrition is not a dimension of current or future inequalities but is also causally related to unequal institutional structures (Walton, 2009). This reinforces the basic premise of this study that institutional factors within the ICDS and NRHM, in addition to economic, social & developmental, are inextricably linked to child malnutrition outcomes.

On Users Engagement with Providers: As per the conceptual framework of the study, accountability relationships manifest through interaction between the user and the provider. Three components that constitute the understanding of accountability are engagement, answerability, and sanctions. The way respondents choose to access a health provider is the first step in understanding the extent of their engagement. Mainstream literature points to a fact that the majority of rural populations, including the poor, choose to access private health providers over public health services mainly because of problems of accessibility, lack of infrastructure and personnel in public health system. Much of the analysis in the literature attributes low access to 'poor supply side' of public health services.

Data revealed that a sizeable number of households in Surli did not access any service of the anganwadi, even once. To note, the anganwadi centre in Surli had a functional toilet, hand washing area, and a separate area for cooking inside its building. Centers looked neat and its walls beautifully were decorated with children's art. Conversely, in Nanduri, almost all households except two, had accessed the anganwadi centres. This is despite the fact that Nanduri anganwadi centres were poorly ventilated with no electricity, un-plastered walls, lacked toilets, and had a general lack of cleanliness.

In addition, households in Nanduri gave the centre a better rating on most counts as compared to those in Surli. The most common reasons for dissatisfaction of anganwadi services in both villages was that quality, variety, and age appropriateness of cooked food, to name a few, were inadequate. However, there were some issues specific to the two villages. In Nanduri, the absence of basic facilities like water, electricity, open space, sanitation and cleanliness, and infrastructure in general were most common issues identified by mothers. In Surli, mothers cited quality related issues like lack of toys, books, play equipment and common medicines etc. as major reasons for their dissatisfaction.

These findings, as discussed in Chapter IV and Chapter V, reveal that mothers in both villages were –

- Aware of optimum services that anganwadi centres should provide for their children, even though there are no 'formal standards' for the same.

- Secondly, although they were aware of the shortcomings prevailing in the services, a higher percentage of households in Nanduri not only accessed anganwadi centre services (as compared to Surli) but also gave better ratings to it. The low presence of private nurseries and tough access to them could be a contributory factor. In the absence of choice, a greater number of households accessed anganwadi centre in Nanduri, as compared to Surli.

- Finally, and most importantly, mothers' responses show that despite being aware of the gaps in services, they do not demand improvements from the anganwadi workers because of the lack of institutional processes for the same. There is no apparent role of mothers in mandated processes like growth charts and the village health nutrition and sanitation committee (VHNSC).

On Barriers to Access: Access to PHC was again low in Surli (33%) while the same was 72.5% in Nanduri, although a higher percentage of households in Surli gave it 'good' rating (45%), as compared to only 26% in Nanduri. A majority of households in Surli opted for private providers for conducting delivery, in contrast to Nanduri where an equal percentage of women delivered in a public facility and a high percentage still delivered at home.

It is interesting to note here that Surli was located merely 3.5 km from its PHC at Wathar which was once a 24x7 PHC with a resident medical officer. In Surli, common reasons for households not accessing or being dissatisfied with PHC included long hours of waiting, inconvenient timings, and the lack of specialist doctors and sonography tests. A common reason for dissatisfaction with the PHC near Nanduri was that it often 'referred' patients to civil or rural hospital. Hence households did not want to approach them, at the first place.

Frontline providers tend to impose demanding 'entry point rituals' or barriers for users in general, with an aim to limit their work burden (Goetz & Jenkins, 2005). Examples of barriers include referring to other facilities, calling at odd timings, and asking to queue-up. Such rituals were reported by respondents largely from non-poor backgrounds. Mothers from the non-poor asset quintiles, especially in Surli, also justified their decision to exit from the ICDS. Reasons for this include the fact that they were not given timely information, or that frontline workers do not conduct home visits to follow-up if their child was absent, or that workers do not pay attention when they visit the centre. Such practices may not be ruled out for the poor too. In absence of alternative choices (like private nursery) for the poor, it is the rich who are discouraged, and finally exit out.

There is evidence in the literature that supports such an observation, that workers use their discretion to limit their workload and constrict client demands which happens when service providers are over-worked and under-motivated (Lipsky, 1980 quoted in Goetz & Jenkins, 2005: 194). In all, mothers from poorer backgrounds were either satisfied with anganwadi services or choose not to comment while those who voiced their concerns were from rich and middle asset category, who had exited out by sending their children to private nursery.

Data revealed that from among the people who visited PHC, the majority of them were either poor, elderly, or women. These form the most vulnerable population. But, politically the weakest, are the ones that are least likely to question or demand better services from this PHC. The rich, productive males and children could simply access private health providers. An explanation for higher utilisation and better rating of public health services in Nanduri can be explained as follows.

When welfare nets in the form of public distribution systems, wage labour, and social security benefits are weak, in addition to weak socio-economic-political capabilities, the poor tend to utilise whatever public services are available even if it is perceived to be of poor quality. This was the case of Nanduri. To note, in Nanduri, there were a higher percentage of households belonging to the poor and lower middle asset quintiles than in Surli. Nanduri village also had a higher population engaged in agricultural labour than those in Surli. On the other hand, in Surli, in spite of perceived good quality of public services, even the poor did not utilise this because of alternative choices available in form of private sector, enabled by higher purchasing capacity of its households. To note, the percentage of households in middle asset quintile was almost double in Surli as compared to that in Nanduri. The study did not factor in these welfare nets but findings on access patterns can be speculatively explain this existing theoretical position.

Role of Exit: There are policy implications for public service delivery when the non-poor exit from public programmes. Humphreys (1998) sees the exit of a section of users from public services as serving the interests of the public providers & its employees. It is because the exit prevents additional work-load within the same remuneration (Humphreys, 1998). Other studies have also shown that when public services are only intended to serve the poor, they tend to rapidly become poor or deteriorate in quality (Kumar, 2007). The exit of large section of middle, upper middle, and rich classes from public services can reduce state commitment and lead to a downward spiral – this is especially perilous in contexts where alternatives exist (ibid.). Evidence from the study also shows that the choice exercised by the non-poor groups to exit out of a public programme is a result of institutional processes and not because of individual decision making alone.

Clearly the consistent argument that 'supply' is a problem in public health service delivery is now questionable. There is evidence in this study, that it is not so. This finding is counter-intuitive since literature on health policy assumes that rural population will use public health facilities if they are accessible and of high quality. Households in both the villages in the study did not conform to this logic. Literature on health seeking behaviour offers explanation towards preference of private providers.

Decisions on the choice of provider is usually made on factors like price of the service, available income, their knowledge of different providers, and their preference for services with different characteristic, particularly relating to quality (Mills et al., 2002). Since Surli village had a growing private health sector around and a higher percentage of upper middle and rich asset households, they used their purchasing power to buy private health services despite a functional PHC nearby. This was not so for Nanduri that had a higher proportion of middle and poor asset category households who accessed and utilised public health services. Most private health providers around Nanduri were available only 18 km away in the nearest town of Tuljapur making it difficult and costly to access.

On Frontline Providers: I asked households in both study villages about few critical aspects of their relationship with the frontline providers, mainly the anganwadi workers - the AWW, ANM and ASHA. The nature of relationship was analysed through concepts like providers' availability, attending community meetings, and finally levels of trust. Of all the providers, the ASHA from Nanduri who elicited maximum trust with 76.8% households felt a 'high' feeling of trust for her. Incidentally, the ASHA worker is neither given an honorarium by the state nor was she paid by the Nanduri VHSC. Yet, she was held in high respect by the community at large.

An alarming observation was that a majority of households in both villages had moderate or low trust in anganwadi workers, which was much lower than scores for the ASHAs or ANMs. This seems to be a bit surprising given a fact that anganwadi worker's position has the potential to command high respect and trust from the local community. The finding of low popularity of anganwadi workers can also be explained by the fact that when poor access services, they are not able to articulate their demands, especially through formal or collective means. The middle class and rich react with indifference, by choosing to exit out of these programs for better alternatives elsewhere.

Bureaucratic surveillance aimed at regulation by means of surprise checks, enumeration, and accountability through maintaining information registers, has created tension and friction between superior officers and anganwadi workers, as well as between anganwadi workers and 'served' population (Gupta, 2001).

The finding conforms with the larger literature which articulates that the processes of NPM with emphasis on surveillance – whether through citizen oversight, new monitoring technologies, public-private partnerships or market-based mechanisms, downplays the importance of building cultures of probity and trusteeship in the public services (Goetz and Jenkins, 2005: 192)

Further, relationship between users and providers in Surli was found to be weak and impersonal, at household level but strong and engaged at the community level. This also matches with the pattern of political engagement in Surli, as discussed in Chapter V. Accountability processes had a role to play in better nutrition outcomes in Surli. Conversely, in Nanduri, a village from a poor HDI ranked district, the relationship between frontline providers and users were inter-personal, trustworthy, and of close engagement, but weak at the community level. Such a conclusion is in line with the political behaviour of households in Nanduri.

Evidence from another study demonstrates similar findings. Similar formal democratic institutions can result in vastly different political processes, forms of electoral competition, and quality of public services, as they interact with local political and social structures (Sebastian, 2007). Where elections are less competitive, there are fewer incentives for elected public officials to perform well. On the contrary, there are incentives for the misallocation of public resources to draw private rents (ibid.). This provides only a part of the whole picture. Besides, this, questions on how this relationship gets enacted and with what implications, also needs to be discussed and this was attempted in Chapter V as presented in the following section.

On Tools of Accountability: Answerability and sanctions are concepts in addition to engagement that are central to study accountability relationships. Two tools that are have been formally institutionalised for demanding explanations between users and providers at the village level for public health services are the growth charts and VHSC. The growth chart is the only link that connects the institution of ICDS, its frontline provider anganwadi worker, and the parents of children. However, the irony of the institution of ICDS is that the weight and height of children is meticulously recorded and extensively shared for bureaucratic monitoring, but the same is not demanded by the mothers or shown to them, defeating its very purpose. It is a common observation that growth-charts are the most under-emphasised, under-utilised and ignored aspect of ICDS from the context of both users and providers.

The issue should not be labelled as 'lack of awareness' among users since anganwadi centres has been in operation for more than a decade in study villages. It is to do with the way existing institutional processes work within the ICDS. The reason for this trend lies within the NPM framework of managerial accountability where, for few activities like 'sharing' growth chart with mothers, there are not any indicators to measure and monitor. So, it is blatantly skipped. It means that the existing processes in ICDS do not provide space for users to use this instrument and ensure their implementation (Goyal

& Sekhar 2015). Because of this, the ICDS has been reduced to a 'dole' as many experts have also voiced earlier. This is one of the central reasons for disinterest and lack of community ownership in ICDS programme, as has also been reiterated in this study.

The state institutionalised a bottom-up accountability and community monitoring mechanism of child nutrition at the village level through Village Health, Sanitation & Nutrition Committee (VHSNC) within the NRHM implementation framework. It is only through the Village Health & Sanitation Committee (VHSC) that the anganwadi centre will be accountable to the gram panchayat (GP) (Husain, 2011). Findings show that the practice, despite the presence of state policy, was grossly under-implemented in the study villages. The VHSC was formed and functioned in Surli as an independent committee, but not within the panchayat.

In fact, households were confused if these were different or the same, as the panchayat had its own water and sanitation committee as well. In Nanduri, its panchayat water & sanitation committee never included nutrition as its mandate nor formed any separate VHSC. Therefore, in both study villages, 'nutrition' was not part of the PRI institution despite the state government policy stipulating that it be so since 2006. The only difference was that in Surli, there was a consensus between the gram panchayat and anganwadi workers on the spending priorities of VHSC funds.

In Surli, grants received by VHSC were used on items like buying chairs/tables for children, paying honorariums to the ASHA, conducting health survey, and addressing sanitation needs. The situation in Nanduri was the opposite where the VHSC was not formed and funds could not be utilised for the anganwadi because of in-fighting between the sarpanch and anganwadi worker. The second difference was that the Surli sarpanch, a woman, often went to the anganwadi centre to taste the food to show solidarity with the workers. It was for this reason, the study argues, that anganwadi centre 'functioned' better in Surli to result in improvements of child malnutrition over a period of time. But the fact that Surli VHSC was a stand-alone committee, not under panchayat's purview defeated its very purpose. Therefore, to conclude, of the two formal institutional tools with users to confront and demand answers,

- The VHSC resulted in community ownership and hence improved services to some extent in Surli.

- The growth chart, a potentially more effective strategy, failed to generate demand and curb exit for ICDS services, equally so in both the villages.

The ability to demand and confront providers is intricately linked to political capability of actors, especially the users. In order to access political capabilities of the people in both the villages, the heads of the households were asked questions on their awareness and nature of participation in community organisations during the household survey. Overall, it is common to see that health and nutrition is not a community issue unlike education, water, and sanitation, despite it being brought together under one roof in the VHSNC.

There is similar evidence in other research that show that health and child nutrition is not an issue at all that draws people to attend gram sabha meetings (Joshi, 2006). There were some distinctive features of political spaces that differed in both villages –

- Surli gram panchayat played an engaged role in its anganwadi centres by contributing funds under heads like rent, miscellaneous fees for the anganwadi, medical help, delivery, and child development.
- Another distinguishing feature of gram panchayat mentioned by households in Surli was that it facilitates anganwadi workers to attend and share their work at the gram sabha meetings.
- In Nanduri, respondents mentioned that its Village Education Committee (VEC) members (and not gram panchayat members) are active in paying visits to the anganwadi centres and also tasting the food, checking supplies etc. Even though, this may be effective to some extent, it falls in the domain of informal and unaccountable practices.

On Formal Versus Informal Institutions for Accountability: Another institution at the village level which is intricately linked to political participation in general and participation in PRIs in particular are political parties. Awareness of local political parties was higher in Surli and a higher percentage of households participated with local political parties than that in Nanduri. Also on average, participation of households in community organisations like the SHGs, gram sabha, bank society, and gram panchayat's water and sanitation committee were higher in Surli than in Nanduri. Political capabilities can also be understood in terms of people's capacity to approach and interact with those in positions of power for common community or personal issues.

This study revealed that households in Nanduri opted for state-related power holders in gram panchayat and bureaucrats, while those in Surli were more inclined towards non-state actors in political parties and politicians.

I explain this observation through the social composition of the two villages. In Surli, a high percentage of rich and upper middle asset quintiles warrants asking and giving favours to local politicians, suggesting a culture of 'benevolent feudalism' (Sekher, 2004).

Such relationships of patronage do not allow confrontations. Hence no narratives, either formal or informal, were shared in Surli. Using present evidence, it is clear that a supposedly well-functioning anganwadi center or a PHC like those for Surli can be explained with local level processes. It was also a result of the large exit of the middle and rich asset class. Smaller numbers remaining are managed by a system of strict top-down bureaucratic monitoring and, to some extent, by participation of PRI institutions or VHSC. These situations were absent in Nanduri.

In Nanduri, higher middle and poor asset households could find no-fringe access to state functionaries. Low community participation of households in local community organisations and high personal political contact with state power holders like panchayat office bearers or bureaucracy at village level in Nanduri points to the practice of paying rents to get one's work done. It shows that personal interests tend to supersede community interest as most approach state power holders for getting work done.

This has implications in the way users confront providers. Nanduri had higher instances of confrontations with the providers, both formal and informal, amid higher utilisation of public services amid their 'perceived' poor quality, especially when compared with Surli. While informal methods of confrontation like rude or violent behaviour lead to immediate results, their long term impact needs to be accessed. Distinct difference in the political participation in both villages has a direct impact in the way users confronted service providers.

The formal institutional mechanisms for eliciting answerability and hence accountability at the frontline of service delivery in a village are elections at various levels of governance including elections, and the Right to Information Act and Citizen Charters. Households in Surli felt that elections had no impact on their lives and on their village as compared to those in Nanduri who attributed infrastructure development to elected representatives. Issues related to improvements in agriculture, healthcare, and school education were hardly identified in relation to elections.

As a counter-intuitive trend, a higher percentage of households in Nanduri were aware about RTI as compared to Surli. Also, a higher percentage of households in Nanduri filed a RTI query (six households) than those in Surli (two households). This finding matches with a previous finding where households in Nanduri preferred state power holders like bureaucrats and panchayat members. Also, to note, Nanduri had three times the number of illiterates and literate-without-schooling as compared to Surli. Main issues on which RTI queries were filed were related to records pertained to land or certificates, schools and anganwadi centers, and corruption at panchayat.

In the relationship of the user and provider, the balance of power usually favours the provider. In such a case, it is unlikely that a user in individual capacities or even as a community will raise their voice or sanction the provider. It is all the more true for health services in the Indian context where social status and professional power distances doctors from poor patients (Hossain, 2010). Respondents were asked six hypothetical open ended questions on instances of poor health and nutrition services. They were asked in an open ended question, that if they were to face these situations, what they would do.

Responses were later categorised in four main categories – 'confrontational', 'exit', 'helplessness or indifference', and finally 'don't know'. Of all the six hypothetical scenarios, in four such situations, a higher percentage of respondents in Nanduri reported to confront the providers. Also, the strategies they used for answerability involved both formal and informal means. The informal forms of confrontations in Nanduri included rough, rude, and violent behaviour, even going as far as naming and shaming in the media. This was not so in Surli. Formal forms included complaints to higher authority, job transfers, and even police action. Surprisingly, neither frontline workers nor respondents reported any formal or informal form of confrontation in Surli.

Incidences of formal sanctions, which are a defining feature in the web of accountability relationship, could be known only from the providers. Some frontline workers from Nanduri revealed few incidents of sanctions. At times, workers become victims of politics of gender hierarchy and face the brunt of sanctions in form of harassment and scrutiny from officials. In cases of food poisoning reported in the media for schemes like mid-day meal or anganwadi, it is the anganwadi worker and cook that are blamed and sanctioned, and rarely the immediate senior.

Frontline workers from Surli denied knowing their colleagues faced sanctions. In health services, medical officers are responsible for ensuring timely health check-ups of all anganwadi children. They are rarely or never held accountable if the service is not delivered. This shows that elite bias and gender bias is prevalent within the bureaucratic hierarchies of the state. Thus, to conclude,

- Relationships of accountability are enacted within local spaces. These spaces could be either formal or informal. Formal ones include institutional spaces mandated in public programmes at the village level like VHSC and PRIs; political parties and street-level bureaucracy and community organisations like bank society and SHGs. Informal spaces are everyday encounters of users with providers at any given space and time.

- The formal spaces have formal instruments of accountability like the elections; RTIs etc; while informal instruments used the agency of the users like a poor patient getting rude with a doctor in a PHC.

The study revealed that the way users used these formal and informal spaces, in turn, impacted people's methods of confrontations in the study villages. In Surli, participation of households, especially the poor in community organisations including panchayat and political parties together with a culture of political patronage, allowed for strengthening of formal institutions of accountability like the VHSC and the panchayat in delivering better child health and nutrition services in the village. Since the poor had an outlet through these formal channels of accountability like the panchayat or VHSC and also through political patronage in non-state actors like local politicians, there was no need for any opportunity to take the route of informal methods like rude or violent forms of accountability. This is a reason that no case of sanction or confrontation was reported by any of the respondents – users and providers in Surli. The finding resonates with Walton (2009),

> *'And with India being called a patronage democracy by Chandra (2004), for politicians and local officials, nutrition is an unattractive source of patronage, in terms of services, as compared to repeatable private goods like wells, house, pension, water tap etc. It is a poor source of corrupt gains. Therefore the core of India's malnutrition puzzle lies in institutional functioning. It also meant that just making the anganwadi centre work better will not work alone to tackle local child malnutrition, in fact such a strategy has failed' (Walton, 2009).*

In context of Surli, this meant that while its anganwadi centre was functioning well, it still fell short of reducing any form of malnutrition which was high from the standards of better HDI ranked district and in fact almost comparable to Nanduri especially at birth. The only difference was that it did prevent any further deterioration to moderate or severe forms of malnutrition through local institutional processes, which were either weak or absent in Nanduri.

The situation was completely opposite in Nanduri. Low participation in community organisations and high contacts with state actors like panchayat members and bureaucrats in Nanduri points to the fact that the poor had few opportunities to participate in formal institutions or to express discontent. It also shows that personal interests superseded community interests because there were hardly any attempts to improve health and nutrition services. In such a case, any lapse in services resulted in individuals either taking the RTI route or taking to the streets to pelt stones at the PHC.

Higher level of contact with state functionaries in Nanduri as compared to Surli made respondents more aware of the formal provisions to demand services from the state institutions.

Users' Choice on Demanding Accountability: Nanduri had many reported cases of both formal methods of demanding answers in the form of RTIs, complaints to higher authorities, and informal methods. Individuals used their agency including rude and violent forms of confrontations to negotiate. However, scholars believe that these informal forms of accountability need not be dismissed. Their impact however is not sustainable and is short lived.

The study findings also revealed that informal methods of accountability were actually counter-productive for Nanduri since its PHC became infamous for shuttling out doctors. In addition, no doctor want to stay in the premises of the PHC. Therefore, formal institutional methods of account giving and answering have a better advantage over the informal forms of accountability in terms of strengthening of local institutions in the long term. This includes also being more sustainable irrespective of the kind of people that may come and go, and finally not being counter-productive or harmful towards the interests of the poor and needy.

One thing that clearly emerges is that role of institutional processes seems to have a stronger influence than socio-economic factors in explaining capacities of the poor to demand accountability in public service delivery. Accountability at the frontline of service delivery works the best through formal institutional spaces, and efforts must be made to strengthen it by encouraging universal inclusion and not selective inclusion. The existing forms of bureaucratic accountability have limits to what it can achieve, and hence needs to be complemented with democratic bottoms-ups local accountability processes.

The Question on Book's cover 'Does Accountability & Local Institution matters?', is answered that yes, accountability matters only when local institution at the frontline of public service delivery are also factored in the design and implementation of programmes.

6.3 Implications for Policy

A work of philosophy like this study cannot be treated as a problem-solving exercise only. The primary objective of this study was to question underlying assumptions and to add new perspectives to existing knowledge paradigms on public service delivery. Policy suggestions can be suggested as a nudge for policy makers to make design corrections. Therefore, ideally, the study is not mandated to offer policy recommendations for current implementations of national programmes like the existing NRHM and ICDS. However, there are few institutional and local processes which if improved, could help limit current challenges which these programmes face.

Firstly, policy implementation needs to make nutrition an inherent part of the VHSC function, and the VHSC in-turn be made a part of the PRIs at the village level.

The state can achieve this either through regulation, by linking the release of panchayat budgetary allocations with a condition that the VHNSC (Village Health Nutrition and Sanitation Committee) be formed at the level of the village panchayat. Alternative the state can turn to incentives like providing some extra grants to those panchayats who have been able to do so. Once the state achieves this, a formal mechanism of local, bottom-up accountability of the institution of anganwadi will be established at the village level.

Although there is no guarantee that state can completely tackle malpractices like the registration of ghost names of children, pilferage of supplies or quality of food, placing such a process in place would make sure that malpractices will entail adverse social costs for the providers. This can act as a strong deterrent. Also, such a process would assure that anganwadi centers work effectively within the institutional constraints which have demonstrated to have some positive impact, if not significant impact, to improve child malnutrition.

Secondly, public agencies entrusted with training of frontline workers like anganwadi workers and ASHAs should explicitly communicate certain ethos of community work to these workers, like the rationalisation of their honorariums, the role for which they are appointed, and the strengths and constraints of being a community worker. These agencies can also facilitate introduction of non-monetary incentives to these workers in the form of honour badges on lines of *esprit de corps*, special brand-building through supplies and materials used at the village level like back-packs for supplies, stationary and books, as well as felicitation at the block and district levels by lower level bureaucrats and community leaders. The last measure would help ease the friction that is often common between these workers and immediate seniors.

These measures are known to increase the self-worth, job satisfaction, and motivation of these workers, thereby building trust between them and the community at large. In the study, the ASHA worker of Nanduri was an example to show that this indeed is possible. There is hardly any evidence, both in theory and in practice, that any increase in community workers' honorariums or converting them to salaried employees has led to improved accountability and their commitment for public services. In fact, the opposite is often true. The state need not see these workers in context of wages in the informal or formal labour market or in context of gender discrimination. Often this argument is made in favour of the fact that these workers are mostly women.

Since the essence of appointing these workers lies in community and voluntary work, a fixed honorarium is institutionally the most appropriate.

The measures suggested here would help instil a feeling of community ownership to such national programmes which are implemented locally. It is here that a momentum can be built for creating a demand especially for tools like growth charts that would make mothers see the benefit of weighing their child and to connect better with the programme. These measures can help create local people as informal agents of accountability especially when formal systems are often captured by local elite and interest groups. Although contexts differ significantly, such practices have been tried in other developing countries of the Global South, like Brazil, and there is scope to learn lessons from the same.

At the institutional level, there are three main policy implications emerging out of this study: -

- Firstly, the study's framework to establish linkages between accountability processes and service delivery outcomes can be adopted to evaluate other development sectors where there exists, public service delivery like education, livelihoods, water and sanitation. This can be one of the most useful applications of the study especially in the field of public programme evaluations and public policy assessments.

- Secondly, the exit of users is neither monitored nor acknowledged within ICDS policy and processes. This was one of the strengths of using the case study design for this study. If I had used representative sample of fixed households from a block, such an exit would never have been revealed. This is a serious gap in the formal accountability processes within ICDS and NRHM institutional framework at the local level. Trends of the exit of users need to be incorporated into the policy frameworks of these national programmes.

- Lastly, focussing on the 'supply' of government service still remains a key strategy for improvements in access and quality for many countries including India. The data from the study show that, in addition to the supply, public policy must also encourage 'demand' for public health services in combination with the regulation of the private health sector. This could be done by making public programmes like the ICDS and NRHM which are 'universal' only on paper, to a one which is actually universal, institutionally.

Therefore, institutional structures need to build common interests between the poor and the better off. Such measures are more likely to lead to quality improvements that are sustainable eventually. Also, existing policy on child nutrition needs to prevent the exit of the middle class as much as it needs to include disadvantaged social groups.

6.4 Scope for Further Research

There are many aspects to the research problem and objectives which the study could not focus, because of constraints of resources and time. The following are some possible and promising areas for further research.

Firstly, the study explores accountability processes at the frontline level of the two programmes of NRHM and ICDS and not at the higher levels of governance like district, state, and country. The reason for this is that, at district, state or national levels, there are already multiple forms of accountability existing, especially the horizontal accountability like the managerial and financial accountability demanded by agencies by CAG and local audit committees.

However, at the level of village or the frontline of service delivery, where there is an interface between the providers, community, and the state, accountability is often diffused. Therefore, studying it at this level has not been attempted before and remains is most pertinent and challenging. In addition the constraints of time, resources and logical difficulties did not allow me to see how the accountability flowed from the frontline to the upper levels of government. It would have helped identify which pathways were used that results in what outcomes for the users or citizens.

Secondly, the study could not capture the field realities of many instruments of social accountability (like community score cards, social audits, and community based monitoring) that may be occurring elsewhere in the state or as a country on the whole. Although there are few assessments-based studies on specific instruments like the CBM experimented in Maharashtra by institutions like SATHI (Shukla et al., 2011). Others also include social audits championed by civil society organisations like Mazdoor Kisan Shakti Sangathan (MKSS) and the Citizen Report Cards popularised by Public Affairs Center (PAC).

Many of the existing studies on these instruments are commissioned by these institutions themselves with few independent assessments. Also, most of these studies are purely assessment oriented and do not include local factors that helped such instruments to strengthen or weaken existing accountability processes and local institutions. In addition, the assumption behind such evaluations is that civil society organisations are apolitical entities working only for social welfare. This is much debatable and contestable. Therefore, there is scope to study these instruments from the perspectives of local institutions especially from prism of the contentious idea of civil society itself.

Thirdly, health and nutrition is a subject with PRIs in many states. The study could have used a devolution index that ranks Indian states on how far they have empowered their Panchayati Raj Institutions (PRIs). The index created by the National Council of Applied Economic Research (NCAER) for the Ministry of Panchayati Raj measures functions, finance, and functionaries of the PRIs, as well as their accountabilities in these institutions to rank Indian states (Oommen, 2009). According to the 2008 Devolution Index, Madhya Pradesh was first in position while Manipur was last at 21. These two states could be compared to understand accountabilities in the PRIs with respect to health and nutrition. The questions under examination of this study however was not limited only to one institution of the PRIs but was intended for community-based institutions like anganwadi, family, and other health providers. Also, since the focus of the study was not decentralisation, such a research design could have limited the scope to only PRIs, a subject that has been heavily studied. However, if such data is available in public domain, this study can form a promising piece of research.

Fourthly, India lacks comprehensive data on citizen satisfaction with public services across states and districts. Few think tanks like the Public Affairs Center (PAC) have conducted a citizen's review or people's audit of five basic public services across few states (Paul, 2006). However, this is only one of the few attempts of citizen voices and such data is not in pubic domain. A study by Sebastian (2007) on accountability and decentralised service delivery in Indonesia had used measures of citizen's perceptions of local public services for Indonesian districts. Such data in Indian context can be a ready indicator to choose cases according to worst or best districts on citizen's responsiveness and compare it with local processes of accountability.

Fifthly, long term impacts of informal accountability mechanisms on local processes of accountability and on service delivery outcomes can be an interesting area of study especially in context of different political contexts. It will also be interesting to see if there is any association between women sarpanch leaders and functioning of local institutions especially in context of the ICDS. These linkages could also be explored in further research.

Lastly, another possible scope for future research is to use a macro comparative framework, by selecting one Indian state and another developing country like Sri Lanka, Bangladesh, or Indonesia to understand how difference in political governance can influence accountability and in-turn influence the implementation of nutrition and health programmes. This could add more variables like the type of political regimes and geographical location that will make the study design complex and resource intensive for doctoral work but can be attempted for institutional research projects.

***

References

1. Baragona, S. (2014, March 26). Rising wealth not enough to raise child health. *Voice of America.* Retrieved March 28, 2014 from http://www.voanews.com.
2. Goetz, A. M., Jenkins, R., & Shaw, T. M. (2005). *Reinventing accountability: making human democracy work for human development* (First). London: Palgrave Macmillan.
3. Goyal, J & Sekher, M. (2015). Accountability, Nutrition and Local Institutions in India. *Development.* Rethinking Democracy, Society for International Development, 58(1), United Kingdom: Palgrave McMillan.
4. Hossain, N. (2010). Rude accountability: Informal pressures on frontline bureaucrats in Bangladesh. *Development and Change*, *41*(5), 907–928.
5. Humphreys, P. C. (1998). *Improving public service delivery.* Dublin: Institute of Public Administration.
6. Husain, Z. (2011). Health of the National Rural Health Mission. *Economic & Political Weekly*, *46*(4), 53.
7. Joshi, A. (2006). Institutions and service delivery in Asia. *IDS Bulletin*, *37*(3), 115–129.
8. Kumar, A. S. (2007). Why are levels of child malnutrition not improving? *Economic and Political Weekly*, *42*(15), 1337–1345.
9. Mills, A., Brugha, R., Hanson, K., & McPake, B. (2002). What can be done about the private health sector in low-income countries? *Bulletin of the World Health Organization*, *80*(4), 325–330.
10. Oommen, M. A. (2009). Limits of a devolution index. *Economic and Political Weekly*, 44(29), 17–21.

11. Parasuraman, S., & Rajaretnam, T. (2011). Agriculture, food security and nutrition in Vidarbha: a household level analysis. *Economic and Political Weekly*, *46*(19), 42–50.

12. Paul, S. (2006). *Who Benefits from India's Public Services? A Peoples Audit of Five Basic Services*. Public Affairs Centre, Bangalore: Academic Foundation.

13. Press Trust of India. (2015). ICDS Scheme Set for Revamp, 13 lakh anganwadis to be Digitised. July 14. New Delhi.

14. Sebastian, E. (2007). Accountability & decentralised service delivery: explaining performance variations across local governments in Indonesia. Institute of Local Public Finance Working Paper 02-2007.

15. Sekher, M. (2004). Indigenous institutions and forest conservation: user-group self-initiatives in India. Working Paper No. 140, Bangalore: Institute for Social and Economic Change.

16. Subramanyam, M. A., Kawachi, I., Berkman, L. F., & Subramanian, S. V. (2011). Is economic growth associated with reduction in child under nutrition in India? *PLoS Med*, *8*(3), e1000424.

17. Vollmer, S., Harttgen, K., Subramanyam, M. A., Finlay, J., Klasen, S., & Subramanian, S. V. (2014). Association between economic growth and early childhood under nutrition: evidence from 121 demographic and health surveys from 36 low-income and middle-income countries. *The Lancet Global Health*, *2*(4), e225–e234.

18. Walton, M. (2009). The political economy of India's malnutrition puzzle. *IDS Bulletin*, *40*(4), 16–24.

APPENDIX I

Table 2.4: Human Development Index (HDI) for Maharashtra, 2001

Human Development Index (HDI) for Districts of Maharashtra, 1999-2001

Districts	*Literacy, 2001*	*Mean Years of schooling, 1999-2000*	*Per Capita Income (PCI), 2000-01 (1993-94 Prices)*	*Infant Mortality Rate (IMR), 2001*	*Education Index*	*PCI Index*	*IMR Index*	*HDI Index, 1999-2001*	*HDI Index, Rank, 1999-2001*
Gadchiroli	60.3	4.9	6829	59	0.72	1.00	0.75	0.18	34
Nandurbar	56.1	3.8	7989	47	0.91	0.95	0.51	0.21	33
Nanded	68.5	3.5	8091	58	0.67	0.95	0.73	0.22	32
Aurangabad	73.6	4.2	11903	72	0.49	0.79	1.00	0.24	31
Parbhani	67.0	3.0	9243	51	0.75	0.90	0.59	0.26	30
Bid	68.5	4.1	9159	55	0.61	0.90	0.67	0.27	27
Osmanabad	70.2	4.2	8537	57	0.56	0.93	0.71	0.27	29
Yavatmal	74.1	4.3	9671	63	0.48	0.88	0.82	0.27	28
Jalna	64.5	2.9	9100	43	0.82	0.90	0.43	0.28	26
Buldhana	76.1	4.3	8709	53	0.43	0.92	0.63	0.34	25
Hingoli	66.9	3.0	9474	32	0.75	0.89	0.22	0.38	24
Chandrapur	73.1	3.8	12507	47	0.54	0.76	0.51	0.40	22
Dhule	71.1	5.6	9075	47	0.40	0.91	0.51	0.40	23
Jalgaon	76.1	5.1	11805	51	0.35	0.79	0.59	0.42	20
Nashik	75.1	4.2	13459	50	0.46	0.72	0.57	0.42	21
Latur	72.3	5.3	8544	39	0.41	0.93	0.35	0.43	19
Gondiya	78.7	6.1	9279	48	0.20	0.90	0.53	0.46	18
Akola	81.8	5.4	9682	46	0.21	0.88	0.49	0.47	16
Bhandara	78.7	6.1	10234	48	0.20	0.86	0.53	0.47	17
Amravati	83.0	5.6	10867	50	0.16	0.83	0.57	0.48	15
Ahmednagar	75.8	4.6	10714	34	0.41	0.84	0.25	0.50	14
Solapur	71.5	4.2	11445	29	0.54	0.81	0.16	0.50	13
Washim	74.0	5.4	10435	35	0.37	0.85	0.27	0.50	12
Raigad	77.3	5.3	17180	50	0.31	0.56	0.57	0.52	11
Wardha	80.5	6.3	11850	43	0.15	0.79	0.43	0.54	10
Nagpur	84.2	6.3	16880	56	0.06	0.58	0.69	0.56	9
Sangli	76.7	5.6	14534	35	0.29	0.68	0.27	0.59	8
Ratnagiri	75.4	4.9	11148	21	0.39	0.82	0.00	0.60	7
Thane	81.0	5.5	17928	41	0.21	0.53	0.39	0.62	6
Kolhapur	77.2	5.8	16169	32	0.26	0.61	0.22	0.64	5
Pune	80.8	5.7	19680	42	0.19	0.46	0.41	0.65	3
Sindhudurg	80.5	6.4	12349	29	0.14	0.77	0.16	0.65	4
Satara	78.5	5.4	13036	22	0.27	0.74	0.02	0.66	2
Mumbai	86.8	5.9	30600	25	0.05	0.00	0.08	0.96	1
Maharashtra	77.3	5.0	15070	48	0.34	0.65	0.53	0.49	-

Note: The HDI values will not be comparable with that given in the Human Development Report Maharashtra, 2002 because at the indactor level the maximum and minimum used are from their respective observation under analysis (see education index, PCI index and IMR index above; in these indices 0 implies minimum failure whereas 1implies maximum failure across districts) and not from a global maximum or minimum. The 2001 IMR estimates for Bhandara, Dhule, Nandurabar and Raigarh are not available. Approximate values are obtained by using 1991 estimates of the district (at times of undivided district) and its variation from the state average.

Sourece: Kumar (2006).

Source: Report on Health Inequities in Maharashtra, 2008. SATHI. (Mishra et al. 2008)

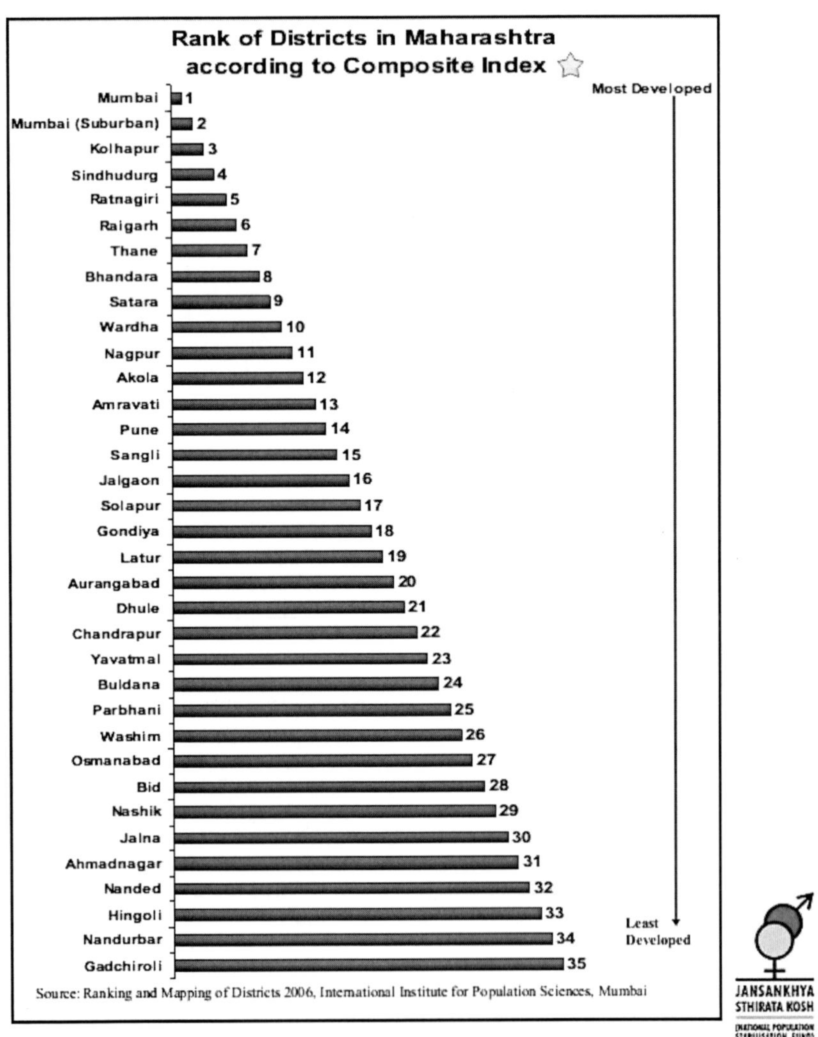

Figure 2.9: Ranking of Districts in Maharashtra, 2006

Source: Jansankhya Sthirta Kosh or National Population Stabilisation Fund 2006. http://www.jsk.gov.in/district_health.asp#a2

Note: Ranking is based upon a 2006 International Institute for Population Sciences, Mumbai report titled "Ranking and Mapping of Districts - Based on Socio -Economic and Demographic Indicators" using the 13 Indicators. This is based on a rural survey and excludes urban area. Indicators used are as follows: Percentage of Population 0-6 Years, Birth Order Three And Above, Birth below Age 20, Complete Immunization Coverage, Dropout from Full Immunization, Female Literacy Rate, Households Using Safe Drinking Water, Households with Toilet Facility, Percentage of Electrified Households, Women Receiving 2 TT Injections, Women Receiving 3 or More ANC Visits, Under 5 Mortality Rate and Contraceptive Prevalence Rate. Composite Index is the average of the above 13 indices.

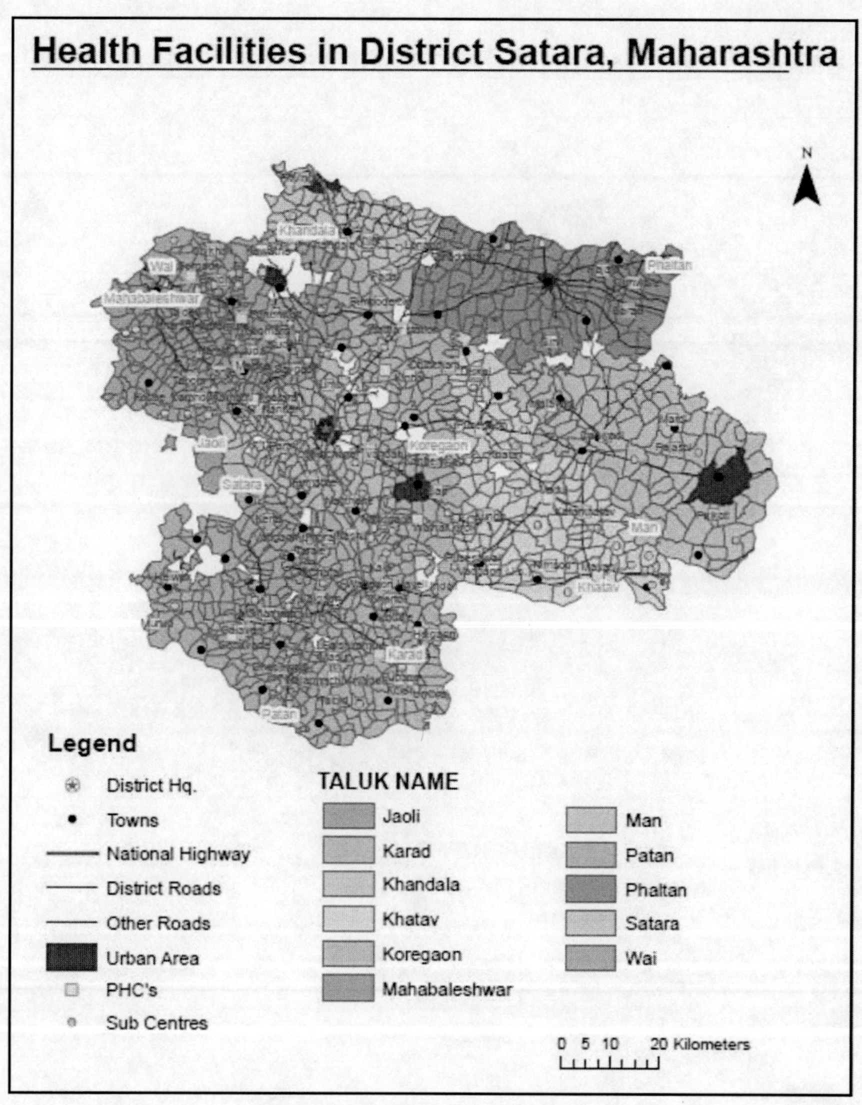

Figure 2.10: Satara District Map

Source: National Population Stabalisation Fund. www.jsk.gov.in

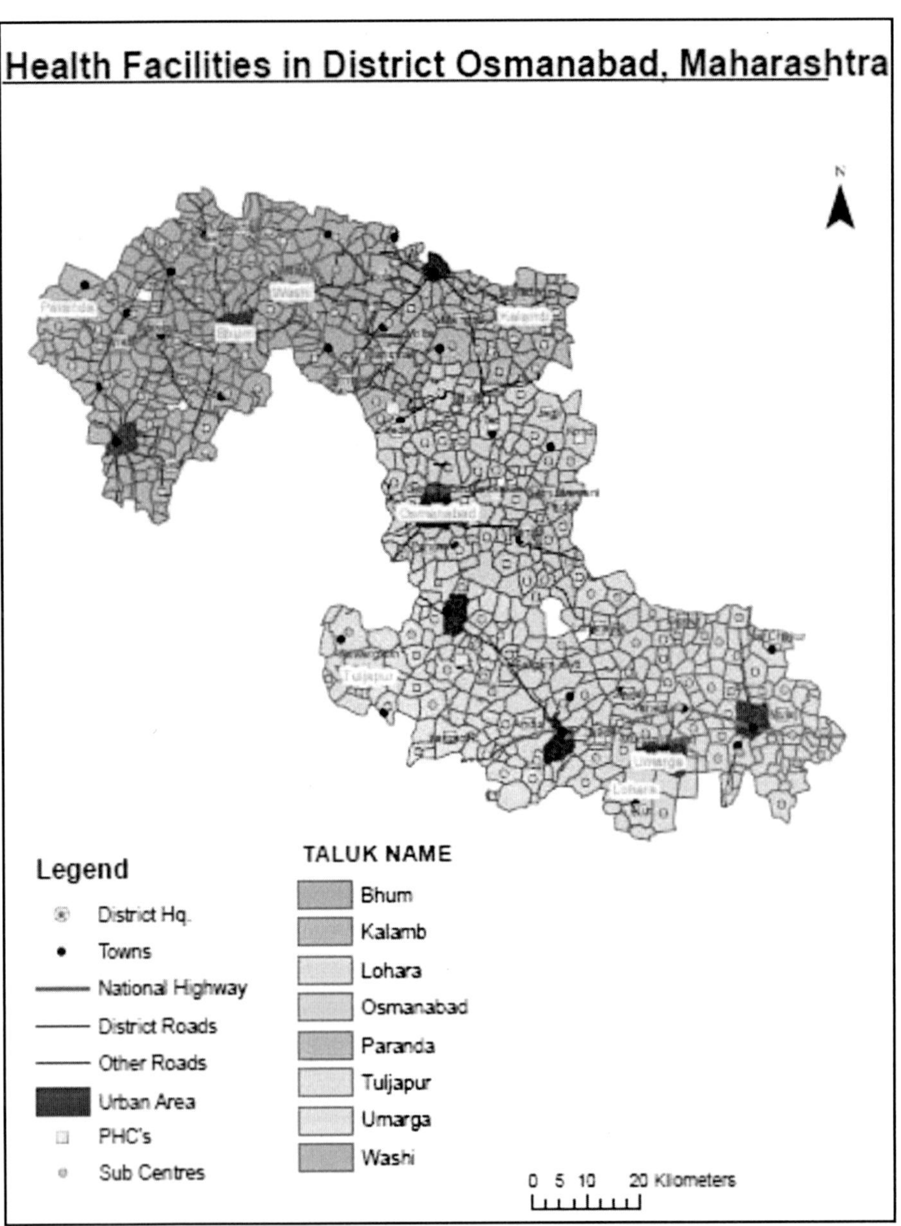

Figure 2.11: Osmanabad District Map

Source: National Population Stabalisation Fund. www.jsk.gov.in

Table 2.5: Monthly Progress Report (MPR) for ICDS Osmanabad, Maharashtra February 2012

Names of Blocks in Osmanabad District	***Nature***	***No. of AWCs / Mini AWCs providing SNP21 days & above***	***Total Population within project (survey figs)***			***Number of Supplementary Nutrition Programme (SNP) Beneficiaries***					***Classification of Nutritional Status of 0 to 5 yr Children***					% Malnourished of total weighed
			Total Pop 0-6year	Prgnant & Lactating Women	Total eligible pop	6m - 3 yr	3 yr - 6 yr	Prgnant & Lactating Women	Total Beneficaries	Percentage Beneficaries	Normal Weight	Modera-tely Underweight	Severly Underweight	Moderate & Severe Underweight	Total Children Weighed	
ALUR (MURUM)	Rural	160	14259	2610	16869	5541	5850	2471	13862	82.17	10284	920	109	1029	11313	9.1
BHOOM	Rural	174	10518	2006	12524	4245	4701	1964	10910	87.11	7602	580	91	671	8273	8.1
KALAMB(O)	Rural	239	18515	3768	22283	7288	7267	3663	18218	81.76	13103	1496	251	1747	14850	11.8
LOHARA	Rural	153	10343	2088	12431	4070	4346	1993	10409	83.73	7581	703	118	821	8402	9.8
OSMANABAD	Rural	197	15123	2934	18057	6036	6454	2487	14977	82.94	10525	1382	224	1606	12131	13.2
OSMANABAD	Urban	67	8218	1145	9363	3038	3203	1090	7331	78.30	4425	846	43	889	5314	16.7
OSMANABAD (TER)-2	Rural	179	14411	2822	17233	5673	5485	2695	13853	80.39	9650	1396	287	1683	11333	14.9
PARANDA	Rural	171	10869	2106	12975	4116	4761	1993	10870	83.78	7530	702	92	794	8324	9.5
TULJAPUR	Rural	239	17642	3428	21070	7391	8404	3420	19215	91.20	12390	1729	331	2060	14450	14.3
UMARGA	Rural	184	13945	2684	16629	5403	5825	2492	13720	82.51	10225	949	127	1076	11301	9.5
WASHI	Rural	133	8575	1713	10288	3581	3746	1650	8977	87.26	6737	380	55	435	7172	6.1
Total		1896	142418	27304	169722	56382	60042	25918	142342	83.87	100052	11083	1728	12811	112863	11.4

* Source: www.icds.gov.in ICDS Maharashtra Commissionerate Women and Child Development Pune.

Table 2.6: Monthly Progress Report (MPR) for ICDS Satara, Maharashtra February 2012

Block	Nature	No. of AWCs / Mini AWCs providing SNP 21 days +	Total Population within project (survey figs)		Total eligible population	Number of Supplementary Nutrition Programme (SNP) Beneficiaries			Total Beneficiaries	Percentage beneficaries from Total Population	Classification of Nutritional Status of 0 to 5 yrs. Children					% Malnourished of total children weighed
			Total Populaion 0 - 6 yrs	Prgnant & Lactating Women		6m - 3 yrs	3 yr - 6 yrs	Pregnant & Lactating Women			Normal	Moderately Underweight	Severly Underweight	Moderate+ Severe	Total Children Weighed	
KHANDALA	Rural	203	12083	2047	14130	4824	4418	2000	11242	79.6	9117	647	120	767	9884	7.8
KHATAV	Rural	235	11916	2137	14053	4854	3881	2090	10825	77.0	8773	710	116	826	9599	8.6
KOREGAON	Rural	228	10761	1817	12578	4051	3833	1734	9618	76.5	7908	589	75	664	8572	7.7
KOREGAON-2	Rural	188	7917	1425	9342	3322	2793	1407	7522	80.5	5874	494	82	576	6450	8.9
MAHABALESHWAR	Rural	127	3744	623	4367	973	1303	390	2666	61.0	2519	398	76	474	2993	15.8
MAN(DAHIWADI)	Rural	250	12219	2121	14340	4896	4416	2121	11433	79.7	8920	696	72	768	9688	7.9
MAN-(DAHIWADIMAHASWA)	Rural	131	6926	1156	8082	2800	2268	1156	6224	77.0	4525	350	44	394	4919	8.0
PATAN	Rural	380	13033	2184	15217	5341	5590	2184	13115	86.2	9423	938	170	1108	10531	10.5
PATAN-2	Rural	299	10935	1827	12762	4532	4270	1827	10629	83.3	7985	718	127	845	8830	9.6
PHALTAN	Rural	232	12490	2099	14589	5053	4756	2099	11908	81.6	9326	883	147	1030	10356	9.9
PHALTAN-2	Rural	212	12484	2069	14553	5111	4415	2069	11595	79.7	9076	1008	132	1140	10216	11.2
SATARA	Rural	331	19912	3047	22959	6890	5960	2698	15548	67.7	14480	1271	141	1412	15892	8.9
SATARA	Urban	115	11100	1071	12171	1828	4028	640	6496	53.4	4901	1400	18	1418	6319	22.4
SATARA-2	Rural	256	11443	1866	13309	3812	3737	1532	9081	68.2	8028	1050	143	1193	9221	12.9
WADUJ	Rural	315	19403	3155	22558	6193	4329	2240	12762	56.6	14103	1310	212	1522	15625	9.7
WAI	Rural	258	12819	2259	15078	4596	4222	2019	10837	71.9	9325	731	125	856	10181	8.4
Total		4645	231874	38170	270044	84250	79264	34212	197726	73.2	165869	15580	2114	17694	183563	9.6

* Source: www.icds.gov.in ICDS Maharashtra Commissionerate Women and Child Development Pune.

Table 2.7: ICDS Koregaon Block, Satara District, Maharashtra, April 2012

Sr. No.	Name of Beat	Centre No.	Survey of 0 - 6 years			Weighed				Normal				Moderate Undernutrition				Severe Undernutrition				Any Malnutrition	
			Boys	Girls	Total	Boys	Girls	Total	%	Boys	Girls	Total	%	Boys	Girls	Total	%	Boys	Girls	Total	%	Total	%
1	Tadvale	37	817	728	1545	781	695	1476	96	693	626	1319	89	82	61	143	10	6	8	14	1	157	10.6
2	Ekambe	44	1109	1017	2126	1097	1004	2101	99	1008	925	1933	92	82	72	154	7	7	7	14	1	169	8.0
3	Koregoan	30	1103	965	2068	1049	933	1982	96	950	836	1786	90	83	84	170	9	13	13	26	1	196	9.9
4	Rahimatpur	44	1022	915	1937	992	900	1892	98	930	845	1775	94	56	50	106	6	6	5	11	1	117	6.2
5	Arvi	33	728	679	1407	677	627	1304	93	615	563	1178	90	50	54	104	8	12	10	22	2	126	9.7
6	Vathar Kiroli	40	840	732	1572	852	704	1556	99	797	668	1465	94	48	30	78	5	6	6	13	1	91	5.8
	TOTAL		5619	5036	10655	5448	4863	10311	97	4993	4463	9456	92	404	351	755	7	51	49	100	1	856	8.3

Source: Data collected from the office of the CDPO, Panchayat Samiti Office, Koregaon Block, Satara, 2012.

Table 2.8: ICDS Tuljapur Block, Osmanabad District, Maharashtra

S. No.	*Activity Description*	*Salgara*	*Kakramba*	*Mangrol*	*Katgaon*	*Savargaon*	*Malumbra*	*Andur*	*Itkal*	*Total*
1	Survey (Rural)									
a	As per 2001 Census Males	9369	8527	12023	10799	10633	10309	13082	10353	85095
	Females	8853	7735	11218	10004	8755	9689	12052	9810	78116
	Total	**18222**	**16262**	**23241**	**20803**	**19388**	**19998**	**25134**	**20163**	**163211**
c	Surveyed Population in project area	16703	20267	21119	22945	19932	19998	24313	22253	167530
	Total population	**16703**	**20267**	**21119**	**22945**	**19932**	**19998**	**24313**	**22253**	**167530**
d	Surveyed child population 0-6 months	187	196	197	179	229	207	257	228	1680
	6 months to 1 year	142	199	171	191	172	134	209	234	1452
	1 year to 3 years	559	688	680	912	706	693	882	811	5931
	3 years to 5 years	517	817	738	785	703	660	881	810	5911
	0 to 5 years total	**1405**	**1900**	**1786**	**2067**	**1810**	**1694**	**2229**	**2083**	**14974**
	5 years to 6 years	239	387	321	368	355	310	372	421	2773
	0 to 6 years total	**1644**	**2287**	**2107**	**2435**	**2165**	**2004**	**2601**	**2504**	**17747**
	Pregnant women	179	198	196	233	210	183	222	229	1650
	Percentage	1.1	1.0	0.9	1.0	1.1	0.9	0.9	1.0	1.0
	Lactating women	187	196	197	179	229	207	257	228	1680
	percentage	1.1	1.0	0.9	0.8	1.2	1.0	1.1	1.0	1.0
	0 to 6 years as a percentage of total population	9.8	11.3	10.0	10.6	10.9	10.0	10.7	11.3	10.6
2a	Weight 0 to 6 years weighed	1580	2242	2054	2369	2103	1957	2513	2387	17205
	Percentage	96.1	98.0	97.5	97.3	97.1	97.7	96.6	95.3	97.0
b	Category Normal wt total number	1277	1913	1621	1932	1670	1692	2126	1937	14168
	Percentage	80.8	85.3	78.9	81.6	79.4	86.5	84.6	81.2	82.3
c	Medium malnutriton total number	258	270	372	388	359	222	316	392	2577
	Percentage	16.3	12.0	18.1	16.4	17.1	11.3	12.6	16.4	15.0
d	Severe malnutrition total number	45	59	61	49	74	43	71	58	460
	Percentage	2.9	2.6	3.0	2.1	3.5	2.2	2.8	2.4	2.7
e	Malnutrition (Moderate & Severe)	303	329	433	437	433	265	387	450	3037
	Percentage	19.2	14.7	**21.1**	18.4	20.6	13.5	15.4	18.9	17.7

Source: Data collected from the office of the CDPO, ICDS Tuljapur Block, Tuljapur city, Osmanabad, 2012.

Table 2.9: Village Level Data Wathar PHC, Koregaon, Satara

Sr. No	Revenue Village Name	AWC No.	Population	Distance from PHC	Children 0-6 years Total surveyed			Children 0-6 yrs Normal Weight				Children 0-6 yrs Moderate Malnourished			Children 0-6 yrs Severe Malnourished			Malnourished (Moderate & Severe)		Total Weighed			
					M	F	Total	M	F	Total	%	M	F	Total	M	F	Total	Total	%	M	F	Total	%
1	Kaloshi	33	164	0-5 km	8	7	15	8	7	15	100.0	0	0	0	0	0	0	0	0.0	7	8	15	100
2	Ki. Roli	37	760	0-5 km	28	20	48	25	18	43	91.5	2	1	3	1	0	1	4	8.5	28	19	47	97.9
	Ki. Roli	38	730	0-5 km	18	17	35	17	16	33	100.0	0	0	0	0	0	0	0	0.0	17	16	33	94.3
	Khaookwasti	243	464	10+ km	28	12	40	26	11	37	100.0	0	0	0	0	0	0	0	0.0	26	11	37	92.5
	Ki. Roli	369	452	0-5 km	29	17	46	17	17	34	94.4	0	0	0	2	0	2	2	5.6	19	17	36	78.3
	Ki. Roli	40	168	0-5 km	4	7	11	4	7	11	100.0	0	0	0	0	0	0	0	0.0	4	7	11	100
	Total		2574		107	73	180	89	69	158	96.3	2	1	3	3	0	3	6	3.7	94	70	164	91.1
3	Targaon	95	424	0-5 km	19	13	32	14	11	25	83.3	3	1	4	1	0	1	5	16.7	18	12	30	93.75
	Targaon	96	662	0-5 km	25	22	47	25	22	47	100.0	0	0	0	0	0	0	0	0.0	25	22	47	100
	Targaon	258	455	0-5 km	30	24	54	30	22	52	67.5	0	0	0	0	1	1	1	1.3	30	23	77	142.6
	Targaon	372	266	0-5 km	16	11	27	15	9	24	96.0	0	1	1	0	0	0	1	4.0	15	10	25	92.6
	Targaon	373	572	0-5 km	22	15	37	22	15	37	100.0	0	0	0	0	0	0	0	0.0	22	15	37	100
	Targaon	11	502	0-5 km	24	15	39	24	15	39	62.9	0	0	0	0	0	0	0	0.0	24	15	62	158.9
	Total		2881		136	100	236	130	94	224	97.0	3	2	5	1	1	2	7	3.0	134	97	231	97.9
4	Riki wadi	166	524	5-10 km	26	18	44	26	18	44	100.0	0	0	0	0	0	0	0	0.0	26	18	44	100
5	Nagjhari	116	512	10+ km	23	18	41	20	17	37	97.4	1	0	1	0	0	0	1	2.6	21	27	38	92.7
	Nagjhari	117	544	10+ km	14	20	34	13	19	32	94.1	1	1	2	0	0	0	2	5.9	14	20	34	100
	Mulikwadi	269	254	5-10 km	14	5	19	10	5	15	83.3	3	0	3	0	0	0	3	16.7	13	5	18	94.8
	Nagjhari	363	452	10+ km	14	21	34	12	17	29	93.5	1	1	2	0	0	0	2	6.5	13	17	31	91.2
	Nagjhari	364	472	10+ km	14	14	34	17	12	29	93.5	2	0	2	0	0	0	2	6.5	19	12	31	91.2
	Total		2234		14	78	162	72	70	142	93.4	8	2	10	0	0	0	10	6.6	80	72	152	93.9
6	Durgalwadi	103	757	0-5 km	14	26	57	30	23	53	94.6	1	2	3	0	0	0	3	5.4	31	25	56	98.3
	Durgalwadi	375	581	0-5 km	14	15	34	15	15	30	93.8	2	0	2	0	0	0	2	6.3	17	15	32	94.2
	Total		1338		14	41	91	45	38	83	94.3	3	2	5	0	0	0	5	5.7	48	40	88	96.7
7	Nalwadewadi	112	553	10+ km	14	28	58	25	24	49	96.1	0	2	2	0	0	0	2	3.9	25	26	51	87.9

Table 2.9: Continued

Sr. No	Revenue Village Name	AWC No.	Population	Distance from PHC	Children 0-6 years Total surveyed			Children 0-6 yrs Normal Weight				Children 0-6 yrs Moderate Malnourished			Children 0-6 yrs Severe Malnourished			Malnourished (Moderate & Severe)		Total Weighed			
	Nalwadewadi	374	431	10+ km	14	16	46	28	15	43	93.5	2	1	3	0	0	0	3	6.5	30	16	46	100
	Total		984		14	44	104	53	39	92	94.8	2	3	5	0	0	0	5	5.2	55	42	97	93.3
8	Surli	210	907	0-5 km	14	25	55	29	23	52	94.5	1	2	3	0	0	0	3	5.5	30	25	55	100
	Surli	211	676	0-5 km	14	17	48	24	17	41	91.1	3	0	3	1	0	1	4	8.9	28	17	45	93.75
	Surli	368	420	0-5 km	14	13	29	14	12	26	89.7	3	0	3	0	0	0	3	10.3	14	15	29	100
	Total		2003		14	55	132	67	52	111	86.0	7	2	9	1	0	1	10	7.8	72	57	129	97.8
9	Kombandchadi	46	438	10+ km	14	16	35	16	13	29	96.7	0	0	0	0	1	1	1	3.3	16	14	30	85.8
10	Wathar Ki	55	678	0-5 km	14	22	51	25	21	46	90.2	4	1	5	0	0	0	5	9.8	29	22	51	100
	Wathar Ki	181	614	0-5 km	14	18	37	18	17	35	100.0	0	0	0	0	0	0	0	0.0	18	17	35	94.6
	Wathar Ki	182	694	0-5 km	14	28	53	24	26	50	94.3	1	2	3	0	0	0	3	5.7	25	28	53	100
	Wathar Ki	183	721	0-5 km	14	32	75	41	28	69	95.8	1	2	3	0	0	0	3	4.2	42	30	72	96
	Wathar Ki	84	773	0-5 km	14	40	70	24	33	57	89.1	2	5	9	0	0	0	9	14.1	26	38	64	91.5
	Wathar Ki	365	421	0-5 km	14	16	35	17	13	30	88.2	2	2	4	0	0	0	4	11.8	19	15	34	97.2
	Wathar Ki	366	436	0-5 km	14	17	33	15	16	31	93.9	1	1	2	0	0	0	2	6.1	16	17	33	100
	Wathar Ki	367	490	0-5 km	14	11	35	23	9	32	94.1	0	2	2	0	0	0	2	5.9	23	11	34	97.2
	Total		4827		14	184	389	187	163	350	93.1	11	15	26	0	0	0	26	6.9	198	178	376	96.7
11	Sathewadi	201	319	10+ km	14	19	36	12	16	28	82.4	3	2	5	1	0	1	6	17.6	16	18	34	94.5
	Sathewadi	266	266	10+ km	14	23	31	7	18	25	89.3	0	2	2	0	1	1	3	10.7	7	21	28	90.4
	Total		585		14	42	67	19	34	53	85.5	3	4	7	1	1	2	9	14.5	23	39	62	92.6
12	Mohitewadi	160	464	10+ km	14	21	49	26	20	46	93.9	2	0	2	1	0	1	3	6.1	29	20	49	100
	Mohitewadi	370	470	10+ km	14	15	34	16	15	31	93.9	1	0	1	1	0	1	2	6.1	18	15	33	97.1
	Total		934		14	36	83	42	35	77	93.9	3	0	3	2	0	2	5	6.1	47	35	82	98.8
13	Dhangarwadi	371	390	5-10 km	14	15	40	21	14	35	94.6	1	1	2	0	0	0	2	5.4	22	15	37	92.5
14	Safarvasti	8	163	5-10 km	14	9	15	6	8	14	100.0	0	0	0	0	0	0	0	0.0	6	8	14	93.4
	Total		1487		14	60	138	69	57	126	94.7	4	1	5	2	0	2	7	5.3	75	58	133	96.4

Source: Data collected from ICDS Supervisor in charge of Wathar Kiroli Beat, Koregaon block, Satara, 2012.

Table 2.10: Village Level Data Mangrol PHC, Tuljapur, Osmanabad

ICDS Mangrol Anganwadi Level Data January 2012																				
Sr. No.	*Revenue Village Name*	*Distance from PHC*	*AWC No.*	*Population*	*Total surveyed (0-6 years children)*			*Normal*				*Moderate Malnutrition*			*Severe Malnutrition*			*Any Malnutrition*		*Total Weighed*	
					M	F	T	M	F	T	%	M	F	T	M	F	T	T	%	T	%
1	Apsinga	5-10 kms	2	4098	48	44	92	38	35	73	82.0	8	8	16	0	0	0	16	18.0	89	96.7
	Apsinga	5-10 kms	3		43	45	88	33	34	67	77.9	7	7	14	2	3	5	19	22.1	86	97.7
	Apsinga	5-10 kms	4		46	45	91	32	27	59	67.0	13	15	28	0	1	1	29	33.0	88	96.7
	Apsinga	5-10 kms	137		59	51	110	37	39	73	68.9	13	17	30	8	5	13	43	40.6	106	96.4
	Apsinga	5-10 kms	226		40	41	81	28	24	52	70.3	10	9	19	1	3	4	23	31.1	74	91.4
	Total			4098	47	45	92	34	32	65	73	10	11	21	2	2	5	26	28.9	89	95.8
2	Katri	0-5 kms	5	1042	59	48	107	40	32	72	72.7	9	8	17	5	4	9	26	26.3	99	92.5
3	Kamtha	0-5 kms	6	1680	45	30	75	31	16	47	66.2	13	9	22	1	1	2	24	33.8	71	94.7
	Kamtha	0-5 kms	227		24	17	41	13	7	20	52.6	7	4	11	2	3	5	16	42.1	38	92.7
	Total			1680	35	24	58	22	12	34	59	10	7	17	2	2	4	20	38.0	55	93.7
4	Bori	0-5 kms	7	737	44	45	89	34	33	67	77.9	9	8	17	2	1	3	20	23.3	86	96.6
5	Sindphal	0-5 kms	15	4197	32	39	71	20	27	47	71.2	10	4	14	1	4	5	19	28.8	66	93.0
	Sindphal	0-5 kms	16		42	39	81	27	28	55	80.9	2	8	10	2	1	3	13	19.1	68	84.0
	Sindphal	0-5 kms	17		58	49	107	48	40	88	84.6	6	7	13	1	2	3	16	15.4	104	97.2
	Sindphal	0-5 kms	18		56	45	101	32	22	54	61.4	14	15	29	2	2	4	33	37.5	88	87.1
	Sindphal	0-5 kms	228		60	59	119	38	31	69	70.4	15	9	24	1	4	5	29	29.6	98	82.4
	Sindphal	0-5 kms	229		32	32	64	15	15	30	52.6	13	9	22	2	3	5	27	47.4	57	89.1
	Total			4197	47	44	91	30	27	57	70	10	9	19	2	3	4	23	29.6	80	88.8
6	Mangrol	0-5 kms	43	5000	56	45	101	42	30	72	72.0	11	10	21	2	5	7	28	28.0	100	99.0
	Mangrol	0-5 kms	44		34	19	53	24	8	32	62.7	6	9	15	3	1	4	19	37.3	51	96.2
	Mangrol	0-5 kms	45		34	35	69	25	18	43	66.2	6	8	14	1	7	8	22	33.8	65	94.2
	Mangrol	0-5 kms	46		46	20	66	35	18	53	80.3	11	2	13	0	0	0	13	19.7	66	100.0
	Mangrol	0-5 kms	230		45	35	80	22	20	42	54.5	14	14	28	6	1	7	35	45.5	77	96.3
	Total			5000	43	31	74	30	19	48	67	10	9	18.2	2.4	2.8	5	23.4	32.9	71.8	97.13784293

Table 2.10: Continued

Sr. No.	*Revenue Village Name*	*Distance from PHC*	*AWC No.*	*Population*	*Total surveyed (0-6 years children)*			*Normal*				*Moderate Malnutrition*			*Severe Malnutrition*			*Any Malnutrition*		*Total Weighed*	
					M	F	T	M	F	T	%	M	F	T	M	F	T	T	%	T	%
7	Khandalkarav	More than 10 kms	142	NA	16	14	30	10	13	23	79.3	4	1	5	1	0	1	6	20.7	29	96.7
8	Sardevadi	0-5 kms	47	386	26	15	41	22	11	33	78.6	4	4	8	1	0	1	9	21.4	42	102.4
9	Dhanegaon	0-5 kms	49	469	21	19	40	20	18	38	95.0	1	1	2	0	0	0	2	5.0	40	100.0
10	Kasai	More than 10 kms	76	1009	55	45	100	32	30	62	73.8	11	7	17	3	2	5	22	26.2	84	84.0
11	Kalegaon	0-5 kms	99	686	33	40	73	18	24	42	70.0	6	7	13	3	2	5	18	30.0	60	82.2
12	Nanduri	5-10 kms	100	1461	30	43	73	27	35	62	84.9	5	3	8	0	0	0	8	11.0	73	100.0
	Nanduri	5-10 kms	231		32	36	68	21	31	52	82.5	6	3	9	2	0	2	11	17.5	63	92.6
13	Khotachiwadi	5-10 kms	203	NA	14	14	28	13	11	24	92.3	0	1	1	0	1	1	2	7.7	26	92.9
14	Vagjaighat	5-10 kms	139	NA	16	11	27	15	10	25	92.6	0	2	2	0	0	0	2	7.4	27	100.0
15	Dipaknagar	5-10 kms	140	NA	15	15	30	14	13	27	90.0	1	2	3	0	0	0	3	10.0	30	100.0
	Total				1159	1025	2184	807	710	1517	73.3	230	208	438	53	54	107	545	26.3	2069	94.7

Source: Data collected from ICDS Supervisor in charge of Mangrol project, Tuljapur block, Osmanabad, 2012

APPENDIX II

एकात्मिक बाल विकास सेवा योजना प्रकल्प, कोरेगाव.

तिमाही कुटुंब सर्व्हे गोषवारा कालावधी –

१) अंगणवाडी केंद्राचे नाव व नंबर – सुर्ली २१०, २११, ३९८.

२) तिमाही गोषवारा कालावधी – एप्रिल, मे, जुन

३) अंगणवाडी क्षेत्रातील एकूण कुटुंबे – ४२८.

४) अंगणवाडी कार्यक्षेत्रातील लोकसंख्या – २००३ पुरुष १०४३ स्त्रिया – ९६० एकूण – २००३

५) अंगणवाडी कार्यक्षेत्रातील कुटुंब संख्या व लागणाऱ्या वर्गीकरणानुसार तपशील

	एकूण कुटुंब	कुटुंबातील संख्या		
		पुरुष	स्त्रिया	एकूण
१) अनुसूचित जाती	49	111	97	208
२) अनुसूचित जमाती	—	—	—	—
३) दारिद्र्य रेषेखालील कुटुंबे	59	121	107	228
४) इतर कुटुंबे १) मा. प्र. ६०००/– पर्यंत उत्पन्न असलेली कुटुंबे	—	—	—	—
२) अत्यल्प भूधारक	—	—	—	—
३) इतर	342	811	756	1567
एकूण –	450	1043	960	2003

सर्व्हेप्रमाणे एकूण लाभार्थी संख्या –

तपशील	अ. जाती		अ. जमाती		दा. रे.		इतर		एकूण	
१) गरोदर स्त्रिया	3		—		—		17		20	
२) स्तनदा माता	2		—		—		13		15	
एकूण –	5						30		35	
	M	F	M	F	M	F	M	F	M	F
३) ० ते ६ महिने	2	–	–	–	–	–	9	4	11	4
४) ६ महिने ते १ वर्ष	–	–	–	–	1	–	4	4	5	4
५) १ वर्ष ते ३ वर्षे	3	–	–	–	2	–	19	20	24	20
६) ३ वर्षे ते ६ वर्षे	2	2	–	–	4	3	33	19	39	24
एकूण बालक	7	2	–	–	7	3	65	47	79	52
७) १५ ते ४५ वयोगटातील स्त्रिया	21				15		152		188	
८) ११ ते १८ वयो. किशोरवर्गीय मुली	12		—		3		75		90	
११ ते १५ वयो.	6		—		1		30		37	
१५ ते १८ वयो.	6		—		2		45		53	
९) १५ ते १८ वयो जी मुले शाळेत जात नाहीत अशा मुलांची संख्या	—		—		—		—		—	

मुख्य सेविका Bhosale अंगणवाडी कार्यकर्ती

Figure 3.3: ICDS Three-monthly Household Survey in Surli

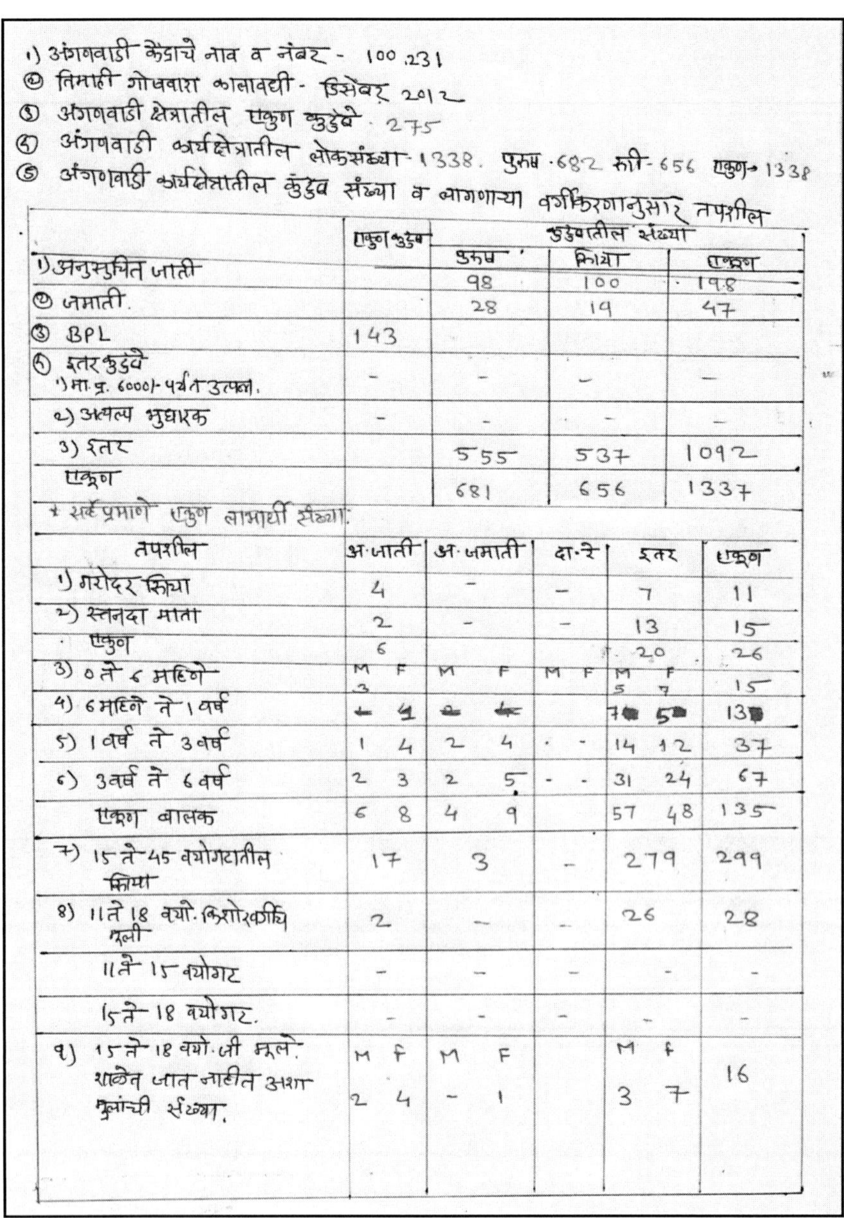

१) अंगणवाडी केंद्राचे नाव व नंबर - 100.231
② तिमाही गोषवारा कालावधी - डिसेंबर 2012
③ अंगणवाडी क्षेत्रातील एकुण कुटुंबे · 275
④ अंगणवाडी कार्यक्षेत्रातील लोकसंख्या · 1338. पुरुष · 682 स्त्री - 656 एकुण → 1338
⑤ अंगणवाडी कार्यक्षेत्रातील कुटुंब संख्या व भागणाऱ्या वर्गीकरणानुसार तपशील

	एकुण कुटुंब	कुटुंबातील संख्या		
		पुरुष	स्त्रिया	एकूण
१) अनुसुचित जाती		98	100	198
② जमाती.		28	19	47
③ BPL	143			
④ इतर कुटुंबे १) मा.प्र. 6000/- पर्यंत उत्पन्न.	-	-	-	-
२) अत्यल्प भुधारक	-	-	-	-
३) इतर		555	537	1092
एकूण		681	656	1337

* सर्वे प्रमाणे एकुण लाभार्थी संख्या:

तपशील	अ.जाती		अ.जमाती		दा.रे		इतर		एकूण
१) गरोदर स्त्रिया	4		-		-		7		11
२) स्तनदा माता	2		-		-		13		15
एकुण	6						20		26
३) ० ते ६ महिने	M 3	F	M	F	M	F	M 5	F 7	15
४) ६ महिने ते १ वर्ष	[illegible]	4	[illegible]	[illegible]			7[illegible]	5[illegible]	13[illegible]
५) १ वर्ष ते ३ वर्ष	1	4	2	4	·	-	14	12	37
६) ३ वर्ष ते ६ वर्ष	2	3	2	5	-	-	31	24	67
एकूण बालक	6	8	4	9			57	48	135
७) १५ ते ४५ वयोगटातील स्त्रिया	17		3		-		279		299
८) ११ ते १८ वयो. किशोरवयीन मुली	2		-		-		26		28
११ ते १५ वयोगट	-		-		-		-		-
१५ ते १८ वयोगट.	-		-		-		-		-
९) १५ ते १८ वयो.जी मुले. शाळेत जात नाहीत अशा मुलांची संख्या.	M 2	F 4	M -	F 1			M 3	F 7	16

Figure 3.5: Compiled Village Population Data from Anganwadis in Nanduri, 2012

Table 3.12: Child Growth Standards (For Boys 0-6 years) by World Health Organisation, 2006

Age in months	*Severe malnutrition Less than minus 3 SD*	*Moderate malnutrition Equal or greater than minus 3 SD to less than minus 2 SD*	*Slight malnutrition Equal to or greater than minus 2 SD*	*Normal weight*	*Age in months*	*Severe malnutrition Less than minus 3 SD*	*Moderate malnutrition Equal or greater than minus 3 SD to less than minus 2 SD*	*Slight malnutrition Equal to or greater than minus 2 SD*	*Normal weight*
0	2.100	2.1 to 2.5	2.500	3.300	17	7.700	7.7 to 8.6	8.600	10.700
1	2.900	2.9 to 3.4	3.400	4.500	18	7.800	7.8 to 8.8	8.800	10.900
2	3.800	3.8 to 4.3	4.300	5.600	19	8.000	8.0 to 8.9	8.900	11.100
3	4.400	4.4 to 5.0	5.000	6.400	20	8.100	8.1 to 9.1	9.100	11.300
4	4.900	4.9 to 5.6	5.600	7.000	21	8.200	8.2 to 9.2	9.200	11.500
5	5.300	5.3 to 6.0	6.000	7.500	22	8.400	8.4 to 9.4	9.400	11.800
6	5.700	5.7 to 6.4	6.400	7.900	23	8.500	8.5 to 9.5	9.500	12.000
7	5.900	5.9 to 6.7	6.700	8.300	24	8.600	8.6 to 9.7	9.700	12.200
8	6.200	6.2 to 6.9	6.900	8.600	30	9.400	9.4 to 10.5	10.500	13.300
9	6.400	6.4 to 7.1	7.100	8.900	36	10.000	10.0 to 11.3	11.300	14.300
10	6.600	6.6 to 7.4	7.400	9.200	42	10.600	10.6 to 12.0	12.000	15.300
11	6.800	6.8 to 7.6	7.600	9.400	48	11.200	11.2 to 12.7	12.700	16.300
12	6.900	6.9 to 7.7	7.700	9.600	54	11.800	11.8 to 13.4	13.400	17.300
13	7.100	7.1 to 7.9	7.900	9.900	60	12.400	12.4 to 14.1	14.100	18.300
14	7.200	7.2 to 8.1	8.100	10.100	66	13.300	13.3 to 15.0	15.000	19.400
15	7.400	7.4 to 8.3	8.300	10.300	72	14.100	14.1 to 15.9	15.900	20.500
16	7.500	7.5 to 8.4	8.400	10.500					

Source: Compiled from ICDS Growth Monitoring Book kept at the Anganwadi center; SD - Standard Deviation; For more information see: www.who.int/childgrowth/publications/en/

Table 3.13: New Child Growth Standards (For Girls 0-6 years) by World Health Organisation, 2006

Age in months	*Severe malnutrition Less than minus 3 SD*	*Moderate malnutrition Equal or greater than minus 3 SD to less than minus 2 SD*	*Slight malnutrition Equal to or greater than minus 2 SD*	*Normal weight*	*Age in months*	*Severe malnutrition Less than minus 3 SD*	*Moderate malnutrition Equal or greater than minus 3 SD to less than minus 2 SD*	*Slight malnutrition Equal to or greater than minus 2 SD*	*Normal weight*
0	2.000	2.0 to 2.4	2.400	3.200	17	7.000	7.0 to 7.9	7.900	10.000
1	2.700	2.7 to 3.2	3.200	4.200	18	7.200	7.2 to 8.1	8.100	10.200
2	3.400	3.4 to 3.9	3.900	5.100	19	7.300	7.3 to 8.2	8.200	10.400
3	4.000	4.0 to 4.5	4.500	5.800	20	7.500	7.5 to 8.4	8.400	10.600
4	4.500	4.5 to 5.0	5.000	6.400	21	7.600	7.6 to 8.6	8.600	10.900
5	4.800	4.8 to 5.4	5.400	6.900	22	7.800	7.8 to 8.7	8.700	11.100
6	5.100	5.1 to 5.7	5.700	7.300	23	7.900	7.9 to 8.9	8.900	11.300
7	5.300	5.3 to 6.0	6.000	7.600	24	8.100	8.1 to 9.0	9.000	11.500
8	5.600	5.6 to 6.3	6.300	7.900	30	8.900	8.9 to 10.0	10.000	12.700
9	5.800	5.8 to 6.5	6.500	8.200	36	9.600	9.6 to 10.8	10.800	13.900
10	5.900	5.9 to 6.7	6.700	8.500	42	10.300	10.3 to 11.6	11.600	15.000
11	6.100	6.1 to 6.9	6.900	8.700	48	10.900	10.9 to 12.3	12.300	16.100
12	6.300	6.3 to 7.0	7.000	8.900	54	11.500	11.5 to 13.0	13.000	17.200
13	6.400	6.4 to 7.2	7.200	9.200	60	12.100	12.1 to 13.7	13.700	18.200
14	6.600	6.6 to 7.4	7.400	9.400	66	12.900	12.9 to 14.6	14.600	19.100
15	6.700	6.7 to 7.6	7.600	9.600	72	13.500	13.5 to 15.3	15.300	20.200
16	6.900	6.9 to 7.7	7.700	9.800					

Source: Compiled from ICDS Growth Monitoring Book kept at the Anganwadi center; SD - Standard Deviation; for more information see: www.who.int/childgrowth/publications/en/

Table 3.14: Price Estimate of Assets owned by Sample Households

Sr. No.	Item	Market value (in Rs.) 2012 price per unit	Sr. No.	Item	Market value (in Rs.) 2012 price per unit
I	Buildings		V	Electric equipment	
	House	As reported		Refrigerator	8,000
	Shops/commercial establishments	As reported		Radio/Tape recorder/Two-in-one	1,500
	Buildings for farm business	As reported		Telephone/Mobile	2,000
II	Livestock			Television / Cable	7,000 / 10,000
	Cow	20,000		Other electrical appliances like Fan / Mixer	600 / 1,500
	Calf	4,000	VI	Furniture	
	Bullocks (pair)	30,000		Cots/beds	4,000
	Buffalo	15,000		Chairs/stools	400
	Hen	150		Tables	500
	Goat	3,000		Almirah/ cupboards/ shelves	3,000
III	Means of production			Sofa sets	6,000
	Plough	2,000		Other furniture (specify)	1000
	Thresher	9,000	VII	Other domestic durable goods	
	Sickle	50		Trunks/boxes/suitcases	1,200
	Axe/Dagger	100		Sewing machine	4,000
	Spade	75		Watches	400
	Tube well and accessories	80,000		Clocks	500
	Diesel pump	8,000		Kerosene stove	400
	Electric pump	15,000		Gas stove	5,000
	Wells	1,00,000		Utensils/kitchen appliances (40)	4,000
	Sprayer	1,300		Pressure cooker	700
	Hammer	100		Gold (1 tola or 10 grams)	30,000
IV	Means of transport			Silver (1 tola or 10 grams)	600
	Bicycle	3,000	VIII	Land Holding	
	Moped	20,000		Dry Land (Surli)	4 lakh/acre
	Scooter/motorcycle	45,000		Irrigable Land (Surli)	8 lakh/acre
	Bullock cart	15,000		Dry Land (Nanduri)	1 lakh/acre
	Tractor	85,000		Irrigable Land (Nanduri)	3 lakh/acre
	Jeep	1,00,000			

Note: Households had reported prices of their assets which varied significantly from one household to another. These prices are indicative and approximately close to prevailing market price.

Table 3.15: Sample Children's Weight and Malnutrition Grade Data (first month till 60th month)

Sr. No.	Household number (Randomly asigned)	Name of the Child	Sex	Age in months	Weight at 1 month (kg)	Grade at 1 month	Weight at 6 months (kg)	Grade at 6 months	Weight at 12 months (kg)	Grade at 12 months	Weight at 18 months (kg)	Grade at 18 months	Weight at 24 months (kg)	Grade at 24 months	Weight at 30 months (kg)	Grade at 30 months	Weight at 36 months (kg)	Grade at 36 months	Weight at 42 months (kg)	Grade at 42 months	Weight at 48 months (kg)	Grade at 48 months	Weight at 54 months (kg)	Grade at 54 months	Weight at 60 months (kg)	Grade at 60 months
1	6	sonali shivaji koli	Female	53	2.500	3	3.100	3	4.000	3	4.400	3	5.000	3	6.000	3	6.800	3	8.000	3	9.000	3	12.100	2		
2	7	aditi mahesh patil	Female	45	3.000	2	3.400	3	4.000	3	4.500	3	5.000	3	5.700	3	6.500	3	7.800	3						
3	8	aishwarya govind pandhare	Female	18	2.700	2	4.000	3	9999.000		9999.000															
4	8	mohini gobinda pandhare	Female	68	2.100	3	2.800	3	4.000	3	5.400	3	7.000	3	8.100	3	9.400	3	10.200	3	10.200	3	10.700	3	11.300	3
5	9	nikita naganath sarade	Female	60	4.000	1	4.500	3	5.500	3	6.500	3	8.000	3	9.300	2	10.100	2	11.300	2	11.700	2	14.000	1	15.700	1
6	12	shreya bhanudas sakhare	Female	24	3.000	2	5.200	2	6.100	3	7.700	2	9.100	1												
7	13	antarali narayan sarade	Female	62	4.000	1	4.900	3	6.500	2	7.800	2	9.300	1	10.500	1	11.700	1	13.300	1	14.100	1	15.200	1	15.500	1
8	15	prathali hrushikesh mule	Female	56	3.500	1	4.500	3	6.000	3	7.500	2	8.100	2	9.400	2	11.000	1	13.000	1	13.500	1	14.200	1		
9	16	shreya pandhurang sakkhare	Female	20	2.500	3	4.500	3	6.900	2	7.900	2														
10	18	sayali satish gade	Female	62	3.400	1	4.500	3	6.000	3	7.600	2	9.100	1	10.000	2	11.000	1	12.500	1	13.300	1	14.400	1	14.800	1
11	20	anita anant rajmane	Female	48	3.500	1	4.000	3	4.900	3	5.600	3	6.700	3	7.800	2	9.400	3	11.000	2	12.500	1				
12	21	gangabai anant bhokare	Female	6	3.000	2	4.800	3																		
13	25	shreya dnyaneshwar roman	Female	18	3.000	2	3.500	3	4.700	3	9999.000															
14	27	laxmi popat sarade	Female	7	2.700	2	4.300	3																		
15	29	kalyani balaji bhokare	Female	12	3.500	1	4.400	3	9999.000																	
16	30	gourav goutam bhokare	Female	53	3.000	2	3.700	3	4.500	3	6.000	3	7.200	3	8.800	3	10.000	2	10.500	2	12.000	2	14.000	1		
17	31	smita yashwant kadam	Female	52	4.000	1	4.700	3	5.700	3	6.500	3	7.300	3	8.000	3	9.000	3	12.000	1	13.000	1				
18	33	arti netaji sarade	Female	18	3.500	1	5.500	2	9999.000		9999.000															
19	34	yogita ramesh surcase	Female	51	2.700	2	3.600	3	4.100	3	5.500	3	6.200	3	6.800	3	7.400	3	8.600	3	9.400	3				
20	39	sanika sudhir sarade	Female	24	5.800	0	9.500	0	9999.000		9999.000		9999.000													
21	39	sayali sudhir sarade	Female	12	3.700	1	4.700	3	9999.000																	
22	41	asmita pandit koli	Female	60	2.500	3	4.100	3	8.100	0	10.900	0	11.100	1	12.100	1	12.700	1	13.400	1	14.100	1	15.000	1	15.900	1
23	42	devyani shrikant koli	Female	60	3.500	1	4.200	3	5.100	3	5.700	3	6.500	3	6.300	3	7.000	3	7.700	3	8.300	3	9.100	3	10.700	3
24	43	mayuri shivraj patil	Female	65	2.700	2	9999.000	9999	3.700	3	4.100	3	4.600	3	4.600	3	5.100	3	7.500	3	8.000	3	9.800	3	11.100	3
25	44	akshara amar rajmane	Female	19	2.500	3	4.000	3	6.200	3	8.400	1														
26	44	anushka amar rajmane	Female	62	9999.000	9999	3.000	3	5.900	3	7.800	2	9.300	1	10.300	1	9.300	3	10.300	2	12.900	1	14.100	1	14.300	1
27	45	bhagyashree datta bhokare	Female	9	3.000	2	9999.000	9999																		
28	45	laxmi datta bhokare	Female	29	3.100	2	5.700	2	7.200	1	9.000	1	10.800	1												
29	47	diksha dnyaneshwar mule	Female	6	3.000	2	7.200	1																		
30	48	shradha narendra sarade	Female	0	3.000	2																				
31	48	manish narendra sarade	Female	11	2.800	2	4.500	1																		
32	50	tanaya prashant gade	Female	17	2.500	3	5.000	1	7.000	1																
33	51	sangeeta shankar sarade	Female	0	2.700	2																				
34	51	sharwari shankar sarade	Female	17	3.000	2	4.500	1	7.300	1																
35	52	shravani sanjay sakhare	Female	24	3.000	2	4.700	1	9999.000		9999.000		9999.000													
36	54	shrawani ganesh gongane	Female	24	3.500	1	6.500	1	8.500	1	9.700	1	11.100	1												
37	57	anjali arjun waghmare	Female	30	4.000	1	5.100	1	6.100	3	9999.000		9999.000		9999.000											
38	57	arti dipak sakhare	Female	48	3.000	2	3.600	1	4.500	3	5.100	3	5.800	3	6.700	3	7.900	3	8.800	3	10.900	2				
39	59	divya kumar jethibhor	Female	56	9999.000	9999	9999.000		9999.000		9999.000		9999.000		9999.000		9999.000				14.000	1	16.500	1		

Table 3.15: Continued

Sr. No.	Household number (Randomly asigned)	Name of the Child	Sex	Age in months	Weight at 1 month (kg)	Grade at 1 month	Weight at 6 months (kg)	Grade at 6 months	Weight at 12 months (kg)	Grade at 12 months	Weight at 18 months (kg)	Grade at 18 months	Weight at 24 months (kg)	Grade at 24 months	Weight at 30 months (kg)	Grade at 30 months	Weight at 36 months (kg)	Grade at 36 months	Weight at 42 months (kg)	Grade at 42 months	Weight at 48 months (kg)	Grade at 48 months	Weight at 54 months (kg)	Grade at 54 months	Weight at 60 months (kg)	Grade at 60 months
40	63	gouri naganath kalsure	Female	60	3.000	2	5.100	2	6.900	2	9.300	1	11.500	0	13.500	0	15.300	0	17.000	0	17.500	0	18.000	0	18.500	0
41	65	mayuri dilip sarade	Female	52	2.300	3	4.900	1	8.500	1	9.400	1	10.400	1	11.500	1	11.700	1	12.300	1	13.700	1				
42	69	shrushti janardhan dhobale	Female	54	3.000	2	3.800	1	5.900	3	6.900	3	7.300	3	8.400	3	9.200	3	10.300	2	11.300	2	12.200	2		
43	40	layba amir shaikh	Female	45	9999.000	9999	6.000	1	6.900	2	7.700	2	9.700	1	10.500	1	11.700	1	12.000	1						
44	1	sarthak pintu dhobale	Male	42	3.200	2	5.400	3	7.100	2	9.100	1	10.100	1	12.000	1	12.900	1	14.100	1						
45	1	ritesh pintu dhobale	Male	71	3.500	1	6.000	2	8.900	1	10.500	1	11.900	1	12.300	1	13.000	1	14.100	1	14.200	1	15.900	1	16.000	1
46	2	omkar yuvraj patil	Male	45	3.500	1	4.200	3	5.000	3	5.400	3	6.500	3	7.800	3	8.400	3	10.000	3						
47	3	shwet santosh sonavne	Male	50	3.500	1	4.300	3	5.300	3	6.200	3	7.000	3	7.700	3	8.600	3	10.300	3	12.400	2				
48	3	sanchet santosh sonavne	Male	68	4.000	1	5.000	3	6.500	3	7.500	3	8.600	2	10.000	2	11.300	2	12.600	1	14.000	1	15.100	1	15.600	1
49	4	parth rajendra roman	Male	20	3.000	2	6.000	2	9.000	1	10.100	1	9999.000													
50	4	hrushikesh rajendra roman	Male	47	2.500	3	4.000	3	6.100	3	6.900	3	7.900	3	8.700	3	10.000	2	10.500	3						
51	5	prasanna vilas sakhare	Male	30	3.000	2	6.300	2	8.300	1	10.000	1	10.200	1	13.100	1										
52	6	chandrakant shivaji koli	Male	12	3.000	2	6.300	2	7.600	2																
53	6	suryakant shivaji koli	Male	28	3.500	1	4.100	3	9999.000	9999	9999.000	9999	9999.000													
54	8	indrajeet vinod pandhare	Male	40	3.500	1	4.400	3	5.500	3	6.700	3	8.100	3	9.500	2	10.100	2								
55	10	krushnant tulsiram jadhav	Male	52	3.500	1	3.700	3	4.800	3	5.900	3	6.500	3	7.000	3	7.900	3	8.000	3	10.100	3				
56	11	harshwardhan hanmant yadav	Male	67	2.000	3	2.800	3	3.500	3	4.600	3	5.800	3	7.000	3	8.400	3	9.500	3	10.700	3	11.300	3	11.800	3
57	13	aditya narayan sarade	Male	26	3.600	1	4.200	3	9999.000		9999.000		9999.000													
58	14	prajwal angad sakhare	Male	13	2.500	3	5.900	2	8.100	1																
59	17	rohan dhanaji sakhare	Male	60	2.500	3	4.900	3	6.900	2	8.500	2	9.700	2	10.900	1	12.200	1	12.900	1	12.900	1	13.700	1	14.100	2
60	19	sambhaji shivaji sarade	Male	12	3.500	1	4.400	3	9999.000																	
61	20	parth anant rajmane	Male	24	3.000	2	4.100	3	9999.000		9999.000		9999.000													
62	22	jayhind dnyaneshwar bhokare	Male	3	3.500	1																				
63	26	prem santaji gongane	Male	29	3.500	1	4.100	3	5.200	3	9999.000		9999.000													
64	27	krushnant popat sarade	Male	7	3.000	2	5.700	2																		
65	29	hari balaji bhokare	Male	36	3.700	1	5.000	3	6.600	3	8.100	2	9.500	2	11.000	1	12.300	1								
66	31	samarth yashwant kadam	Male	36	2.700	3	3.700	3	4.500	3	6.000	3	8.000	3	10.400	2	11.900	1								
67	32	arman basu shaikh	Male	18	3.500	1	5.000	3	9999.000		9999.000															
68	33	atharav netaji sarade	Male	49	3.700	1	5.000	3	6.200	3	6.900	3	8.200	3	9.700	2	11.200	2	12.700	1	13.900	1				
69	35	prasad padmakar patil	Male	42	3.500	1	4.700	3	5.800	3	7.000	3	7.000	3	8.600	3	10.600	2	12.700	1						
70	36	prathmesh kanteshwar mule	Male	36	3.000	2	4.300	3	5.700	3	7.300	3	8.800	2	10.300	2	11.500	1								
71	36	tushar krushnath patil	Male	36	3.300	2	4.400	3	6.000	3	7.400	3	9.400	2	10.300	2	11.500	1								
72	37	pratik shesherao patil	Male	40	2.500	3	3.500	3	5.000	3	6.300	3	8.000	3	9.600	2	9.800	3								
73	38	soham dayanand rajmane	Male	6	3.500	1	6.200	2																		
74	38	sangam dayanand rajmane	Male	48	3.500	1	5.500	3	7.900	1	8.300	2	9.000	2	9.200	3	9.700	3	11.000	2	12.000	2				
75	43	prathmesh shivraj patil	Male	42	3.000	2	6.100	2	8.500	1	10.000	1	9.800	1	11.500	1	14.100	1	15.100	1						
76	45	parmeshwar ashok bhokare	Male	13	3.200	2	5.600	3	9.500	1																
77	46	shivraj sanjay karale	Male	66	2.500	3	5.100	3	7.300	2	8.500	2	9.500	2	9.500	2	10.900	2	11.500	2	12.900	1	14.300	1	14.000	2
78	46	samarth sanjay karale	Male	43	2.300	3	2.700	3	5.400	3	6.200	3	8.100	3	10.300	2	11.400	1	14.100	1						
79	50	prathmesh prashant gade	Male	48	3.400	1	6.700	1	8.600	1	9.700	1	10.300	1	11.700	1	12.800	1	13.300	1	14.300	1				
80	55	shlok sunil sarade	Male	11	3.100	2	6.700	1																		
81	55	sanskar sunil sarade	Male	42	3.200	2	5.300	3	7.200	2	10.300	1	11.500	1	11.900	1	12.500	1	14.100	1						
82	60	amir karim shaikh	Male	6	3.000	2	5.700	2																		

Table 3.15: Continued

Sr. No.	Household number (Randomly asigned)	Name of the Child	Sex	Age in months	Weight at 1 month (kg)	Grade at 1 month	Weight at 6 months (kg)	Grade at 6 months	Weight at 12 months (kg)	Grade at 12 months	Weight at 18 months (kg)	Grade at 18 months	Weight at 24 months (kg)	Grade at 24 months	Weight at 30 months (kg)	Grade at 30 months	Weight at 36 months (kg)	Grade at 36 months	Weight at 42 months (kg)	Grade at 42 months	Weight at 48 months (kg)	Grade at 48 months	Weight at 54 months (kg)	Grade at 54 months	Weight at 60 months (kg)	Grade at 60 months
83	61	suresh sunil roman	Male	6	3.500	1	6.000	2																		
84	61	yash sunil roman	Male	36	3.000	2	5.400	3	7.300	2	9.500	1	12.100	1	13.000	1	13.900	1								
85	62	omkar vishwanath roman	Male	50	3.000	2	5.700	2	8.300	1	10.000	1	9999.000	9999	14.100	0	14.100	1	14.000	1	14.500	1				
86	63	gourav naganath kalsure	Male	36	3.200	2	5.400	3	7.300	2	10.000	1	11.700	1	13.800	0	14.400	0								
87	64	abhijeet balaji sarade	Male	30	3.000	2	6.000	2	8.000	1	9.700	1	12.100	1	15.000	0										
88	65	prathmesh dilip sarade	Male	11	3.100	2	6.200	2																		
89	65	pruthviraj dilip sarade	Male	27	3.200	2	6.000	2	8.000	1	10.300	1	12.200	0												
90	66	pradhunya yogesh bhokare	Male	7	3.000	2	5.100	3																		
91	67	aditya mohan mule	Male	30	3.500	1	4.400	3	5.000	3	6.200	3	7.400	3	9.700	2										
92	68	yash dnyaneshwar koli	Male	11	2.300	3	5.300	3																		
93	68	vithal dnyaneshwar koli	Male	71	2.300	3	4.000	3	7.000	2	8.100	2	8.000	3	8.500	3	9.800	3	10.000	3	10.500	3	10.500	3	11.100	3
94	49	shree dayanand patil	Male	6	2.900	3	5.100	3																		
95	372	sayali rajendra pawar	Female	35	2.500	3	6.000	1	7.300	1	8.200	1	8.900	2	10.000	1										
96	574	saniya ahamad sayyed	Female	67	3.000	2	5.500	2	8.000	1	9.500	1	9.100	1	9.900	2	10.800	1	11.200	2	12.300	1	13.000	1	14.000	1
97	776	shradha sachin bhosale	Female	33	3.000	2	6.200	1	7.500	1	7.400	2	8.800	2	9.300	2										
98	776	snehal sachin bhosale	Female	60	3.000	2	5.500	2	8.100	1	9.200	1	10.600	1	11.200	1	12.200	1	12.600	1	13.500	1	14.600	1	15.100	1
99	877	madhura umesh randive	Female	8	3.200	2	5.500	2	8.000	1																
100	1281	sanchita tanaji bhosale	Female	57	9999.000	9999	5.500	2	8.100	1	9.400	1	10.400	1	12.700	0	11.800	1	12.500	1	13.600	1	14.300	1		
101	1483	arti mahadev shinde	Female	49	3.000	2	5.600	2	6.500	2	9.700	1	10.200	1	10.800	1	12.400	1	11.700	1	12.800	1				
102	1483	kirti mahadev shinde	Female	71	3.000	2	5.500	2	8.000	1	9.000	1	10.200	1	9.600	2	10.400	2	11.400	2	13.400	1	13.100	1	13.200	2
103	1786	akshara swarup pandit	Female	8	9999.000	9999	5.800	1																		
104	1887	payal nitin jadhav	Female	22	3.000	2	6.500	1	9.500	0	10.600	0														
105	2291	Utkarsha atul kadam	Female	24	3.500	1	6.000	1	7.900	1	8.800	1	8.700	2												
106	2291	Shravani Atul Kadam	Female	10	3.000	2	5.800	1	8.500	1																
107	2392	shivanjali ganesh jangam	Female	37	2.000	3	6.000	1	7.800	1	9.300	1	9.000	1	10.500	1	11.400	1								
108	2392	sidhi ganesh jangam	Female	8	2.400	3	6.000	1	8.000	1																
109	2493	shrutika mahesh kadam	Female	13	2.700	2	6.400	1	8.500	1																
110	10233	damini amit bhosale	Female	64	9999.000	9999	5.100	2	6.500	2	7.800	2	10.000	1	9.800	1	10.700	2	11.900	1	12.800	1	13.300	1	14.300	1
111	10334	pari ramraje bhosale	Female	14	3.700	1	6.500	1	9.000	0																
112	10435	samrudhi ajeet chavan	Female	3	3.500	1																				
113	10738	swaranjali somnath pawar	Female	26	9999.000	9999	5.700	2	9.500	0	10.500	0	11.500	0												
114	10738	shivanjali rahul pawar	Female	30	3.500	1	7.900	0	9.400	0	11.000	0	12.900	0	13.400	0										
115	10940	sanskruti sandip rakshe	Female	23	2.700	2	6.000	1	7.700	1	8.600	1	9.300	1												
116	11647	anushka pitambar kadam	Female	43	9999.000	9999	7.900	0	9.500	0	10.300	0	12.300	0	12.700	0	13.300	1	14.300	1						
117	11647	swaranjali pitambar kadam	Female	25	9999.000	9999	6.000	1	7.000	2	8.000	2	9.000	1												
118	11950	sweta pramod bhosale	Female	41	3.000	2	6.400	1	9.800	0	10.400	0	11.200	1	11.500	1	12.400	1								
119	12354	shreya jaysingh kadam	Female	42	9999.000	9999	6.200	1	7.500	1	7.900	2	9.000	1	9.500	2	10.500	2	11.500	2						
120	12758	aditi kishor kadam	Female	23	9999.000	9999	6.300	1	8.500	1	10.200	0	11.500	0												
121	170	sumeet sanjay yadav	Male	55	2.500	3	5.500	3	8.800	1	9.300	1	9.000	2	10.700	1	11.500	1	13.000	1	14.000	1	14.900	1		
122	271	pranav ravindra rakshe	Male	43	3.500	1	5.600	3	7.800	1	10.500	1	10.200	1	12.500	1	14.300	0	13.200	1						
123	372	rohan rajendra pawar	Male	69	9999.000	9999	3.400	3	7.000	2	8.500	2	9.500	2	10.400	1	11.000	2	12.500	1	13.100	1	14.400	1	15.000	1
124	473	raj amol kadam	Male	49	2.500	3	5.500	3	6.300	3	8.800	1	10.400	1	11.000	1	12.700	1	13.500	1	14.100	1				
125	675	atharv manoj bhosale	Male	43	3.500	1	8.200	0	12.500	0	13.100	0	13.000	0	13.800	0	16.000	0	16.600	0						

Table 3.15: Continued

Sr. No.	Household number (Randomly asigned)	Name of the Child	Sex	Age in months	Weight at 1 month (kg)	Grade at 1 month	Weight at 6 months (kg)	Grade at 6 months	Weight at 12 months (kg)	Grade at 12 months	Weight at 18 months (kg)	Grade at 18 months	Weight at 24 months (kg)	Grade at 24 months	Weight at 30 months (kg)	Grade at 30 months	Weight at 36 months (kg)	Grade at 36 months	Weight at 42 months (kg)	Grade at 42 months	Weight at 48 months (kg)	Grade at 48 months	Weight at 54 months (kg)	Grade at 54 months	Weight at 60 months (kg)	Grade at 60 months
126	776	shubham sachin bhosale	Male	36	2.500	3	5.500	3	7.200	2	7.500	3	8.600	2	10.400	2	10.100	2								
127	877	karan umesh randive	Male	25	3.600	1	6.500	1	7.000	2	9.200	1	9.800	1												
128	978	yash dhanaji pawar	Male	57	9999.000	9999	6.900	1	9.800	0	10.600	1	10.900	1	12.900	1	13.100	1	13.500	1	14.200	1	14.500	1		
129	1180	vedant ajit bhosale	Male	57	9999.000	9999	6.100	2	8.400	1	9.200	1	10.400	1	11.900	1	11.900	1	13.500	1	14.200	1	14.500	1		
130	1281	sangram tanaji bhosale	Male	31	9999.000	9999	6.500	1	8.100	1	9.300	1	10.000	1	10.600	1										
131	1382	harshwardhab sandip bhosale	Male	9	9999.000	9999	5.900	2																		
132	1483	soham mahadev shinde	Male	10	3.000	2	5.000	3																		
133	1584	atharv vikas bhosale	Male	60	9999.000	9999	7.800	1	9.800	0	10.600	1	12.900	0	12.700	1	13.500	1	14.200	1	15.500	1	16.000	1	16.900	1
134	1584	shreyash somnath bhosale	Male	4	3.000	2																				
135	1685	vedant jayshing shinde	Male	31	3.000	2	7.500	1	9999.000	9999	9.300	1	10.000	1	10.300	2										
136	1988	shivraj indrajeet shirke	Male	2	3.000	2																				
137	2089	amar manoj rakshe	Male	62	9999.000	9999	6.650	1	9999.000	9999	10.100	1	10.800	1	11.100	1	11.900	1		9999		9999		9999		9999
138	2089	aditya manoj rakshe	Male	45	9999.000	9999	6.200	2	6.500	1	8.200	2	9.400	2	10.800	1	11.300	1	11.700	2						
139	2190	rehan ayub sayyed	Male	28	9999.000	9999	6.500	1	8.500	1	10.800	1	11.200	1												
140	2493	om mahesh kadam	Male	50	3.500	1	7.500	1	9.000	1	9.000	1	10.700	1	11.900	1	11.700	1	15.500	0	16.100	1				
141	2695	hrushikesh ashok kokare	Male	45	3.500	1	5.000	3	8.900	1	11.200	0	11.800	1	12.100	1	13.500	1	14.700	1						
142	2796	prajwal arun kadam	Male	59	3.500	1	6.800	1	8.300	1	12.300	0	12.200	0	13.200	1	13.700	1	15.000	1	15.500	1	17.000	1		
143	2897	arnav pankaj bansode	Male	4	9999.000	9999	5.200	3																		
144	3099	atharv sachin pawar	Male	49	3.000	2	5.500	3	8.500	1	10.100	1	11.600	1	12.300	1	12.100	1	13.000	1	13.700	1				
145	10132	boy amol bhosale	Male	2	3.500	1																				
146	10233	sumeet amit bhosale	Male	52	9999.000	9999	5.700	2	7.900	1	8.100	2	9.300	2	10.400	2	11.900	1	12.500	1	13.500	1				
147	10738	samarth rahul pawar	Male	17	9999.000	9999	6.100	2	9.500	1	11.500	0														
148	10738	sairaj somnath pawar	Male	5	3.300	9999	5.700	2																		
149	10839	aryan shashikant yadav	Male	28	3.000	2	5.900	2	8.700	1	9.500	1	10.200	1												
150	10839	sahil shashikant yadav	Male	12	2.800	3	8.000	0	9.700	0																
151	11041	akshay umesh rakshe	Male	54	9999.000	9999	9999.000	9999	9999.000	9999	9999.000	9999	12.600	0	12.600	1	12.900	1	13.900	1	14.500	1	15.500	1		
152	11142	karan rajendra yadav	Male	24	3.000	2	6.500	1	8.500	1	9.700	1	10.400	1												
153	11243	yash samadhan kadam	Male	20	3.000	2	7.000	1	10.200	0	11.200	0														
154	11344	vedant rajendra chavan	Male	48	9999.000	9999	9999.000	9999	9999.000	9999	9999.000	9999	9999.000	9999	9999.000	9999	9999.000	9999		9999		9999				
155	11748	saransh pramod ghadage	Male	3	3.200	2	9999.000	9999																		
156	11849	samarth mahesh sankapal	Male	12	3.500	1	7.000	1	8.800	1																
157	12253	devraj suhas pandit	Male	26	2.800	3	5.900	2	7.400	2	8.000	2	8.900	2												

Source: Author's data collection during fieldwork in 2012

Notes: This is the actual data used for analysis in section 3.3.3. It is the reference data set for Tables 3.8 to Table 3.13. Weight data for birth was missing for many children, therefore first month weights was taken as a starting point. Also since most children after 5th year joins a formal play school; they are out of the anganwadi system. Their weights were also not available. Weights were converted into Grades using WHO Child Growth Standards, 2006. Weights and Grades at an interval of 6 months were used as that would have allowed analysing change in the grade of malnutrition. Cells that are blank means that child has not reached that age; Cells with values of 0999 or 9999.000 indicate missing or unavailable data and had to be differentiated from blank cells. In order to protect the identity of the children, their village information is hidden.

Grades of Malnutrition (as per WHO Child Growth Standards 2006: 0 (Normal Weight for Age); 1 Slight malnutrition (Equal to or greater than minus 2 standard deviation); 2 Moderate malnutrition (equal or greater than minus 3 standard deviation to less than minus 2 standard deviation); 3 Severe malnutrition (Less than minus 3 standard deviation)